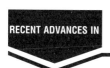RECENT ADVANCES IN

Blood Coagulation

Look out for *Recent Advances in Blood Coagulation 6* in March 1993

You can place your order from July 1992 by contacting your local medical bookseller or The Sales Promotion Department, Churchill Livingstone, Robert Stevenson House, 1–3 Baxter's Place, Leith Walk, Edinburgh EH1 3AF, UK

Tel: (031) 556 2424; Telex: 727511 LONGMN G; Fax: (031) 558 1278

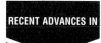
RECENT ADVANCES IN

Blood Coagulation

Edited by

L. Poller DSc, MD, FRCPath

Director, National (UK) Reference Laboratory for Anticoagulant Reagents and Control
(WHO collaborating centre for quality assessment in blood coagulation testing); Consultant
Haematologist, Withington Hospital, Manchester; Honorary Lecturer, University of
Manchester, UK

NUMBER FIVE

CHURCHILL LIVINGSTONE
EDINBURGH LONDON MELBOURNE NEW YORK AND TOKYO 1991

CHURCHILL LIVINGSTONE
Medical Division of Longman Group Limited

Distributed in the United States of America by
Churchill Livingstone Inc., 1560 Broadway,
New York, N.Y. 10036, and by associated companies,
branches and representatives throughout the world.

First published 1991

ISBN 0-443-04343-4

ISSN 0143-6740

British Library Cataloguing in Publication Data
Recent advances in blood coagulation. — No. 5
   1. Blood — Coagulation, Disorders of
   616.1'57'005   RC647.C55   76-42237

Produced by Longman Singapore Publishers Pte Ltd
Printed in Singapore

Preface

Advances in our knowledge of the mechanisms of blood coagulation haemostasis and thrombosis have proceeded at an ever increasing rate since the previous issue of *Recent Advances in Blood Coagulation*. This new issue covers the greater understanding which has been acquired in recent years, including an improved knowledge of the basic pathways of clotting. The topics covered include developments in molecular biology which have had a growing impact, the purification and amino acid sequencing of clotting factors and their synthesis by recombinant techniques. These have important implications.

In fibrinolysis recent developments have included the isolation of tissue plasminogen activator (tPA), the production of recombinant tPA and the demonstration of the importance of plasminogen activator inhibitors (PAI-1 and PAI-2).

The search for alternative drugs equal in effectiveness to heparin in the prevention and treatment of thrombosis but with reduced risk of bleeding has continued. Thus low molecular weight heparins, recombinant hirudin and dermatan sulphate are considered.

Deep vein thrombosis and concomitant pulmonary embolism are among the most common and serious complications in hospitalized patients. The relative effectiveness of the various alternative forms of prophylaxis are reviewed. The true value of thrombolytic therapy which has been available for over 30 years, has only recently become recognized, particularly after myocardial infarction. The vitamin K cycle and the inhibitory effects of warfarin on the vitamin K dependent clotting factor are now better understood.

The application of the INR system of reporting prothrombin time results for anticoagulant control has provided a basis for agreement on optimal therapeutic range for the different clinical states.

A new development in the present issue is the inclusion of a collection of reviews selected by the authors of the respective chapters covering one or two important papers which have appeared in their field.

Thanks must be expressed to the contributors of the various chapters of their promptness in producing their manuscripts and for their painstaking efforts to maintain the standards set by previous writers in the earlier issues of the series. The editor is also particularly indebted to Yvonne O'Leary and other staff at Churchill Livingstone involved in *Recent Advances* for their great efficiency and helpful advice which have greatly reduced the burden of the preparation of this issue.

Manchester 1991 L.P.

Contributors

Bruce Bennett MD FRCP FRCPath
Reader in Medicine, University of Aberdeen; Honorary Consultant
Physician, Aberdeen Royal Infirmary, Aberdeen, UK

Arthur L. Bloom MD FRCP FRCPath
Professor of Haematology, University of Wales College of Medicine,
Cardiff, UK

Edwin G. Bovill MD FACP FRCS
Associate Professor of Pathology, University of Vermont College of
Medicine, Burlington, Vermont, USA

P Brakman MD PhD
Director, Gaubius Institute TNO, Leiden; Professor of Medicine, Leiden
University, The Netherlands

E. J. P. Brommer MD PhD
Senior Investigator, Gaubius Institute TNO, Leiden, The Netherlands

P. Close MD
International Project Leader, Clinical Research and Development, Ciba-
Geigy Ltd, Basle, Switzerland

P. Desnoyers
Laboratoire Central d'Hématologie, Hôtel-Dieu, Paris, France

Kazuo Fujikawa PhD
Research Professor, Department of Biochemistry, University of
Washington, Seattle, Washington, USA

Michael Greaves MD MRCPath FRCP FRCP (Ed)
Reader and Consultant in Haematology, and Honorary Consultant
Physician, Royal Hallamshire Hospital, Sheffield, UK

Bernard Hoet MD
Research Associate, Centre for Thrombosis and Vascular Research,
University of Leuven, Leuven, Belgium

Gordon D. O. Lowe MD FRCP
Senior Lecturer and Consultant Physician, University Department of Medicine, Royal Infirmary, Glasgow, UK

K. G. Mann PhD
Professor and Chairman, Department of Biochemistry, University of Vermont College of Medicine, Burlington, Vermont, USA

John H. McVey BSc PhD
Post-doctoral Research Scientist, Clinical Research Centre, Harrow, Middlesex, UK

Derek Ogston MD DSc FRCP FRSE
Professor of Medicine, University of Aberdeen, Aberdeen, UK

Jonathan K. Pattinson MA MB BS MRCP
Clinical Scientist, Clinical Research Centre, Harrow, Middlesex, UK

Ian R. Peake BSc PhD
Professor of Molecular Medicine, University of Sheffield Medical School, Sheffield, UK

Leon Poller MD DSc FRCPath
Honorary Lecturer, University of Manchester; Director, UK Reference Laboratory for Anticoagulant Reagents and Control; Consultant Haematologist, Withington Hospital, Manchester, UK

F. E. Preston MD MRCP FRCPath
Professor of Haematology, University of Sheffield Medical School and Royal Hallamshire Hospital, Sheffield, UK

J. A. Sadowski PhD
Scientist I: USDA Human Nutrition Research Center on Aging, Tufts University, Boston, Massachusetts, USA

Meyer M. Samama MD
Professor, Laboratoire Central d'Hématologie, Hôtel-Dieu, Paris, France

Koji Suzuki PhD
Division of Enzyme Cytology, Institute for Enzyme Research, University of Tokushima, Tokushima, Japan

Edward G. D. Tuddenham MD FRCP FRCPath
Director, Haemostasis Research Group, MRC Clinical Research Centre, Harrow, Middlesex; Honorary Consultant Haematologist, Northwick Park Hospital and Royal Postgraduate Medical School, Harrow, Middlesex

Alexander G. G. Turpie MB ChB FRCP FACP FRCPC
Professor of Medicine, McMaster University, Hamilton, Ontario, Canada

Orhan N. Ulutin MD
Professor of Medicine, Cerrahpasa Medical School of Istanbul University, Istanbul, Turkey

Jos G. Vermylen MD
Professor of Internal Medicine, University of Leuven, Leuven, Belgium

Marc Verstraete MD FRCP FACP
Professor of Medicine, Centre for Medicine and Centre for Thrombosis and Vascular Research, University of Leuven, Leuven, Belgium

Contents

1

Blood coagulation mechanism

D. Ogston   B. Bennett

Blood loss following injury to blood vessels is normally minimized by the coordinated responses of the vessel wall, the blood platelets and the blood coagulation mechanism leading to the formation of a haemostatic plug.

The coagulation mechanism is concerned with the formation of thrombin which converts fibrinogen into insoluble fibrin, allowing stabilization of aggregated platelets at injury sites. The process requires initiation at the appropriate site, undergoes amplification through a number of sequential proteolytic reactions, is subjected to modification and enhancement by feedback reactions, and there are mechanisms to control enzyme formation and function to prevent clotting beyond the site of injury.

The last few years has witnessed the continued rapid advance in the elucidation of the molecular structure of the blood coagulation system components. In addition, further interactions between coagulation factors, their inhibitors, vascular endothelium and platelets have been documented, but their importance and relevance in the coagulation mechanism or haemostatic process have, in many cases, not been determined.

This review considers some of the newer findings relating to the coagulation system in the light of previous knowledge.

THE CONTACT ACTIVATION SYSTEM

The contact activation system, which initiates the intrinsic coagulation mechanism, involves the interaction of factor XII (Hageman factor), prekallikrein and high-molecular-weight kininogen (HMW kininogen) with a negatively charged surface. The activated form of factor XII which is generated (factor XIIa) proceeds to activate factor XI. The structures of human factor XI and prekallikrein have been determined and found to have a high degree of amino acid sequence homology (Fujikawa et al 1986). The biological functions of the two proteins, however, are distinct; kallikrein is not able to activate factor IX while factor XIa has only weak factor XII-activating activity.

The precise mechanism for the initiation of the contact system has remained elusive, and neither the mechanism for the accelerating influence of an anionic surface nor the mechanism for the initial activation of factor

1

XII has been established (for review see Kaplan & Silverberg 1987). It is clear, however, that reciprocal activation between factor XII and prekallikrein becomes the major pathway when both are surface-bound. HMW kininogen functions as a cofactor in the reciprocal activation by augmenting the attachment of prekallikrein and factor XI, with which it circulates in plasma as a complex, to negatively charged surfaces and facilitating their cleavage by factor XIIa.

The significance of the contact activation system in the coagulation mechanism is speculative. Deficiency of factor XII, prekallikrein and HMW kininogen are not associated with a haemorrhagic tendency, while only around a half of factor XI-deficient patients suffer from bleeding. The bleeding in these patients appears to be determined by factors, presently unidentified, other than the plasma factor XI level (Ragni et al 1985).

Platelets are not essential for contact activation, but provide a surface on which factors XII and XI can be activated (Walsh & Griffin 1981). In recent years further data have been provided on the possible involvement of platelets in the contact activation system. Platelets have been shown to contain HMW kininogen which can be expressed on the surface of activated platelets (Schmaier et al 1986). In addition, unstimulated and activated platelets possess further binding sites for HMW kininogen (Gustafson et al 1986). The binding of HMW kininogen to platelets requires zinc ion. Factor XIa binds reversibly to high-affinity sites on platelets, distinct from those for the zymogen: HMW kininogen is required for binding of both factor XI and XIa to platelets, but zinc ion is not required for this, suggesting that the platelet binding site for factor XIa is not HMW kininogen. Platelet-bound factor XIa is protected from inactivation by its major plasma inhibitor, α_1-protease inhibitor, and is capable of activating factor IX at a similar rate to the unbound enzyme (Walsh et al 1986).

Endothelial cells have also been shown to be capable of synthesizing HMW kininogen and to possess binding sites for HMW kininogen on their external membrane (Schmaier et al 1988, van Iwaarden et al 1988). It was suggested that the binding of HMW kininogen to endothelial cells and platelets may provide sites for the localization and activation of prekallikrein and factor XI on physiological surfaces.

ACTIVATION OF FACTOR IX

The importance of factor IX in the coagulation mechanism is underlined by the severe haemorrhagic tendency which results from its deficiency. The activation of factor IX is achieved through the action of factor XIa or the factor VIIa–tissue factor complex. Its activation by factor XIa involves a calcium-dependent two-step reaction. Each light chain of factor XIa contains a catalytic site, while the heavy chain contains the substrate binding site which is distinct from the HMW kininogen binding site (Baglia et al 1989). It has been proposed that the binding of calcium ion to factor IX induces a conformational change in the molecule which allows it to bind to the site on the heavy chain of the factor XIa, essential for optimal rates of factor IX activation (Sinha et al 1985, 1987).

THE INTERACTION BETWEEN FACTORS IXa, VIIIa AND X
(The Intrinsic Factor X-Activating Complex)

Activation of factor X through the intrinsic coagulation system is achieved by an enzyme complex of factor IXa, thrombin-modified factor VIII, negatively charged phospholipid and calcium ions. Factor X is activated to factor Xa by the cleavage of a single peptide bond (Arg_{191}–Ile_{192}) in the zymogen, the enzymatic activity of the complex residing in factor IXa.

Factor VIII is synthesized as a single-chain molecule with M_r of approximately 280 000, comprising a heavy chain 200-kD polypeptide in a metal ion-stabilized complex with a light chain 80-kD polypeptide. It circulates in plasma as an inactive cofactor tightly bound to von Willebrand factor which mediates platelet adhesion to the subendothelium at sites of vascular injury and supports the platelet interactions necessary for the formation of platelet aggregates. Von Willebrand factor stabilizes factor VIII in the circulation and may serve additionally to localize the coagulant activity to sites of platelet adhesion. The factor VIII binding domain has been shown to reside in a 272 amino acid fragment from the amino-terminus of the von Willebrand factor polypeptide (Foster et al 1987).

Factor VIII requires proteolytic modification in order to fulfil its cofactor function. Activation of factor VIII by thrombin or factor Xa is associated with cleavage at Arg_{740} in the heavy chain region to generate a 90-kD polypeptide that is subsequently cleaved at Arg_{372} to yield fragments of 50 and 43 kD. There is simultaneous cleavage of the light chain 80-kD polypeptide at Arg_{1689} to yield a 73-kD fragment. Both the heavy and light chain cleavages at residues 372 and 1689 are required for the activation of factor VIII (Eaton et al 1986, Pittman & Kaufman 1988). Activation of factor VIII by factor Xa requires either phospholipid or platelets, while factor VIII activated by thrombin is more active in factor X activation than that activated by factor Xa (Neuenschwander & Jesty 1988). Factor VIII can also be activated by factor IXa; this is a relatively inefficient reaction, but may have a function in the initial production of active enzymes.

In the presence of phospholipid and calcium ion proteolytically modified factor VIII greatly enhances the rate of activation of factor X by factor IXa. Gilbert and colleagues (1990) have demonstrated that human factor VIII binds to phospholipid vesicles and that the presence of the anionic phosphatidylserine, which becomes available at the surface of platelets after their activation, is required for the binding.

Factor VIII interacts specifically and reversibly with a limited number of binding sites on human platelets, the expression of these sites being dependent upon platelet activation. The binding sites for factor VIII are distinct from those for factor V. It is likely that the platelet binding domain of factor VIII is specifically associated with its light subunit (Nesheim et al 1988).

Factor VIIIa is inactivated by activated protein C through limited proteolysis, $Arg_{336}-Met_{337}$ being proposed as the cleavage site (Eaton et al 1986). The binding to factor IXa of factor VIIIa protects the cofactor from inactivation by activated protein C.

Activated platelets possess specific, high-affinity binding sites for factor IXa; the presence of factor VIIIa and factor X has been found to increase the affinity of factor IXa binding to activated platelets (Ahmad et al 1989). It remains to be established whether, analogous to the role of factor Va in factor Xa binding, factor VIIIa comprises the binding site for factor IXa.

In addition to the formation of the intrinsic factor X-activating complex on a negatively charged phospholipid surface, endothelium has been shown to provide a specific binding site for factor IX/IXa. The binding site has been identified and found to consist of a membrane protein of $M_r \simeq 140\,000$ which preferentially binds factor IXa in the presence of factors VIII and X. This protein may promote assembly of the factor IXa/VIIIa/X complex on the endothelial cell surface and it has been proposed that it could function as a vessel-localized focus capable of propagating coagulation (Stern et al 1985a, Rimon et al 1987).

EXTRINSIC COAGULATION MECHANISM (Tissue factor-dependent coagulation)

The extrinsic coagulation mechanism involves the formation of a complex composed of factor VII associated with the membrane-bound tissue factor in the presence of calcium ions. This complex has the ability to activate both factor X and factor XI, thereby initiating two pathways for the formation of thrombin (Fig. 1.1). The association of tissue factor with factor VIII may well be the crucial reaction in the initiation of coagulation following injury (Nemerson 1988).

Factor VII is a single-chain glycoprotein of 406 amino acids (Hagen et al 1986). The conversion to factor VIIa involves the cleavage of an Arg–Ile bond resulting in a light chain and a heavy chain containing the active site, linked by two disulphide bonds. In contrast to the zymogens of other serine proteases, factor VII possesses significant catalytic activity and coagulation can be initiated by the association of factor VII with membrane-bound tissue factor. The complex generates activated factor X which catalyses the conversion of factor VII to its active two-chain form, increasing its coagulant activity by around an additional 100-fold (Rao et al 1986).

The tissue factor molecule contains three domains: a 219-residue extracellular domain, with a highly hydrophilic amino-terminal region; a hydrophobic transmembrane region of 23 amino acids; and a cytoplasmic domain consisting of 21 residues (Scarpati et al 1987, Spicer et al 1987).

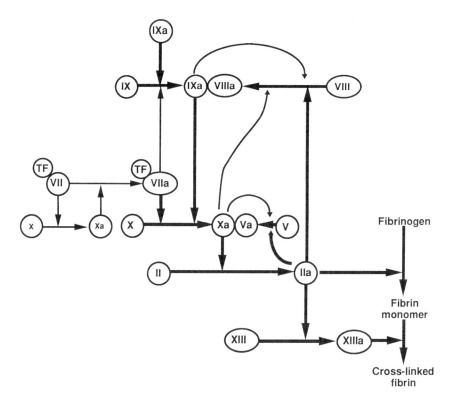

Fig. 1.1 Formation and action of thrombin. TF, tissue factor; → major reactions; →
minor reactions.

Studies have suggested that tissue factor is present on cell surfaces as a
dimer composed of two identical subunits with interacting enzyme binding
sites. Binding of factor VII to tissue factor is believed to exhibit positive
cooperativity, binding to the first site on tissue factor perturbing the receptor
permitting easier binding of the second factor VII molecule (Bach et al
1986, Fair & MacDonald 1987).

Nemerson & Gentry (1986) have proposed that the reaction between
factor VIIa, tissue factor and the substrates factor IX and factor X follows
an ordered addition model. Factor VIIa binds to tissue factor; this complex
then combines with the substrate producing a conformational change in the
factor VIIa so that it binds more tightly to tissue factor. In this way
dissociation of factor VIIa from tissue factor is precluded while significant
concentrations of substrate are present.

Anionic phospholipids enhance the ability of low concentrations of factor

Xa to activate factor VII; experimental data have been produced that the surface of platelets can provide this cofactor activity (Rao & Rapaport 1988).

To achieve coagulation through the intrinsic pathway in vivo factor VII must be delivered from the bloodstream to the membrane-bound tissue factor. Using a continuous-flow reactor consisting of microcapillaries coated with a phospholipid bilayer containing immobilized tissue factor Gemmell and associates (1988) have evaluated the effects of factor VII/VIIa concentration, factor X concentration and wall shear rate on factor Xa formation. They showed that steady-state catalytic activity in this system is independent of factor VIIa concentration, but the time required to attain steady state factor Xa formation was a function of the factor VIIa concentration. The delay in reaching steady state was reduced when shear rate increased. It was suggested that these findings could explain why patients with moderate decreases in factor VII level do not bleed.

THE INTERACTION BETWEEN FACTORS Xa, Va AND PROTHROMBIN

Thrombin is formed from its zymogen prothrombin through two proteolytic cleavages in a reaction catalysed by an enzyme complex termed prothrombinase, composed of factor Xa, thrombin-modified factor V, negatively charged phospholipid and calcium ion. A detailed review has been prepared by Mann and colleagues (1988).

Factor V is a single-chain glycoprotein with a molecular weight of about 286 000 (Kane & Davie 1988). It consists of four major domains, the heavy and light-chain regions corresponding to two of these and a connecting region corresponding to the remaining two (Dahlback 1985).

Factor V circulates in plasma in an essentially inactive state and requires activation by thrombin in order to function as a cofactor in the prothrombinase complex (see Fig. 1.1). This reaction involves three specific enzymatic cleavages. During its activation by thrombin, factor V loses its central connecting region and consists of a heavy and a light chain (Jenny et al 1987).

Factor Xa is also capable of activating factor V; this is achieved through a different set of bond cleavages, but less efficiently than by thrombin and requiring anionic phospholipid. This pathway for the formation of factor Va, however, may be of physiological significance by providing some prothrombinase activity and the formation of small amounts of thrombin. Counter to this hypothesis, however, Pieters and associates (1989) have reported that thrombin rather than factor Xa is responsible for the activation of factor V in plasma activated with thromboplastin: they suggest that factor Xa is able by itself, albeit at a low rate, to convert prothrombin to thrombin which is then able to activate factor V (and factor VIII).

It is the light chain of factor Va which is responsible for the binding of the cofactor to the platelet membrane and there is evidence from the use of a lipophilic, photoactivable probe that the factor Va penetrates into the lipid bilayer (Lecompte et al 1987). There is also evidence for the direct binding of factor Xa to factor Va in the absence of phospholipid or platelets (Annamalai et al 1987) and direct binding of factor Va through a site on its heavy chain to prothrombin (Guinto & Esmon 1984, Lucknow et al 1989). There has been, therefore, further validation of the concept that factor Va serves as a receptor for factor Xa and its substrate prothrombin on membrane surfaces.

Human prothrombinase consists of a $1:1$ stoichiometric complex of factor Xa and factor Va assembled on a phospholipid surface in the presence of calcium ions. The complex is capable of catalysing the activation of prothrombin through the cleavage of the Arg_{322}–Ile_{323} bond with the formation of an intermediate termed meizothrombin, followed by cleavage at the Arg_{273}–Thr_{274} bond to yield α-thrombin. In the absence of factor Va prothrombin activation proceeds via the cleavage of the Arg_{273}–Thr_{274} bond to produce prethrombin 2, followed by its slow conversion to α-thrombin (Krishnaswamy et al 1987).

Since both factor Xa and thrombin generation involves a phospholipid surface it is feasible that the reactions of the coagulation mechanism involved in their formation take place on the same cell surface. The alternative possibility is that the factor Xa formed dissociates to become free in solution before taking part in the prothrombinase complex with factor Va. The latter hypothesis is supported by experiments reported by Hemker and associates (1989); using a synthetic pentasaccharide which inhibits only free factor Xa they have concluded that free factor Xa plays a rate-limiting role in both the intrinsic and extrinsic coagulation pathways.

Regulation of the cofactor activity of factor Va is achieved through the catalytic action of activated protein C which induces proteolytic cleavages in both chains of factor Va. Cleavage of the heavy chain of the cofactor by activated protein C results in a reduction in its ability to interact with prothrombin or factor Xa (Guinto & Esmon 1984), whereas cleavage of the light chain does not affect its biological activity (Odegaard & Mann 1987).

Platelet factor V

Around 20% of the total factor V in blood is located in the α-granules of platelets, and is secreted on platelet activation. Human platelet factor V appears to be stored in platelets as a partially fragmented procofactor that can be activated by thrombin to yield platelet factor Va indistinguishable from plasma factor Va (Viskup et al 1987).

The importance of platelet factor V is suggested by the report of a family afflicted with a bleeding tendency whose affected members had grossly abnormal platelet factor V function, but normal plasma factor V level and function (Tracy et al 1984). Additionally, Nesheim and colleagues (1986) have described a patient who developed a plasma factor V inhibitor without the appearance of a haemorrhagic tendency: the factor V in the platelets appeared to be relatively inaccessible to the antibody.

Thrombin

Human α-thrombin is a serine protease composed of a 36 aminoacyl residue A chain linked via a disulphide bond to a 259 aminoacyl residue B chain which contains the specific catalytic site.

Thrombin represents the culmination of the coagulation cascade with a number of actions in the coagulation mechanism in addition to the conversion of fibrinogen to fibrin. These include the activation of factors V and VIII, the activation of factor XIII and the activation of protein C (Figs 1.1 and 1.2).

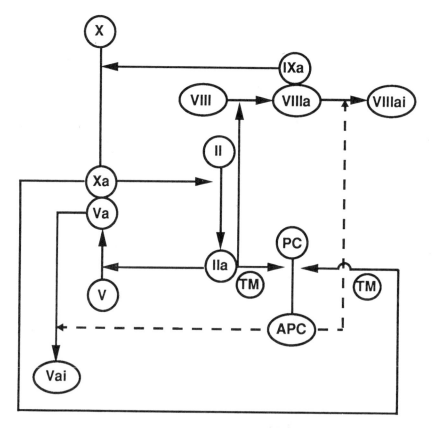

Fig 1.2   Modulation of coagulation mechanism by thrombin feedback reactions – activation of factors V and VIII, and activation of protein C which inactivates factors Va and VIIIa. PC, protein C; APC, activated protein C; TM, thrombomodulin; Vai, inactivated factor Va; VIIIai, inactivated factor VIIIa.

Thrombin has further influences on the haemostatic mechanism; it has an important role in the activation of platelets, while thrombin binding to the endothelium results in the release of von Willebrand factor, prostacyclin, adenosine diphosphate and plasminogen activator inhibitor.

Bar-Shavit and colleagues (1989) have shown recently that thrombin can also interact with the subendothelial basement membrane and thereby contribute to its thrombogenic properties: thrombin was found to bind specifically with the subendothelial extracellular cell matrix, retaining functional catalytic sites, but protected from inactivation by antithrombin III.

The importance of thrombin as a mediator of platelet-dependent haemostatic plug formation (and acute high-shear thrombosis) has been demonstrated in experiments reported by Hanson & Harker (1988) using a synthetic antithrombin and a baboon model of arterial graft thrombosis.

Regulation of thrombin activity to accord with the requirement for its various roles in the coagulation mechanism is ill understood. A contribution has been made by the demonstration of the effects of complexes of thrombin, fibrin II monomer and polymer and heparin (Hogg & Jackson 1990). Thrombin in a complex with heparin and fibrin II, fibrin from which both fibrinopeptide A and B have been romoved, was shown to have an altered reactivity to some of its substrates and inhibitors – the rate of cleavage of prothrombin and the rate of inactivation by antithrombin III are reduced whereas its ability to convert fibrinogen to fibrin is uninfluenced. Experimental data suggested that the effects of heparin and fibrin on the actions of thrombin would diminish as the fibrin polymerized. It is suggested, therefore, that in the earlier stages of clotting, when there is a higher concentration of fibrin monomer, inactivation of thrombin by inhibitors is reduced. As polymerization proceeds and the requirement for thrombin activity or fibrinogen is reduced, the binding of thrombin in the ternary complex becomes weaker, allowing inhibition to proceed.

INHIBITION OF THE COAGULATION SYSTEM

A number of inhibitors acting on different stages of the coagulation system have been identified, including antithrombin III, protein C, α_1-protease inhibitor and extrinsic pathway inhibitor. The functional importance of antithrombin III and protein C is underscored by the high incidence of venous thrombosis at an early age in patients with hereditary deficiencies of either inhibitor.

Antithrombin III

Antithrombin III, its activity enhanced by binding to heparin, inhibits both thrombin and factor Xa and contributes to the localization of coagulation by rapidly inhibiting thrombin and factor Xa released into the circulation.

In contrast, factor Xa bound to factor Va on a phospholipid surface is not susceptible to inhibitors. Additionally, antithrombin III is bound to the luminal surface of the endothelium by heparin-like proteoglycans which enhance its anticoagulant activity; this may contribute to the prevention of activation of the coagulation system on the vessel wall (Stern et al 1985b).

Platelet factor 4 and histidine-rich glycoprotein are known to be capable of neutralizing the anticoagulant activity of heparin. More recently protein S, the major inhibitor of the membrane-attack complex assembly of complement, has also been shown to counteract the heparin-catalysed inhibition of thrombin by antithrombin III (Preissner & Muller-Berghaus, 1986).

Protein C

Protein C in its activated form inactivates factors Va and VIIIa through proteolytic cleavage in a reaction requiring a cofactor termed protein S, an anionic surface and calcium. Activated protein C is formed from its zymogen by a complex of α-thrombin and the endothelial cell surface protein thrombomodulin. When bound to thrombomodulin α-thrombin has a 1000-fold greater ability to activate protein C compared with α-thrombin alone. The binding of thrombin to thrombomodulin alters its procoagulant properties so that it is no longer capable of converting fibrinogen to fibrin, activating factor V or inducing platelet aggregation. In this way thrombomodulin imparts a natural anticoagulant surface to the endothelium and, by binding thrombin released at the site of injury, plays a part in protecting the microvasculature downstream.

Factor Xa in the presence of phospholipid and calcium ion has also been found to be able to activate protein C, thrombomodulin again serving as a cofactor in the factor Xa-catalysed reaction (Haley et al 1989).

Extrinsic pathway inhibitor

An inhibitor of the catalytic activity of the factor VIIa/tissue factor complex has been identified and characterized as a Kunitz-type proteinase inhibitor which requires factor Xa as a cofactor (Broze & Miletich 1987, Rao & Rapaport 1987). Through this relationship the factor Xa formed during coagulation can initiate a regulating mechanism that inhibits further factor VIIa/tissue factor-catalysed generation of factor Xa (Fig. 1.3). The inhibitor has recently been isolated from human plasma and partially characterized (Novotny et al 1989). It has been termed the extrinsic pathway inhibitor (Rao & Rapaport 1987) or the lipoprotein-associated coagulation inhibitor (Broze et al 1988).

The inhibition of factor VIIa/tissue factor activity appears to involve the formation of an inhibitor/factor Xa complex followed by a calcium-dependent

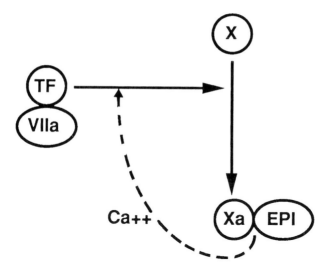

Fig. 1.3   Formation and action of extrinsic pathway inhibitor activity. TF, tissue factor; EPI, extrinsic pathway inhibitor.

quaternary inhibitor/factor Xa/factor VIIa/tissue factor complex (Broze et al 1988).

A functionally and antigenically similar inhibitor is released from stimulated platelets (Novotny et al 1988).

THE FORMATION OF FIBRIN

Fibrinogen participates in the haemostatic process both by supporting, with von Willebrand factor, the platelet–platelet interactions required for platelet aggregation, and in the stabilization of the platelet aggregates following its conversion to fibrin.

Human fibrinogen is composed of three pairs of non-identical polypeptide chains (Aα, Bβ and γ). Its conversion to fibrin is initiated through limited proteolysis of the two Aα-chains by thrombin to release fibrinopeptide A and form fibrin I monomer. The fibrin I monomers become fibrin I profibrils through rapid end-to-end assembly. Lateral association of the profibrils to form thicker fibrin fibres takes place following thrombin-catalysed proteolysis of the Bβ chain to release fibrinopeptide B.

Stabilization of the fibrin fibres is achieved through the formation of γ-glutamyl-ε-lysine peptide cross-links between adjacent fibrin units, a reaction catalysed by factor XIIIa. Plasma factor XIII is a tetramer composed of two a and two b subunits; the a subunit possession factor XIIIa enzymatic activity after activation by thrombin in the presence of calcium ions. The b subunit functions as a carrier for the a subunit. The complete amino acid sequence of both a and b subunits of human factor XIII has been determined (Ichinose et al 1986a, 1986b).

Investigations have continued to elucidate the domains involved in the fibrinogen–thrombin interaction and the other biological activities of fibrinogen. All three fibrinogen chains have been shown to interact with thrombin, the amino-terminal domain of the γ-chain having an important role in recognizing thrombin (Kaczmarek & McDonagh 1988). Varadi & Scheraga (1986) have provided data to indicate that the γ-chain 356/357–411 region is essential for the maintenance of a polymerization site, and the platelet receptor recognition site has been localized to the sequence of 12 amino acid residues at the carboxy-terminal end of the γ-chain (Kloczewiak et al 1984).

Fibrin may have an additional function in the haemostatic mechanism. It has been shown to be capable of inducing the release of von Willebrand factor from endothelial cells (Ribes et al 1987). Cleavage of fibrinopeptide B from fibrinogen is required for the von Willebrand-releasing activity of fibrin, indicating that a site including the amino-terminus of the β-chain is involved (Ribes et al 1989).

KEY POINTS FOR CLINICAL PRACTICE

1. A haemorrhagic tendency occurs in a proportion of factor XI-deficient patients, but the bleeding is determined by factors other than the plasma factor XI level.
2. A bleeding tendency may result from a platelet factor V abnormality, even in the presence of a normal plasma factor V level and function.

REFERENCES

Ahmad S S, Rawala-Sheikh R, Walsh P N 1989 Comparative interactions of factor IX and factor IXa with human platelets. J Biol Chem 264: 3244–3251
Annamalai A E, Rao A K, Chiu H C et al 1987 Epitope mapping of functional domains of human factor Va with human and murine monoclonal antibodies: evidence for the interaction of heavy chain with factor Xa and calcium. Blood 70: 139–146
Bach R, Gentry R, Nemerson Y 1986 Factor VII binding to tissue factor in reconstituted phospholipid vesicles: induction of cooperativity by phosphatidylserine. Biochemistry 25: 4007–4020
Baglia F A, Sinha D, Walsh P N 1989 Functional domains in the heavy-chain region of factor XI: a high molecular weight kininogen-binding site and a substrate-binding site for factor IX. Blood 74: 244–251
Bar-Shavit R, Eldor A, Vlodavsky I 1989 Binding of thrombin to subendothelial extracellular matrix. J Clin Invest 84: 1096–1104
Broze G J Jr, Miletich J P 1987 Characterisation of the inhibition of tissue factor in serum. Blood 69: 150–155
Broze G J Jr, Warren L A, Novotny W F et al 1988 The lipoprotein-associated coagulation inhibition that inhibits the factor VII-tissue factor complex also inhibits factor Xa: insight into its possible mechanism of action. Blood 71: 335–343
Burke R L, Pachl C, Quiroga M et al 1986 The functional domains of coagulation factor VIII:C. J Biol Chem 261: 12574–12578

Dahlback B 1985 Ultrastructure of human coagulation factor V. J Biol Chem 260: 1347–1349

Eaton D, Rodriguez H, Vehar G A 1986 Proteolytic processing of human factor VIII: correlation of specific cleavages by thrombin, factor Xa and activated protein C with activation and inactivation of factor VIII coagulant activity. Biochemistry 25: 505–512

Fair D S, MacDonald M J 1987 Cooperative interaction between factor VII and cell surface-expressed tissue factor. J Biol Chem 262: 11692–11698

Foster P A, Fulcher C A, Marti T et al 1987 A major factor VIII binding domain resides within the amino-terminal 272 amino acid residues of von Willebrand factor. J Biol Chem 262: 8443–8446

Fujikawa K, Chung D W, Hendrickson L E, Davie E W 1986 Amino acid sequence of human factor XI, a blood coagulation factor with four tandem repeats that are highly homologous with plasma prekallikrein. Biochemistry 25: 2417–2424

Gemmell C H, Turitto V T, Nemerson Y 1988 Flow as a regulator of the activation of factor X by tissue factor. Blood 72: 1404–1406

Gilbert G E, Furie B C, Furie B 1990 Binding of human factor VIII to phospholipid vesicles. J Biol Chem 265: 815–822

Guinto E R, Esmon C T 1984 Loss of prothrombin and of factor Xa-factor Va interactions upon inactivation of factor Va by activated protein C. J Biol Chem 259: 13986–13992

Gustafson E J, Schutsky D, Knight L C, Schmaier A H 1986 High molecular weight kininogen binds to unstimulated platelets. J Clin Invest 78: 310–318

Hagen F S, Gray C L, O'Hara P et al 1986 Characterisation of a cDNA coding for human factor VII. Proc Natl Acad Sci USA 83: 2412–2416

Haley P E, Doyle M F, Mann K G 1989 The activation of bovine protein C by factor Xa. J Biol Chem 264: 16303–16310

Hanson S R, Harker L A 1988 Interruption of acute platelet-dependent thrombosis by the synthetic antithrombin D-phenylalanyl-L-arginyl chloromethyl ketone. Proc Natl Acad Sci USA 85: 3184–3188

Hemker H C, Choay J, Beguin S 1989 Free factor Xa is on the main pathway of thrombin generation in clotting plasma. Biochim Biophys Acta 992: 409–411

Hogg P J, Jackson C M 1990 Formation of a ternary complex between thrombin, fibrin monomer, and heparin influences the action of thrombin on its substrates. J Biol Chem 265: 248–255

Ichinose A, Hendrickson L E, Fujikawa K, Davie E W 1986a Amino acid sequence of the a subunit of human factor XIII. Biochemistry 25: 6900–6906

Ichinose A, McMullen B A, Fujikawa K, Davie E W 1986b Amino acid sequence of the b subunit of human factor XIII, a protein composed of ten repetitive segments. Biochemistry 25: 4633–4638

Jenny R J, Pittman D D, Toole J J 1987 Complete cDNA and derived amino acid sequence by human factor V. Proc Natl Acad Sci USA 84: 4846–4850

Kaczmarek E, McDonagh J 1988 Thrombin binding to the Aα, Bβ and γ chains of fibrinogen and to their remnants contained in fragment E. J Biol Chem 263: 13896–13900

Kane W H, Davie E W 1988 Blood coagulation factors V and VIII: structural and functional similarities and their relationship to haemorrhagic and thrombotic disorders. Blood 71: 539–555

Kaplan A P, Silverberg M 1987 The coagulation-kinin pathway of human plasma. Blood 70: 1–15

Kloczewiak M, Timmons S, Lukas T J, Hawiger J 1984 Platelet receptor recognition site on human fibrinogen: synthesis and structure–function relationship of peptides corresponding to the carboxy-terminal segment of the γ chain. Biochemistry 23: 1767–1774

Krishnaswamy S, Church W R, Nesheim M E, Mann K G 1987 Activation of human prothrombin by human prothrombinase. J Biol Chem 262: 3291–3299

Lecompte M-F, Krishnaswamy S, Mann K G et al 1987 Membrane penetration of bovine factor V and Va detected by labelling with 5-iodonaphthalene-1-azide. J Biol Chem 262: 1935–1937

Lucknow E A, Lyons D A, Ridgeway T M et al 1989 Interaction of clotting factor V heavy chain with prothrombin and prethrombin 1 and role of activated protein C in regulating this interaction: analysis by analytical ultracentrifugation. Biochemistry 28: 2348–2354

Mann K G, Jenny R J, Krishnaswamy S 1988 Cofactor proteins in the assembly and expression of blood clotting enzyme complexes. Annu Rev Biochem 57: 915–956

Nemerson Y 1988 Tissue factor and hemostasis. Blood 71: 1–8

Nemerson Y, Gentry R 1986 An ordered addition, essential activation model of the tissue factor pathway of coagulation: evidence for a conformational cage. Biochemistry 25: 4020–4033

Nesheim M E, Nichols W L, Cole T L et al 1986 Isolation and study of an acquired inhibitor of human coagulation factor V. J Clin Invest 77: 405–415

Nesheim M E, Pittman D D, Wang J H et al 1988 The binding of ^{35}S-labeled recombinant factor VIII to activated and unactivated human platelets. J Biol Chem 263: 16467–16470

Neuenschwander P, Jesty J 1988 A comparison of phospholipid and platelets in the activation of human factor VIII by thrombin and factor Xa, and in the activation of factor X. Blood 72: 1761–1770

Novotny W F, Girard T J, Miletich J P, Broze G J Jr 1988 Platelets secrete a coagulation inhibitor functionally and antigenetically similar to the lipoprotein associated coagulation inhibitor. Blood 72: 2020–2025

Novotny W F, Girard T J, Miletich J P, Broze G J Jr 1989 Purification and characterization of the lipoprotein-associated coagulation inhibitor from human plasma. J Biol Chem 264: 18832–18837

Odegaard B, Mann K 1987 Proteolysis of factor Va by factor Xa and activated protein C. J Biol Chem 262: 11233–11238

Pieters J, Lindhout T, Hemker H C 1989 In situ-generated thrombin is the only enzyme that effectively activates factor VIII and factor V in thromboplastin-activated plasma. Blood 74: 1021–1024

Pittman D, Kaufman RJ 1988 Proteolytic requirement for thrombin activation of anti-hemophilic factor (factor VIII). Proc Natl Acad Sci USA 85: 2429–2433

Preissner K T, Muller-Berghaus G 1986 S protein modulates the heparin-catalyzed inhibition of thrombin by antithrombin III. Eur J Biochem 156: 645–650

Ragni M V, Sinha R D, Seaman F et al 1985 Comparison of bleeding tendency, factor XI coagulant activity and factor XI antigen in 25 factor XI-deficient kindreds. Blood 65: 719–724

Rao V M, Rapaport S I 1987 Studies of a mechanism inhibiting the initiation of the extrinsic pathway of coagulation. Blood 69: 645–651

Rao L V M, Rapaport S I 1988 The effect of platelets upon factor Xa-catalyzed activation of factor VII in vitro. Blood 72: 396–401

Rao L V M, Rapaport S I, Bajaj S P 1986 Activation of human factor VII in the initiation of tissue factor-dependent coagulation. Blood 68: 685–691

Ribes J A, Francis C W, Wagner D D 1987 Fibrin induces release of von Willebrand factor from endothelial cells. J Clin Invest 79: 117–123

Ribes J A, Ni F, Wagner D D, Francis C W 1989 Mediation of fibrin-induced release of von Willebrand factor from cultured endothelial cells by the fibrin β chain. J Clin Invest 84: 435–442

Rimon S, Melamed R, Savion N et al 1987 Identification of a factor IX/IXa binding protein on the endothelial cell surface. J Biol Chem 262: 6023–6031

Scarpati E M, Wen D, Broze G J Jr et al 1987 Human tissue factor: cDNA sequence and chromosome localization of the gene. Biochemistry 26: 5234–5238

Schmaier A H, Smith P M, Purdon A D et al 1986 High molecular weight kininogen: localization in the unstimulated and activated platelet and activation by a platelet calpain(s). Blood 67: 119–130

Schmaier A H, Kuo A, Lundberg D et al 1988 The expression of high molecular weight kininogen on human umbilical vein endothelial cells. J Biol Chem 263: 16327–16333

Sinha D, Koshy A, Seaman F S, Walsh P N 1985 Functional characterization of human blood coagulation factor XIa using hybridoma antibodies. J Biol Chem 260: 10714–10719

Sinha D, Seaman F S, Walsh P N 1987 Role for calcium ions and heavy chain of factor XIa in the activation of human coagulation factor IX. Biochemistry 26: 3768–3775

Spicer E K, Horton R, Bloem L et al 1987 Isolation of cDNA clones coding for human tissue factor: primary structures of the protein and cDNA. Proc Natl Acad Sci USA 84: 5148–5152

Stern D M, Nawroth P P, Kisiel W et al 1985a The binding of factor IXa to cultured bovine aortic endothelial cells. J Biol Chem 260: 6717–6722

Stern D M, Nawroth P, Marcum J et al 1985b Interaction of antithrombin III with bovine aortic seguments: role of heparin in binding and enhanced anticoagulant activity. J Clin Invest 75: 272–279

Tracy P B, Giles A R, Mann K G et al 1984 Factor V (Quebec): a bleeding diathesis associated with a qualitative platelet factor V deficiency. J Clin Invest 74: 1221–1228

van Iwaarden F, de Groot P G, Bouma B N 1988 The binding of high molecular weight kininogen to cultured human endothelial cells. J Biol Chem 263: 4698–4703

Varadi A, Scheraga H A 1986 Localization of segments essential for polymerization and for calcium binding in the γ-chain of human fibrinogen. Biochemistry 25: 519–528

Viskup R W, Tracy P B, Mann K G 1987 The isolation of human platelet factor V. Blood 69: 1188–1195

Walsh P N, Griffin J H 1981 Contributions of human platelets to the proteolytic activation of blood coagulation factors XII and XI. Blood 57: 106–118

Walsh P N, Sinha D, Koshy A et al 1986 Functional characterization of platelet-bound factor XIa: retention of factor XIa activity on the platelet surface. Blood 68: 225–230

2

Developments in fibrinolysis

E.J.P. Brommer,   P. Brakman

During the last ten years or so, fibrinolysis has come to the fore in clinical medicine mainly through the success of thrombolytic treatment of acute myocardial infarction. Promising results have coincided with the isolation of human tissue-type plasminogen activator (t-PA) and the commercial production of the recombinant enzyme, rt-PA, which has nurtured both thrombolytic therapy and fibrinolytic research. This has in turn stimulated the development of commercial test kits: nowadays an array of test kits is available for the measurement of fibrinolytic enzymes, inhibitors and reaction products in blood and other body fluids. Small wonder that interest in fibrinolysis penetrated into almost every hospital.

Outside cardiology, however, the practical implications of the growing knowledge of fibrinolysis are still limited. Thrombolytic therapy is only hesitatingly used in deep vein thrombosis and pulmonary embolism. Indications for diagnostic fibrinolytic tests are slow to emerge, concomitant with the recognition of the consequences for treatment. The main clinical applications of the acquired knowledge remain within the treatment of thrombosis and bleeding disorders, although the role of fibrinolysis or just plasminogen activation in tissue repair, chronic disease and tumour growth, the scenes of the pioneers in fibrinolysis, makes a comeback, for the time being mainly experimentally.

In this chapter the major acquisitions of knowledge of fibrinolysis over the last few years will be reviewed, with particular focus on the clinical applications. For more detailed information on biochemistry and experimental data, as well as to literature before 1987, the reader is referred to other recent reviews and *Recent Advances in Blood Coagulation 4.*

THE FIBRINOLYTIC SYSTEM

The ensemble of proteins in blood, urine and body fluids involved in the dissolution of fibrin strands, or in the inhibition of lysis, is commonly referred to as the fibrinolytic system. Understandably, this imaginary system gradually expands as our techniques detect more enzymes, inhibitors, stimulators or other modifiers of fibrinolysis. There is an obvious overlap with other conceptual systems, e.g. the coagulation system, the contact activation or the complement system. The principal sources of fibrinolytic components of circulating blood are the liver (e.g. plasminogen and the main inhibitor of plasmin: α_2-antiplasmin) and the vascular wall (e.g. tissue-type plasminogen activator, t-PA). The main plasminogen activator inhibitor, PAI-1, although produced to a large extent by the vascular endothelium, is also present in circulating blood platelets (Kruithof et al 1987) and consequently accrues to a high concentration in platelet-rich thrombi.

According to the simplest scheme, plasmin, the enzyme responsible for the degradation of fibrin, is formed by partial cleavage of plasminogen by one of the recognized plasminogen activators: tissue-type (t-PA) and/or urokinase-type (u-PA). The reaction seems to take place preferentially upon the fibrin surface, which offers sites for an optimal contact between plasminogen and its activators. This stimulatory effect of fibrin results in a relatively fibrin-specific action, at least in the case of t-PA. Fibrin-bound t-PA initiates fibrin degradation by activating fibrin-bound plasminogen; certain new high-affinity binding sites for plasminogen become available which induce conformational changes in the plasminogen molecules; these attract pro-urokinase or single-chain u-PA (scu-PA) which cooperates in this way with t-PA in breaking down the fibrin structure (Gurewich 1989). An alternative explanation is that the conversion of single-chain u-PA to two-chain u-PA is an essential step (Lijnen et al 1989). It is not known whether the removal of fibrin from an arteriosclerotic arterial wall, from glomerular tufts in nephritis or from other inflammatory sites, proceeds in an identical manner to the removal of fibrin from a haemostatic plug or a thrombus. Lytic enzymes from granulocytes and mononuclear leucocytes are active in inflammatory areas and within tissues in general, probably more so than enzymes supplied by the blood. However, for the dissolution of fibrin some of these enzymes seem to need plasminogen. Mononuclear cells can secrete u-PA when in contact with fibrin (Ghezzo et al 1986). In other circumstances monocytes can be stimulated to produce t-PA, for instance by lipopolysaccharide or interleukin-4 (Hart et al 1989). There are, however, a number of other leucocyte enzymes which might break down fibrin. In areas of inflammation, as for example in the inflamed appendix, the endothelial cells may also contain u-PA, whereas in normal circumstances only t-PA can be found (Grøndahl-Hansen et al 1989). The implications of this change are not fully understood. Although fibrin may accomplish an important function in inflammatory processes, eventual removal of extravascular fibrin is regarded as useful. Fibrin deposition between serous membranes during peritonitis and the ensuing propensity to abscess formation can be prevented by t-PA, at least in animal models (Doody et al 1989, Dörr et al 1990).

Local inflammation may induce changes in circulating components of the fibrinolytic system through an acute phase reaction. The most dramatic changes are seen in the level of PAI-1 (Kluft et al 1988a). The purpose of this acute and short-lasting rise in the PAI activity of the blood is not clear. Presumably, it protects against the hazardous action of proteolytic enzymes, released during the septic state.

Apart from removing fibrin, proteolysis which is induced by free or cell-bound plasmin may contribute to various physiological and pathological processes, such as keeping ducts open, homing of tumour metastasis, infiltration of inflammatory cells in tissues and activation of proenzymes, such as procollagenase.

Important new insight has been gained in the regulation of fibrinolysis upon cell membranes. Receptors for plasminogen (Miles & Plow 1988) and others for plasminogen activators (Blasi 1988) detected upon endothelial cells, upon platelets and upon monocytes migrating into areas of inflammation, enhance plasminogen activation in contact with the cell membrane, which can result in a localized fibrinolytic potential. Receptor-bound u-PA is catalytically twice as active as fluid-phase u-PA and is inhibited only by a 20 times higher molar concentration of a second type of PAI, produced by monocytes, PAI-2, not by PAI-1 (Kirchheimer & Remold 1989). Meanwhile, the extracellular matrix of the endothelium should be protected from plasmin action. One of the defence mechanisms is activated by the plasminogen activator inhibitor, PAI-1, which, bound to the matrix, might prevent plasmin formation upon the matrix by binding t-PA and by presenting t-PA to plasmin formed elsewhere which splits this complexed t-PA (Knudsen & Nachman 1988).

Free t-PA is rapidly neutralized by endothelial plasminogen activator inhibitor (PAI-1) and, to a smaller extent, by a complement inhibitor, C1INH (Booth et al 1987) and by α_2-antiplasmin (Lucore & Sobel 1988). Whether this also occurs in vivo is not certain. In the presence of clotting fibrinogen, free t-PA is incorporated into the clot where it can activate bound plasminogen. This activation of fibrin-bound plasminogen is greatly enhanced by polymerization of fibrin (Koopman et al 1986, Suensen & Petersen 1986). This might explain impaired fibrinolysis with resultant thrombosis in several cases of dysfibrinogenaemia.

On pre-formed clots, single-chain t-PA is converted into two-chain t-PA by traces of plasmin, which allows for binding to a larger number of low-affinity binding sites. Cross-linking of fibrin by factor XIIIa, itself in turn activated by thrombin, results in the masking of high-affinity binding sites that are present in non-cross-linked fibrin (Husain et al 1989). Thus, excessive thrombin action, as for instance in antithrombin III deficiency or in some dysfibrinogenaemias (Haverkate et al 1986), may counteract fibrinolysis and may also predispose to thrombosis through this pathway.

Even on the fibrin surface, t-PA is inhibited by fibrin-bound PAI. There is evidence that free t-PA competes with t-PA/PAI-1 complexes for common binding sites (Wagner et al 1989). Presumably, high concentrations of t-PA can oust these complexes from binding sites on fibrin. Conversely, high PAI-1 levels may suppress fibrinolysis at this level: in rabbits, the infusion of reactivated recombinant PAI-1 normalized the prolonged bleeding time induced by the combination of rt-PA and aspirin (Vaughan et al 1989). Regulation of the blood level of plasminogen activators is crucial for an adequate removal of fibrin from the circulation, from damaged vessel walls and, probably, from the luminal part of haemostatic plugs. A circadian fluctuation of fibrinolytic activity had already been observed; and it has recently been shown that the rise in activity during the day was primarily a result of a decrease in the PAI level (Kluft et al 1988b).

Notwithstanding a decrease in t-PA antigen, t-PA activity rises during the day, due to a relatively large decrease in PAI-1 (Kluft et al 1988b, Grimaudo et al 1988, Angleton et al 1989). It has been surmised that the peak in the incidence of myocardial infarctions in the morning hours is related to this diurnal rhythm (Andreotti et al 1989, Angleton et al 1989). With regard to patients with thrombophilia having normal fibrinolytic activity in the morning, one might ask whether PAI activity in these patients actually drops during the day (Grimaudo et al 1988).

Obviously it is important to identify the mechanism behind these regulations. A number of physiological stimuli have been detected, but their relevance is not known. For instance, physiological variations of vasopressin concentrations in the blood induce changes in t-PA activity, leaving PAI-1 antigen unchanged (Hariman et al 1989). Physical exercise can raise t-PA activity acutely, possibly mediated through liberation of adrenaline from the adrenal glands into the circulation. After the stimulus, free t-PA is present in the blood, overshadowing PAI for a short period of time. Mental stress appears to do the same (Jern et al 1989). In case of a labile equilibrium between coagulation and fibrinolysis, as for instance in coagulation factor deficiencies, this might cause bleeding episodes. Plasma u-PA levels seemed to be stable under the above-mentioned conditions when measured with old, crude techniques, but with a recently developed biological immunoassay (BIA) a significant rise has been observed after infusion of desmopressin (DDAVP) (Levi et al 1989). Clinicians hope to find anomalies which might disclose the secret of the physiological regulation of the fibrinolytic activity at least in the blood. This partly explains their interest in disturbances in fibrinolysis in their patients.

DISTURBANCES OF FIBRINOLYSIS IN HUMAN PATHOLOGY

The efficacy of fibrinolysis depends on the amount and on the constitution of its substrate, fibrin. A high fibrinogen level creates a predisposition to cardiovascular disease, coronary atherosclerosis (Meade et al 1986, Handa et al 1989), peripheral arterial disease (Kannel et al 1987) and stroke (Di Minno & Mancini 1990), although it is possible that other processes are responsible, rather than just hampered fibrinolysis. Hypercoagulability, increased platelet aggregation and hyperviscosity have also been suggested as contributory factors. Abnormal fibrinogen molecules may induce a greater than normal risk of thrombosis (see above) or arteriosclerosis (Gandrille et al 1988a). Again, various different mechanisms may be envisaged, among which are decreased binding of thrombin, of plasminogen or of plasminogen activator to the abnormal fibrinogen molecule, reduced stimulation of plasminogen activation, increased cross-linking or anchoring of fibrin onto platelets and other structures. Occasionally, resistance of fibrin clots to plasmin degradation is observed.

Most dysfibrinogenaemias are detected by chance and are not associated with clinical manifestations. Acquired polymerization defects, even when causing delayed fibrin digestion, e.g., in nephrotic syndrome (Gandrille et al 1988b) can exist without a thrombotic or haemorrhagic diathesis. The same holds true for the inhibition of fibrin polymerization induced by circulating Bence-Jones protein, observed in a case of amyloidosis (Shigekiyo et al 1989). Increased post-translational glycosylation of fibrinogen due to high blood glucose levels in diabetes mellitus may cause impaired α-cross-linking with a higher than normal susceptibility to plasmin degradation (Lütjens et al 1988).

As for plasminogen, a genetic polymorphism has been discovered. Most variants are 'silent' (Skoda et al 1988). Genetically low plasminogen levels may be associated with thrombophilia (Hach-Wunderle et al 1988, Liu et al 1988) as are some abnormal plasminogens (Scharrer et al 1988). Non-enzymatic glycosylation of plasminogen in diabetes mellitus may induce functional abnormalities such as exaggerated substrate inhibition (Geiger & Binder 1986) or increased activation by streptokinase (Lütjens et al 1991).

Acquired α_2-antiplasmin deficiency with ensuing haemorrhagic tendency is seen in severe liver failure, after L-asparaginase therapy and after infusion of thrombolytic agents. The level of α_2-antiplasmin may be dramatically reduced in disseminated intravascular coagulation and in acute promyelocytic leukaemia (Williams 1989). It has now also been described in secondary amyloidosis (Clyne & Caldwell 1987).

Evidence for a reduced release of t-PA after adequate stimulation as a cause of clinical thrombosis remains scanty. On the other hand, a decrease in available t-PA as a sequela of its complexing with PAI, which may occur in an abnormally high concentration in the blood, is noticed in an increasing number of diseases (Kruithof et al 1988).

In the first place, a high PAI activity is associated with coronary heart disease (Hamsten et al 1987, Korninger et al 1988, Olofsson et al 1989) and with early peripheral atherosclerosis (Aronson et al 1989). A causal relationship, however, is difficult to prove.

In the second place, as had been proposed earlier, high PAI is possibly causally related to venous thrombosis; new evidence has been provided (Jørgenson & Bonnevie-Nielsen 1987, Sloan & Firkin 1989, Tabernero et al 1989). Among patients with a circulating lupus anticoagulant, those who failed to respond to venous occlusion with a rise in t-PA activity, despite a normal rise in t-PA antigen activity, experienced thrombosis

(Francis et al 1988). A high PAI level was regarded as responsible for the inability to raise the fibrinolytic activity of the blood. The high PAI level in patients with a lupus anticoagulant has been confirmed by Tsakiris et al (1989).

In some cases of thrombophilia, the elevated PAI activity seemed to be the exponent of a familial disorder, but in a nation-wide study, comprising 203 probands with venous thrombophilia, in none of the cases could thrombophilia be attributed to a hereditary, persistent elevation of the blood level of PAI (Engesser et al 1989).

In part, the rise in PAI activity might be the consequence of smoking (Haire et al 1989) or of a diet: even a moderate fish intake increases PAI activity (Emeis et al 1989). Furthermore, PAI activity is correlated with serum triglyceride levels, at least in young survivors of acute myocardial infarction (Hamsten et al 1987) and in obese women (Juhan-Vague et al 1987b). Some investigators have found a similar correlation in healthy volunteers (Crutchley et al 1989), dependent on the nutritional status (Sundell et al 1988).

Chronic disease and malignancy are often associated with high PAI activity in the blood (De Jong et al 1987, Páramo et al 1987, Kirchheimer et al 1987), which may be a consequence of a chronic stimulation, comparable with the acute phase reaction. It has to be noted that in chronic diseases high PAI levels are often accompanied by elevated plasma concentrations of t-PA antigen (De Jong et al 1987), presumably reflecting a high concentration of complexes of t-PA with PAI. Glomerular fibrin deposits and renal microthrombosis have been attributed to a severe impairment of fibrinolysis in patients with chronic obstructive jaundice, most of them suffering from carcinoma; PAI levels were significantly elevated and could account for impaired fibrinolysis (Colucci et al 1988).

High PAI activity has been reported in pregnancy (De Boer et al 1988, Wright et al 1988) and especially in pre-eclampsia (Estellés et al 1989). It is tempting to relate the vascular obstructions in the spiral arteries, in the placenta and in renal glomeruli to the suppression of fibrinolysis. A second, 'placenta-type' inhibitor, identical to the inhibitor secreted by monocytes, PAI-2, but immunologically distinguishable from PAI-1, is detectable in the blood during pregnancy (Lecander et al 1988). In pre-eclampsia, PAI-2 levels remain below those in normal pregnancy despite the overall rise in PAI activity. Interestingly, the level of PAI-2 antigen correlates with placenta weight and with birth weight, and actually may reflect placental function (De Boer et al 1988, Estellés et al 1989). After parturition, PAI-1 activity returns to normal, within a couple of hours, whereas PAI-2 remains detectable for a few days afterwards (Reith et al 1989).

It is difficult to establish how far PAI-3, a third plasminogen activator inhibitor, identical to protein C inhibitor, influences the PAI activity of plasma in vivo. PAI-3 is stimulated by heparin-like substances which are attached to the vessel wall (Geiger 1988).

Other causes of high PAI activity are hyperinsulinaemia (Juhan-Vague et al 1989a), and obesity (Sundell et al 1989). In insulin-dependent diabetes mellitus, the high PAI may contribute, together with a concomitant hypertriglyceridaemia, to the vascular complications (Juhan-Vague et al 1989b). The elevated PAI levels in bacteraemia and sepsis (Páramo et al 1988) are attributed to direct or indirect stimulation by endotoxins (Suffredini et al 1989). When measured on admission of patients with septic shock, PAI-1 antigen levels appear to have a predictive value for mortality (Pralong et al 1989). Apparently, the PAI level reflects the gravity of the disease, rather than protecting the patient.

The influence of androgenic steroids on the PAI level and the relationship between PAI and testosterone levels (Caron et al 1989) suggest an association with sex hormones and their binding proteins. Indeed, a discrete binding protein for PAI has been found by Wiman and coworkers (1988). However, there is no evidence that the level of PAI is regulated through changes in the concentration of this binding protein, which is identified as a multimer of vitronectin (Declerck et al 1988).

A high PAI level is regarded as harmful as it may predispose to thrombosis or atherosclerosis, while too low a PAI activity, as observed in a patient with antibodies directed against PAI (Francis et al 1986), or an abnormally functioning PAI (Schleef et al 1989) may cause a severe bleeding tendency. Presumably, in these cases t-PA or u-PA are not prevented from activating fibrin-bound plasminogen in haemostatic plugs.

The haemostatic disturbance in disseminated intravascular coagulation with fibrinolysis (DIC) is complex. With regard to fibrinolysis, mean t-PA antigen levels are higher than normal, whereas t-PA activity may be low (Francis & Seyfert 1987) or high (Bennett et al 1989). High PAI antigens are expected to be found. The same holds true for thrombotic thrombocytopenic purpura, although the pathogenesis of this syndrome is quite different. As a matter of fact, not only high t-PA values, but exceedingly high PAI-1 antigen values, have been measured in this disorder (Kakishita et al 1989).

In severe hepatic insufficiency, a disease often complicated by DIC, comparable disturbances of fibrinolysis can be found (Carr 1989, Tran-Thang et al 1989). Reduction of the synthesis of a number of coagulation factors, fibrinolytic components and inhibitors, viz. antithrombin III, α_2-antiplasmin and histidine-rich glycoprotein (Leebeek et al 1989), adds to the complexity of haemostatic disturbances in hepatic insufficiency. Partly, the elevated concentration of t-PA in liver disease can be ascribed to impairment of clearance (Brommer et al 1988). This is mimicked by the anhepatic phase during liver transplantation (Porte et al 1989). Administration of ε-aminocaproic acid in the anhepatic stage produced favourable results (Kang et al 1987). This is an argument for a proteolytic state in this condition. Evidence for plasmin formation even in the blood of non-surgical patients with severe liver disease has been provided by Takahashi et al (1989).

The notorious haemorrhagic diathesis accompanying acute promyelocytic leukaemia has often been ascribed to primary fibrinogenolysis. Recently, our earlier observation of elastase activity during treatment of blastic crisis in this disease (Sterrenberg et al 1985) has been confirmed (Saito et al 1989). However, Bennett et al (1989) ascribed the characteristic depression of the α_2-antiplasmin level (with normal antithrombin III concentration) to plasmin activity; in their two patients with acute promyelocytic leukaemia, plasminogen had been activated by u-PA, released from the malignant promyelocytes. Suppression of plasmin activity with ε-aminocaproic acid (Schwartz et al 1986) or tranexamic acid (Avvisati et al 1989) reduces haemorrhagic episodes and transfusion requirement in acute promyelocytic leukaemia, without giving rise to thromboembolic complications.

With recently available monoclonal antibodies differentiation can be made between fibrinolysis and fibrinogenolysis: fibrin degradation products (FbDP) and fibrinogen degradation products (FgDP) can be determined separately and specifically, even in plasma (instead of serum) (Nieuwenhuizen 1988). This may help to unravel these complicated disturbances of haemostasis. For example, in most cases of DIC a mixture of FbDP and FgDP is found in roughly equal amounts (Prisco et al 1989), whereas after thrombolytic therapy with streptokinase, FgDP are found in excess of FbDP (Brommer et al 1987). For the purpose of comparison, when fibrin is being dissolved in an enclosed space, as for example in an arthritic joint, only FbDP are detected in the majority of synovial fluid samples (Jespersen et al 1989).

Extravascular fibrinolysis may be important to prevent fibrin deposition in a variety of tissues, including the aqueous humour of the eye (Tripathi et al 1988) and alveolar secretions in the lung. In a high percentage of patients with adult respiratory distress syndrome (ARDS) absence of fibrinolytic activity in bronchoalveolar lavage was observed (Idell et al 1989). The depressed fibrinolytic activity, together with an increase in coagulation factors in the same samples, may have promoted the persistence of fibrin deposits.

The function of the relatively high urokinase level in urine is still unknown. A relationship with urolithiasis is conjectured (Charlton & Osmond 1986). In contrast to earlier observations by others, Takada et al (1986) found higher than normal amounts of urokinase in the urine of patients with mild glomerulonephritis, which did not correlate with protein excretion. They deduce that mild nephritis stimulates urokinase production by tubular cells. In severe SLE or proliferative glomerulonephritis, urokinase levels were less high. Fibrin degradation products in the urine of patients with glomerulonephritis seem to indicate crescentic lesions (Kamitsuji et al 1988) rather than impaired excretory function (Taira et al 1989).

In a variety of skin diseases, fibrin deposits occur in and around small cutaneous blood vessels. Efforts have been made – with some success – to demonstrate reduced blood fibrinolysis in patients with vasculitis (including systemic lupus erythematosus, SLE), venous liposclerosis, psoriasis, atopic dermatitis, atrophie blanche and others. Histochemical investigations have revealed that t-PA and u-PA are present in keratinocytes (Grøndahl-Hansen et al 1987, Hashimoto et al 1989). A role for plasminogen activators in the pathogenesis of pemphigus Wilkinson et al 1989) and dystrophic epidermolysis bullosa (Kaneko et al 1989) has been surmised.

DIAGNOSTIC CONSEQUENCES

The notion of a circadian rhythm of the fibrinolytic parameters in the blood, with the most brisk changes during the morning and evening hours, should lead to a strictly standardized time of the day for collection of blood. Perhaps, estimation of the circadian amplitude is necessary for establishing a relationship between thrombophilia or persistence of fibrin elsewhere, and a disturbance of the fibrinolytic system (Andreotti et al 1989, Grimaudo et al 1988).

The instability of t-PA in vitro, especially in cases of high PAI activity, necessitates the prevention of the complex formation between t-PA and PAI-1 even during the collection of blood for assay of t-PA activity. Acidification, originally proposed by Wiman, seems to be the favoured method (Rånby et al 1989).

Serum, prepared in a routine manner, contains about three to five times the concentration of PAI found in carefully prepared citrated plasma, due to leakage from platelets. For the preparation of plasma for fibrinolytic assays, collection of blood in a proper mixture of anticoagulant and antiplatelet agents is recommended (Juhan-Vague et al 1987a). In order to avoid ongoing proteolysis after withdrawal of blood during thrombolytic therapy, it should be collected in antibodies that protect against activation of plasminogen by plasminogen activators (Holvoet et al 1986), or else in a solution of the synthetic inhibitor of serine proteases, PPACK (Mohler et al 1986, Seifried & Tanswell 1987).

Assay of local fibrinolytic activity in affected organs might, in certain diseases, give more insight into the pathogenesis of the disease than just measuring blood levels of activators and inhibitors. However, the diagnostic procedure is much more complicated both for the clinician and for the laboratory and, last but not least, for the patient. A few examples are available: fibrinolytic activity of renal biopsies (Bergstein et al 1988), superficial vein biopsies (Smokovitis et al 1989) and skin biopsies (Lotti et al 1989).

The question of whether venous occlusion or DDAVP infusion has any clinical relevance in defining an abnormal fibrinolytic potential is still open. Quite a number of new diagnostic possibilities in the field of fibrinolysis have appeared, comprising immunological assays of activators, various inhibitors, complexes between activators and inhibitors and other reaction products.

The last years have seen a flare-up of interest in fibrin(ogen) degradation products, thanks to the introduction of monoclonal antibodies, specific against epitopes upon either (cross-linked) fibrin or fibrinogen degradation products, which do not interact with the native molecule (Nieuwenhuizen 1988). An array of diagnostic kits, based on monoclonals, have come to light.

THERAPEUTIC CONSEQUENCES

The therapeutic arsenal consists of two classes of drugs and revision of diet or life style. The first class of drug consists of isolated components of the fibrinolytic system and artificial substitutes, especially of inhibitors. Thrombolytic agents belong to this class, but are dealt with in another chapter. Purified plasminogen has been infused ancillary to thrombolytic treatment, and as the sole drug in acute renal failure (Seitz et al 1989). Favourable effects of ε-aminocaproic acid or tranexamic acid have recently been reported in immune and non-immune thrombocytopenia (Bartholomew et al 1989), Kasabach–Meritt syndrome (Ortel et al 1988), in acute promyelocytic leukaemia (Schwartz et al 1986, Avvisati et al 1989) and in gastrointestinal haemorrhage (Staël et al 1987, Henry & O'Connell 1989). Local application in mouthwash after oral surgery has proved to be successful (Sindet-Pedersen et al 1989).

A comparable effect can be attributed to the protease inhibitor aprotinin. When administered during cardiovascular bypass surgery it is supposed to suppress either kallikrein or elastase activity with favourable effects on platelet number and blood loss (Van Oeveren et al 1987, Bidstrup et al 1989).

The second class comprises agents that influence the production and/or release of endogenous fibrinolytic and other factors from endothelial cells or perhaps from smooth muscle cells (G. Sperti, personal communication) in the vascular wall. DDAVP, is the major drug in this class. By its effect upon the von Willebrand factor, it reduces the bleeding tendency in a variety of conditions after intravenous infusion and it has been administered to hundreds of patients on this indication (Mannucci 1988). Subcutaneous injection of a more concentrated preparation seems to be equally successful (Köhler et al 1989). Obviously, the release of t-PA does not interfere with its haemostatic action. Also worthy of mention among this class of drugs is stanozolol, which increases the plasminogen level apart from its effect on PAI activity (Mannucci et al 1986), and oestrogens with a more complex action. The use of contraceptive pills causes a rise in plasminogen and a decrease in histidine-rich glycoprotein, resulting in a higher free plasminogen level; oral contraceptives also lower PAI activity (Gevers Leuven et al 1987, Siegbahn & Ruusuvaara 1988). The effects seem to depend on the oestrogen content of the pill (Gevers Leuven et al 1987).

Dietary and life-style influences upon fibrinolytic components of the blood include those reducing hyperlipoproteinaemia and obesity (Juhan-Vague et al 1987b, Sundell et al 1989), apart from previously recommended measures, such as abandoning excessive use of alcohol and tobacco, and promoting exercise.

CONCLUSION

In this chapter, the emphasis has been laid upon clinical medicine. Although perhaps preventive medicine is our ultimate goal, application of our knowledge to the patient and the improved treatment of diseases can be regarded as the primary purpose to accomplish. The selected literature in this article shows that recent years have seen a steady rise of interest in fibrinolysis in clinical medicine. Apart from thrombolytic therapy attention has been focused on the involvement of fibrinolysis in inflammatory processes, the search for the cause of thrombophilia and atherosclerosis, the unravelling of the complex mechanisms of disseminated intravascular coagulation with secondary fibrinolysis and primary fibrinogenolysis. We have witnessed cautious attempts to apply rational therapy for the haemorrhagic tendency occurring in promyelocytic leukaemia and in hepatic failure. In other areas, application of biochemists' achievements to clinical medicine serves to illustrate the validity of their concepts.

REFERENCES

Andreotti F, Davies G J, Maseri A, Kluft C 1989 Inhibition of fibrinolysis in blood: circadian fluctuation and possible relevance to coronary artery disease. In: Von Arnim Th et al (eds) Predisposing conditions for acute ischemic syndromes. Steinkopff Verlag, Darmstadt, pp 20–32

Angleton P, Chandler W L, Schmer G 1989 Diurnal variation of tissue-type plasminogen activator and its rapid inhibitor (PAI-1). Circulation 79: 101–106

Aronson D C, Ruys T, Van Bockel J H et al 1989 A prospective survey of risk factors in young adults with arterial occlusive disease. Eur J Vascular Surg 3: 227–232

Avvisati G, Ten Cate J W, Büller H R, Mandelli F 1989 Tranexamic acid for control of haemorrhage in acute promyelocytic leukaemia. Lancet 2: 122–124

Bartholomew J R, Salgia R, Bell W R 1989 Control of bleeding in patients with immune and nonimmune thrombocytopenia with aminocaproic acid. Arch Int Med 149: 1959–1961

Bennett B, Booth N A, Croll A, Dawson A A 1989 The bleeding disorder in acute promyelocytic leukaemia: fibrinolysis due to u-PA rather than defibrination. Br J Haematol 71: 511–517

Bergstein J M, Riley M, Bang N U 1988 Analysis of the plasminogen activator activity of the human glomerulus. Kidney Int 33: 868–874

Bidstrup B P, Royston D, Taylor K M, Sapsford R N 1989 Reduction in blood loss and blood use after cardiopulmonary bypass with high dose aprotinin (Trasylol). J Thorac Cardiovasc Surg 97: 364–372

Blasi F 1988 Surface receptors for urokinase plasminogen activator. Fibrinolysis 2: 73–84

Booth N A, Walker E, Maughan R, Bennett B 1987 Plasminogen activator in normal subjects after exercise and venous occlusion: t-PA circulates as complexes with C1-inhibitor and PAI-1. Blood 69: 1600–1604

Brommer E J P, Engbers J, Van der Laarse A, Nieuwenhuizen W 1987 Survival of fibrinogen degradation products in the circulation after thrombolytic therapy for acute myocardial infarction. Fibrinolysis 1: 149–153

Brommer E J P, Derkx F H M, Schalekamp M A D H, Dooijewaard G, Van der Klaauw
M M 1988 Renal and hepatic handling of endogenous tissue-type plasminogen activator
(t-PA) and its inhibitor in man. Thromb Haemostasis 59: 404–411

Caron P, Bennet A, Camare R, Louvet J P, Boneu B, Sié P 1989 Plasminogen activator
inhibitor in plasma is related to testosterone in men. Metabolism 38: 1010–1015

Carr J M 1989 Disseminated intravascular coagulation in cirrhosis. Hepatology
10: 103–110

Charlton C A C, Osmond C 1986 Deficient urinary fibrinolysis in renal stone disease. Br
Med J 292: 1239–1240

Clyne L P, Caldwell A B 1987 Acquired alpha-2 anti-plasmin deficiency secondary to
amyloidosis. Thromb Haemostasis 58: 797

Colucci M, Altomare D F, Chetta G, Triggiani R, Cavallo L G, Semeraro N 1988
Impaired fibrinolysis in obstructive jaundice: evidence from clinical and experimental
studies. Thromb Haemostasis 60: 25–29

Crutchley D J, McPhee G V, Terris M F, Canossa-Terris M A 1989 Levels of three
haemostatic factors in relation to serum lipids: monocyte pro-coagulant activity, tissue
plasminogen activator, and type-1 plasminogen activator inhibitor. Arteriosclerosis
9: 934–939

De Boer K, Lecander I, Ten Cate J W, Borm J J J, Treffers P E 1988 Placental-type
plasminogen activator inhibitor in preeclampsia. Am J Obstet Gynaecol 158: 518–522

Declerck P J, De Mol M, Alessi M-C, Baudner S, Pâques E-P, Preissner K T, Müller-
Berghaus G, Collen D 1988 Purification and characterization of a plasminogen activator
inhibitor 1 binding protein from human plasma: identification as a multimeric form of S
protein (Vitronectin). J Biol Chem 263: 15454–15461

De Jong E, Knot E A R, Piket D, Iburg A H C, Rijken D C, Veenhof K H N,
Dooijewaard G, Ten Cate J W 1987 Increased plasminogen activator inhibition levels in
malignancy. Thromb Haemostasis 57: 140–143

Di Minno G, Mancini M 1990 Measuring plasma fibrinogen to predict stroke and
myocardial infarction. Arteriosclerosis 10: 1–7

Doody K J, Dunn R C , Buttram V C Jr 1989 Recombinant tissue plasminogen activator
reduces adhesion formation in a rabbit uterine horn model. Fertil Sterility 51: 509–512

Dörr J P J, Vemer H M, Brommer E J P, Willemsen W N P, Veldhuizen R W, Rolland R
1990 Prevention of postoperative adhesions by tissue-type plasminogen activator (t-PA)
in the rabbit. Eur J Obstet Gynaecol Reprod Biol 37: 287–291

Emeis J J, Van Houwelingen A C, Van den Hoogen C M, Hornstra G 1989 A moderate
fish intake increases plasminogen activator inhibitor type-1 in human volunteers. Blood
74: 233–237

Engesser L, Brommer E J P, Kluft C, Briët E 1989 Elevated plasminogen activator
inhibitor (PAI), a cause of thrombophilia? A study in 203 patients with familial or
sporadic venous thrombophilia. Thromb Haemostasis 62: 673–680

Estellés A, Gilabert J, Aznar J, Loskutoff D J, Schleef R R 1989 Changes in the plasma
levels of type 1 and type 2 plasminogen activator inhibitors in normal pregnancy and in
patients with severe preeclampsia. Blood 74: 1332–1338

Francis R B Jr, Seyfert U 1987 Tissue plasminogen activator antigen and activity in
disseminated intravascular coagulation: clinicopathologic correlations. J Lab Clin Med
110: 541–547

Francis R, Liebman H, Koehler S, Feinstein D 1986 Accelerated fibrinolysis in
amyloidosis: specific binding of tissue plasminogen activator inhibitor by an
amyloidogenic monoclonal IgG. Blood 68: 333a

Francis R B Jr, McGehee W G, Feinstein D I 1988 Endothelial-dependent fibrinolysis in
subjects with the lupus anticoagulant and thrombosis. Thromb Haemostasis
59: 412–414

Gandrille S, Priollet P, Capron L, Roncato M, Fiessinger J N, Aiach M 1988a Association
of inherited dysfibrinogenaemia and protein C deficiency in two unrelated families. Br J
Haematol 68: 329–337

Gandrille S, Jouvin M H, Toulon P, Remy P, Fiessinger J N, Roncato M, Moatti N, Aiach
M 1988b A study of fibrinogen and fibrinolysis in 10 adults with nephrotic syndrome.
Thromb Haemostasis 59: 445–450

Geiger M 1988 Protein C inhibitor/plasminogen activator inhibitor 3. Fibrinolysis
2: 183–188

Geiger M, Binder B R 1986 Nonenzymatic glucosylation as a contributing factor to defective fibrinolysis in diabetes mellitus. Haemostasis 16: 439–446

Gevers Leuven J A, Kluft C, Bertina R M, Hessel L W 1987 Effects of two low-dose oral contraceptives on circulating components of the coagulation and fibrinolytic systems. J Lab Clin Med 109: 631–636

Ghezzo F, Savoca P, Vallero P, Bellone G 1986 Interaction between leukocytes and serum plasminogen: an essential mechanism in peripheral blood fibrinolytic activity. Am J Haematol 22: 233–239

Grimaudo V, Hauert J, Bachmann F, Kruithof E K O 1988 Diurnal variation of the fibrinolytic system. Thromb Haemostasis 59: 495–499

Grøndahl-Hansen J, Ralfkiær E, Nielsen L S, Kristensen P, Frentz G, Danø K 1987 Immunohistochemical localization of urokinase- and tissue-type plasminogen activators in psoriatic skin. J Invest Dermatol 88: 28–32

Grøndahl-Hansen J, Kirkeby L T, Ralfkiær E, Kristensen P, Lund L R, Danø K 1989 Urokinase-type plasminogen activator in endothelial cells during acute inflammation of the appendix. Am J Pathol 135: 631–636

Gurewich V 1989 The sequential, complementary and synergistic activation of fibrin-bound plasminogen by tissue plasminogen activator and pro-urokinase. Fibrinolysis 3: 59–66

Hach-Wunderle V, Scharrer I, Lottenberg R 1988 Congenital deficiency of plasminogen and its relationship to venous thrombosis. Thromb Haemostasis 59: 277–280

Haire W D, Goldsmith J C, Rasmussen J 1989 Abnormal fibrinolysis in healthy male cigarette smokers: role of plasminogen activator inhibitors. Am J Haematol 31: 36–40

Hamsten A, De Faire U, Walldius G, Dahlén G, Szamosi A, Landou C, Blombäck M, Wiman B 1987 Plasminogen activator inhibitor in plasma: risk factor for recurrent myocardial infarction. Lancet 2: 3–9

Handa K, Kono S, Saku K, Sasaki J, Kawano T, Sasaki Y, Hiroki T, Arakawa K 1989 Plasma fibrinogen levels as an independent indicator of severity of coronary atherosclerosis. Atherosclerosis 77: 209–213

Hariman H, Grant P J, Hughes J R, Booth N A, Davies J A, Prentice C R M 1989 Effect of physiological concentrations of vasopressin on components of the fibrinolytic system. Thromb Haemostasis 61: 298–300

Hart P H, Burgess D R, Vitti G F, Hamilton J A 1989 Interleukin-4 stimulates human monocytes to produce tissue-type plasminogen activator. Blood 74: 1222–1225

Hashimoto K, Wun T-C, Baird J, Lazarus G S, Jensen P J 1989 Characterization of keratinocyte plasminogen activator inhibitors and demonstration of the prevention of pemphigus IgG-induced acantholysis by a purified plasminogen activator inhibitor. J Invest Dermatol 92: 310–315

Haverkate F, Koopman J, Kluft C, D'Angelo A, Cattaneo M, Mannucci P M 1986 Fibrinogen Milano II: a congenital dysfibrinogenaemia associated with juvenile arterial and venous thrombosis. Thromb Haemostasis 55: 131–135

Henry D A, O'Connell D L 1989 Effects of fibrinolytic inhibitors on mortality from upper gastrointestinal haemorrhage. Br Med J 298: 1142–1146

Holvoet P, Lijnen H R, Collen D 1986 A monoclonal antibody preventing binding of tissue-type plasminogen activator to fibrin: useful to monitor fibrinogen breakdown during t-PA infusion. Blood 67: 1482–1487

Husain S S, Hasan A A K, Budzynski A Z 1989 Differences between binding of one-chain and two-chain tissue plasminogen activators to non-cross-linked and cross-linked fibrin clots. Blood 74: 999–1006

Idell S, James K K, Levin E G, Schwartz B S, Manchanda N, Maunder R J, Martin T R, McLarty J, Fair D S 1989 Local abnormalities in coagulation and fibrinolytic pathways predispose to alveolar fibrin deposition in the adult respiratory distress syndrome. J Clin Invest 84: 695–705

Jern Ch, Erikson E, Tengborn L, Risberg B, Wadenvik H, Jern S 1989 Changes of plasma coagulation and fibrinolysis in response to mental stress. Thromb Haemostasis 62: 767–771

Jespersen J, Brommer E J P, Haverkate F, Nieuwenhuizen W 1989 Degradation products of fibrin and of fibrinogen in synovial fluid and in plasma of patients with rheumatoid arthritis. Fibrinolysis 3: 183–186

Jørgenson M, Bonnevie-Nielsen V 1987 Increased concentration of the fast-acting plasminogen activator inhibitor in plasma associated with familial venous thrombosis. Br J Haematol 65: 175–180

Juhan-Vague I, Alessi M C, Fossat C, Declerck P J, Kruithof E K O 1987a Plasma determination of plasminogen activator inhibitor 1 antigen must be performed in blood collected on antiplatelet/anticoagulant mixture. Thromb Haemostasis 58: 1096

Juhan-Vague I, Vague P, Alessi M C, Badier C, Valadier J, Aillaud M F, Atlan C 1987b Relationship between plasma insulin, triglyceride, body mass index, and plasminogen activator inhibitor 1. Diabete Metab 13: 331–336

Juhan-Vague I, Alessi M C, Joly P, Thirion X, Vague P, Declerck P J, Serradimigni A, Collen D 1989a Plasma plasminogen activator inhibitor-1 in angina pectoris: influence of plasma insulin and acute-phase response. Arteriosclerosis 9: 362–367

Juhan-Vague I, Roul C, Alessi M C Ardissone J P, Heim M, Vague P 1989b Increased plasminogen activator inhibitor activity in non insulin dependent diabetic patients: relationship with plasma insulin. Thromb Haemostasis 61: 370–373

Kakishita E, Koyama T, Higuchi M, Kunitomi O, Oura Y, Nagai K 1989 Fibrinogenolysis in thrombotic thrombocytopenic purpura. Am J Haematol 32: 14–19

Kamitsuji H, Matsunaga K, Taira K, Nakajima M, Whitworth J A, Kinkaid-Smith P 1988 Urinary cross-linked fibrin degradation products in glomerular disease with crescents. Clin Nephrol 29: 124–128

Kaneko F, Tsukinaga I, Ando M, Ohkawara A, Oguchi H, Oikawa K, Nagai M 1989 Studies on two siblings with recessive dystrophic epidermolysis bullosa (Hallopeau–Siemens) and the plasminogen activator and its inhibitor in the lesion. Dermatologica 178: 156–163

Kang Y, Lewis J H, Navalgund A, Russell M W, Bontempo F A, Niren L S, Starzl T E 1987 Epsilon-aminocaproic acid for treatment of fibrinolysis during liver transplantation. Anesthesiology 66: 766–773

Kannel W B, Wolf P A, Castelli W P, D'Agostino R B 1987 Fibrinogen and risk of cardiovascular disease: the Framingham study. JAMA 258: 1183–1186

Kirchheimer J C, Remold H G 1989 Functional characteristics of receptor-bound urokinase on human monocytes: catalytic efficiency and susceptibility to inactivation by plasminogen activator inhibitors. Blood 74: 1396–1402

Kirchheimer J C, Huber K, Wagner O, Binder B 1987 Pattern of fibrinolytic parameters in patients with gastrointestinal carcinomas. Br J Haematol 66: 85–89

Kluft C, De Bart A C W, Barthels M, Sturm J, Möller W 1988a Short term extreme increases in plasminogen activator inhibitor 1 (PAI-1) in plasma of polytrauma patients. Fibrinolysis 2: 223–226

Kluft C, Jie A F H, Rijken D C, Verheijen J H 1988b Daytime fluctuations in blood of tissue-type plasminogen activator (t-PA) and its fast-acting inhibitor (PAI-1). Thromb Haemostasis 59: 329–332

Knudsen B S, Nachman R L 1988 Matrix plasminogen activator inhibitor: modulation of the extracellular proteolytic environment. J Biol Chem 263: 9476–9481

Köhler M, Hellstern P, Tarrach H, Bambauer R, Wenzel E, Jutzler G A 1989 Subcutaneous injection of desmopressin (DDAVP): evaluation of a new, more concentrated preparation. Haemostasis 1: 38–44

Koopman J, Engesser L, Nieveen M, Haverkate F, Brommer E J P 1986 Fibrin polymerization associated with tissue-type plasminogen activator (t-PA) induced glu-plasminogen activation. In: Müller-Berghaus G et al (eds) Fibrinogen and its derivatives. Elsevier, Amsterdam, pp 315–318

Korninger C, Jäger R, Huber K, Lechner K 1988 Levels of plasminogen activator inhibitor in patients with angina pectoris. Klin Wochenschr 66(suppl XII): 59–61

Kruithof E K O, Nicolosa G, Bachmann F 1987 Plasminogen activator inhibitor 1: development of a radioimmunoassay and observations on its plasma concentration during venous occlusion and after platelet aggregation. Blood 70: 1645–1653

Kruithof E K O, Gudinchet A, Bachmann F 1988 Plasminogen activator inhibitor 1 and plasminogen activator inhibitor 2 in various disease states. Thromb Haemostasis 59: 7–12

Lecander I, Nilsson I M, Åstedt B 1988 Depression of plasminogen activator activity during pregnancy by the placental inhibitor PAI 2. Fibrinolysis 2: 165–167

Leebeek F W G, Kluft C, Knot E A R, De Maat M P M 1989 Histidine-rich glycoprotein is elevated in mild liver cirrhosis and decreased in moderate and severe liver cirrhosis. J Lab Clin Med 113: 493–497

Levi M, Ten Cate J W, Dooijewaard G, Sturk A, Brommer E J P, Agnelli G 1989 DDAVP induces systemic release of urokinase-type plasminogen activator. Thromb Haemostasis 62: 686–689

Lijnen H R, Van Hoef B, De Cock F, Collen D 1989 The mechanism of plasminogen activation and fibrin dissolution by single chain urokinase-type plasminogen activator in a plasma milieu in vitro. Blood 73: 1864–1872

Liu Y, Lyons R M, McDonagh J 1988 Plasminogen San Antonio: an abnormal plasminogen with a more cathodic migration, decreased activation and associated thrombosis. Thromb Haemostasis 50: 49–53

Lotti T, Battini M L, Brunetti L, Fabbri P, Panconesi E 1989 Plasminogen activators and antiplasmin activity in atopic dermatitis. Int J Dermatol 28: 457–459

Lucore C L, Sobel B E 1988 Interactions of tissue-type plasminogen activator with plasma inhibitors and their pharmacologic implications. Circulation 77: 660–669

Lütjens A, Jonkhoff-Slok T W, Sandkuijl C, Van der Veen E A, Van der Meer J 1988 Polymerisation and crosslinking of fibrin monomers in diabetes mellitus. Diabetologica 31: 825–830

Lütjens A, Sanderson-Sellmeijer H, Van der Veen E A, Van der Meer J 1991 Fibrinogen and plasminogen isolated from diabetic patients: consequences for fibrinolysis. Diabetologia

Mannucci P M 1988 Desmopressin: a nontransfusional form of treatment for congenital and acquired bleeding disorders. Blood 72: 1449–1455

Mannucci P M, Kluft C, Traas D W, Seveso P, D'Angelo A 1986 Congenital plasminogen deficiency associated with venous thromboembolism: therapeutic trial with stanozolol. Br J Haematol 63: 753–759

Meade T W, Mellows S, Brozovic M et al 1986 Haemostatic function and ischaemic heart disease: principal results of the Northwick Park heart study. Lancet ii: 533–537

Miles L A, Plow E F 1988 Plasminogen receptors: ubiquitous sites for cellular regulation of fibrinolysis. Fibrinolysis 2: 61–71

Mohler M A, Refino C J, Chen S A, Chen A B, Hotchkiss A J 1986 D-Phe-Pro-Arg-chloromethylketone: its potential use in inhibiting the formation of in vitro artifacts in blood collected during tissue-type plasminogen activator thrombolytic therapy. Thromb Haemostasis 56: 160–164

Nieuwenhuizen W 1988 New strategies in the determination of fibrin and fibrin(ogen) derivatives by monoclonal antibodies. Blut 57: 285–291

Olofsson B O, Dahlén G, Nilsson T K 1989 Evidence for increased levels of plasminogen activator inhibitor and tissue plasminogen activator in plasma of patients with angiographically verified coronary artery disease. Eur Heart J 10: 77–82

Ortel T L, Onorato J J, Bedrosian C L, Kaufman R E 1988 Antifibrinolytic therapy in the management of the Kasabach Merritt syndrome. Am J Hematol 29: 44–48

Páramo J A, Campbell W, Cuesta B, Gómez C, Aranda A, Rocha E 1987 Fibrinolytic response in malignancy. Fibrinolysis 1: 195–199

Páramo J A, Fernández-Diaz F J, Rocha E 1988 Plasminogen activator inhibitor activity in bacterial infection. Thromb Haemostasis 59: 451–454

Porte R J, Bontempo F A, Knot E A R, Lewis J H, Kang Y G, Starzl T E 1989 Tissue-type-plasminogen-activator-associated fibrinolysis in orthotopic liver transplantation. Transplantation Proc 21: 3542

Pralong G, Calandra T, Glauser M-P, Schellekens J, Verhoef J, Bachmann F, Kruithof E K O 1989 Plasminogen activator inhibitor 1: a new prognostic marker in septic shock. Thromb Haemostasis 61: 459–462

Prisco D, Paniccia R, Bonechi F, Francalanci I, Abbate R, Gensini G F 1989 Evaluation of new methods for the selective measurement of fibrin and fibrinogen degradation products. Thromb Res 56: 547–551

Rånby M, Sundell I B, Nilsson T K 1989 Blood collection in strong acidic citrate anticoagulant used in a study of dietary influence on basal tPA activity. Thromb Haemostasis 62: 917–922

Reith A, Bennett B, Moore N R, Walker I D, Mackkinnon S, Booth N A 1989 Changes in circulating plasminogen activator inhibitors in labour and the puerperium. Br J Haematol 73: 437 (abstract)

Saito M, Asakura H, Uotani C, Jokaji H, Kumabashiri I, Matsuda T 1989 Quantitative estimation of elastase-α_1-proteinase inhibitor (E-α_1PI) complex in leukaemia: marked elevation in cases of acute promyelocytic leukaemia. Thromb Res 53: 163–171

Scharrer I, Hach-Wunderle V, Wohl R C, Sinio L, Boreisha I, Robbins K C 1988 Congenital abnormal plasminogen, Frankfurt I, a cause for recurrent venous thrombosis. Haemostasis 18(suppl 1): 77–86

Schleef R R, Higgins D L, Pillemer E, Levitt L J 1989 Bleeding diathesis due to decreased functional activity of type 1 plasminogen activator inhibitor. J Clin Invest 83: 1747–1752

Schwartz B S, Williams E C, Conlan M G, Mosher D F 1986 Epsilon-aminocaproic acid in the treatment of patients with acute promyelocytic leukemia and acquired alpha-2-plasmin inhibitor deficiency. Ann Int Med 105: 873–877

Seifried E, Tanswell P 1987 Comparison of specific antibody, D-Phe-Pro-Arg-CH$_2$Cl and aprotinin for prevention of in vitro effects of recombinant tissue-type plasminogen activator on haemostasis parameters. Thromb Haemostasis 58: 921–926

Seitz R, Karges H E, Wolf M, Egbring R 1989 Reduced fibrinolytic capacity and its restoration by plasminogen substitution in acute renal failure. Int J Tissue React 11: 39–46

Shigekiyo T, Kosaka M, Shintani Y, Azuma H, Iishi Y, Saito S 1989 Inhibition of fibrin monomer polymerization by Bence Jones protein in a patient with primary amyloidosis. Acta Haematol 81: 160–165

Siegbahn A, Ruusuvaara L 1988 Age dependence of blood fibrinolytic components and the effects of low-dose oral contraceptives on coagulation and fibrinolysis in teenagers. Thromb Haemostasis 60: 361–364

Sindet-Pedersen S, Ramström G, Bernvil S, Blombäck M 1989 Haemostatic effect of tranexamic acid mouthwash in anticoagulant-treated patients undergoing oral surgery. N Engl J Med 320: 840–843

Skoda U, Goldman S F, Händler C, Hummel K, Lechner E, Lübcke I, Mauff G, Meyer-Börnecke D, Pesch S, Pulverer G 1988 Plasminogen hemizygosity: detection of a silent allele in 7 members of a family by determination of plasminogen phenotypes, antigenic levels, and functional activity. Vox Sang 54: 210–214

Sloan I G, Firkin B G 1989 Impaired fibrinolysis in patients with thrombotic or haemostatic defects. Thromb Res 55: 559–567

Smokovitis A A, Kokolis N A, Alexaki E, Binder B R 1989 Demonstration of plasminogen activator activity in the intima and media of the normal human aorta and other large arteries: immunological identification of the plasminogen activator(s). Thromb Res 55: 259–265

Staël von Holstein C C, Eriksson S B, Källén R 1987 Tranexamic acid as an aid to reducing blood transfusion requirements in gastric and duodenal bleeding. Br Med J 294: 7–10

Sterrenberg L, Haak H L, Brommer E J P, Nieuwenhuizen W 1985 Evidence of fibrinogen breakdown by leukocyte enzymes in a patient with acute promyelocytic leukaemia. Haemostasis 15: 126–133

Suenson E, Petersen L C 1986 Fibrin and plasminogen structures essential to stimulation of plasmin formation by tissue-type plasminogen activator. Biochem Biophys Acta 870: 510–519

Suffredini A F, Harpel P C, Parrillo J E 1989 Promotion and subsequent inhibition of plasminogen activation after administration of intravenous endotoxin to normal subjects. N Engl J Med 320: 1165–1172

Sundell I B, Nilsson T K, Hallmans G, Nygren C 1988 The effect of body build, diet and endocrine factors on the extrinsic fibrinolytic system in healthy young women. Scand J Clin Lab Invest 48: 557–564

Sundell I B, Dahlgren S, Rånby M, Lundin E, Stenling R, Nilsson T K 1989 Reduction of elevated plasminogen activator inhibitor levels during modest weight loss. Fibrinolysis 3: 51–53

Tabernero M D, Estellés A, Vicente V, Alberca I, Aznar J 1989 Incidence of increased plasminogen activator inhibitor patients with deep venous thrombosis and/or pulmonary embolism. Thromb Res 56: 565–570

Taira K, Matsunaga T, Kawahara S, Sakamoto S, Kamitsuji H 1989 Fragments of urinary fibrin/fibrinogen degradation products and cross-linked fibrin degradation products in various renal diseases. Thromb Res 53: 367–377

Takada A, Sakakibara K, Nagase M, Shizume K, Takada Y 1986 Determination of urokinase in the urine of healthy volunteers and patients with renal diseases. Thromb Res 44: 867–873

Takahashi H, Tatewaki W, Wada K, Yoshikawa A, Shibata A 1989 Thrombin and plasmin generation in patients with liver disease. Am J Hematol 32: 30–35

Tran-Thang C, Fasel-Felley J, Pralong G, Hofstetter J-R, Bachmann F, Kruithof E K O 1989 Plasminogen activators and plasminogen activator inhibitors in liver deficiencies caused by chronic alcoholism or infectious hepatitis. Thromb Haemostasis 62: 651–653

Tripathi R C, Park J K, Tripathi B J, Millard C B 1988 Tissue plasminogen activator in human aqueous humor and its possible therapeutic significance. Am J Ophthalmol 106: 719–722

Tsakiris D A, Marbet G A, Makris P E, Settas L, Duckert F 1989 Impaired fibrinolysis as an essential contribution to thrombosis in patients with lupus anticoagulant. Thromb Haemostasis 61: 175–177

Van Oeveren W, Jansen N J G, Bidstrup B P, Royston D, Westaby S, Neuhof H, Wildevuur C R H 1987 Effects of aprotinin on hemostatic mechanisms during cardiopulmonary bypass. Ann Thorac Surg 44: 640–645

Vaughan D E, Declerck P J, De Mol M, Collen D 1989 Recombinant plasminogen activator inhibitor-1 reverses the bleeding tendency associated with the combined administration of tissue-type plasminogen activator and aspirin in rabbits. J Clin Invest 84: 586–591

Wagner O F, De Vries C, Hohmann C, Veerman H, Pannekoek H 1989 Interaction between plasminogen activator inhibitor type 1 (PAI-1) bound to fibrin and either tissue-type plasminogen activator (t-PA) or urokinase-type plasminogen activator (u-PA): binding of t-PA/PAI-1 complexes to fibrin mediated by both the finger and the kringle-2 domain of t-PA. J Clin Invest 84: 647–655

Wilkinson J E, Smith C A, Suter M M, Falchek W, Lewis R M 1989 Role of plasminogen activator in pemphigus vulgaris. Am J Pathol 134: 561–569

Williams E C 1989 Plasma α_2-antiplasmin activity: role in the evaluation and management of fibrinolytic states and other bleeding disordered. Arch Int Med 149: 1769–1772

Wiman B, Lindahl T, Almquist A 1988 Evidence for a discrete binding protein of plasminogen activator inhibitor in plasma. Thromb Haemostasis 59: 392–395

Wright J G, Cooper P, Åstedt B, Lecander I, Wilde J T, Preston F E, Greaves M 1988 Fibrinolysis during normal human pregnancy: complex inter-relationships between plasma levels of tissue plasminogen activator and inhibitors and the euglobulin clot lysis time. Br J Haematol 69: 253–258

3

Cellular coagulant and anticoagulant proteins

K. Fujikawa   K. Suzuki

TISSUE FACTOR AND FACTOR VII

Tissue factor (TF), a membrane-bound glycoprotein, potentiates the enzyme activity of factor VIIa to a great extent, when it binds to factor VIIa. TF/factor VIIa complex exhibits a strong catalytic activity to convert the zymogens of factor X and factor IX to their active forms to initiate the extrinsic and intrinsic pathways of blood coagulation. This complex is formed when latent TF is exposed to circulating blood at trauma sites. Recent progress in molecular and cellular biology led to an understanding of the molecular mechanism of the TF/factor VIIa complex formation, which implied the initial event of fibrin formation under physiological conditions.

Purification of TF apoprotein

The tissue factor activity is detected in various tissues, such as brain, placenta and lung, and its purification was attempted by a number of investigators employing conventional chromatographic media. The purification, however, was difficult probably due to the low concentration and insoluble nature of TF. It was not successful until affinity chromatographies were recently introduced into the purification steps. Bovine brain TF was first purified to a homogenous state by using an immobilized polyclonal antibody column. Human brain TF was then purified by essentially the same steps except that factor VII was used for an affinity ligand. Acetone powder of human brain was solubilized with 2% Triton X-100 and the sample was applied on the factor VII–agarose column in the presence of $CaCl_2$ (the binding of TF with factor VII requires Ca^{2+}). After the column was extensively washed, bound TF was eluted with ethylenediaminetetraacetic acid (EDTA). TF was finally purified by gel filtration to a homogenous state (Broze et al 1985, Guha et al 1986). Since the lipid component, which non-covalently bound to TF, was removed from the protein portion during the purification, both purified bovine and human TF were apoproteins and had little or no procoagulant activity. The purified human TF apoprotein contained less than 1 mol of lipid per mole of protein. The procoagulant activity was restored by incorporation of the apoproteins into lipid vesicles. When human TF apoprotein was mixed with increasing concentrations of a mixture of rabbit brain phospholipid and cholesterol, the procoagulant activity was restored concomitantly with the lipid concentration and a 5000-fold increase of the activity was obtained at a lipid/protein weight ratio of >600/1.

The purified human and bovine TF apoprotein have similar characteristics in molecular weights and amino acid compositions. Their molecular weights are 44 000–47 000 under reduced or non-reduced conditions, indicating the apoproteins are composed of a single polypeptide chain. The amino-terminal sequence of human TF apoprotein was found to be Ser-X-Asn-Thr-Val-Ala-Val-Tyr- (X refers to an unidentified residue).

The structure of human TF apoprotein

The primary structure of TF apoprotein was elucidated by cDNA cloning. cDNA of human TF apoprotein was isolated by four research groups almost simultaneously in 1987 (Morrissey et al 1987, Scarpati et al 1987, Spicer et al 1987, Fisher et al 1987). The isolated TF cDNA clone consisted of 2147 base pairs (b.p.) including 5'- and 3'- end non-coding regions. The deduced amino acid sequence from the cDNA agreed with those of the amino-terminus of TF apoprotein as well as the peptide fragments produced from purified TF apoprotein. The deduced sequence showed the presence of a leader peptide of 32 residues followed by the mature protein of 295 residues. The leader peptide is removed by a signal peptidase during post-translational events to produce the mature apoprotein.

Hydropathy analysis showed the presence of two hydrophobic segments in the molecule, one in residues from −32 to −1 and the second between 243 and 263. The first one corresponded to the leader peptide and the second was located at the carboxyl-terminal area of the mature apoprotein. The latter segment is thought to be a membrane-spanning domain, which likely anchors TF in cell membranes. The TF molecule is composed of three domains in the order from the amino terminus; extracelluar, membrane-spanning and cytoplasmic domains (Fig. 3.1). This molecular organization is similar to membrane-bound receptor proteins. Three potential sites for carbohydrate attachment are present in the extracellular domain. Recombinant human TF apoprotein, expressed in human kidney cells, had the same molecular weight as the natural protein, while the apoprotein expressed in *Escherichia coli* had a molecular weight of 33 000 and lacked carbohydrate. These two products had the full procoagulant activity after reassociation with lipid vesicles, indicating that the carbohydrate chains did not have in vitro functional activities (Paborsky et al 1989).

The disulphide bond structure of TF apoprotein was thoroughly studied by Back et al (1988). Four half-Cys residues present in the extracellular

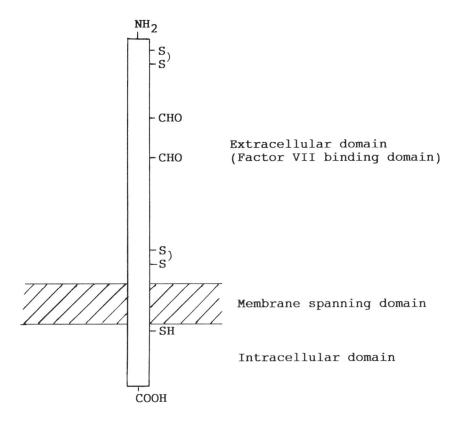

Fig. 3.1 Schematic structure of human tissue factor. — CHO represents N-linked carbohydrate chains.

domain forms two disulphide bonds between Cys_{49}–Cys_{57} and Cys_{186}–Cys_{209}. Reduction of these disulphide bonds causes the total loss of the functional activity of TF. Half-Cys_{245} in the cytoplasmic domain causes artefacts. In some preparations of human TF apoprotein, two bands, 58 kD and dimeric form, were observed on a non-reduced sodium dodecyl sulphate – polyacrylamide gel electrophoresis (SDS–PAGE) gel in addition to the major 47-kD TF apoprotein. On reduction, the dimer was converted into the monomer and the 58-kD band was separated into two bands, 47-kD apoprotein and a polypeptide of 12.5 kD, which was identified as α-chain of haemoglobin. In a separate experiment, acylation by palmitate and stearate on Cys_{245} was demonstrated in TF apoprotein produced by cultured human lung fibroblast cells. If these fatty acid residues were removed by treating with hydroxamine, the dimer was spontaneously formed by oxidation, showing that the dimer was formed through a disulphide bridge between Cys_{245} residues of the two molecules. The 58-kD species was also likely formed between half-Cys_{245} and one free half-Cys present in the haemoglobin molecule. A mutant molecule in which half-Cys_{245} was replaced by serine by site-directed mutagenesis showed the full coagulant activity and the purified preparation of the mutant protein was contaminated by a significantly lower content of the dimeric form. Therefore, the 58-kD species and the dimer were likely artefacts, which were formed during the purification. The presence of the fatty acid residues in the isolated TF preparations is not known.

The TF gene and regulation of its expression

The gene of human TF apoprotein, which locates in chromosome 1, spans 12.4 kb.p. and its complete sequence including the promoter region and downstream of the polyadenylation signal site has been sequenced (Mackman et al 1989). Adenine (numbered as position 1), identified as the major start site for transcription (cap site), is located 123 b.p. upstream from the initiation site for translation. The gene is organized by six exons and five introns. Intron 5 begins with GT and ends with AG, and each exon/intron boundary has the consensus nucleotide sequence for correct RNA splicing. Each exon encodes the following residues: exon 1 encodes from the cap site to the amino-terminal Ser residue including the leader peptide; exon 2 from Gly_2 to Ser_{39}, exon 3 from Thr_{40} to Glu_{105}, exon 4 from Thr_{106} to Lys_{165}, exon 5 from Lys_{166} to Arg_{218}, exon 6 from Glu_{219} to Ser_{263}. A TATA sequence, consensus for a promoter component, is located 26 b.p. upstream from the cap site. A number of putative transcription factor binding sites are present in the promoter region. Cytokines, interleukin-1, tumour necrosis factor (TNF), and endotoxin (bacterial lipopolysaccharide), are known to induce TF expression in monocytes and vascular endothelial cells (Gregory et al 1989). The binding sites of these transcription factors, however, remain to be elucidated.

When monocytes were treated with endotoxin, the level of TF-mRNA increased and reached the maximum level in 4 hours (Gregory et al 1989). During this period, the TF antigen, which was synthesized in parallel with the increase of TF-mRNA, appeared mostly on the cell surface. After the transcript was ceased by treating the cells with actinomycin, TF-mRNA decayed rapidly with an apparent half-life of 1.5 hours. The expression of TF on the surface of monocytes or endothelial cells by stimuli may be related with fibrin formation in sepsis or disseminated intravascular coagulation.

Cellular distribution of TF

With cDNA and antibodies specific to TF apoprotein being available, the cellular distribution of TF was examined by in situ hybridization and immunohistochemistry (Wilcox et al 1989). Normal endothelial cells in any vessel were negative in both analyses. This observation indicates that normal endothelial cells do not synthesize or store TF; TF is not exposed to the bloodstream under normal physiological conditions. On the other hand, TF-mRNA and TF-antigen were detected in tunica media of the saphenous vein and adventitial fibroblast. These results are consistent with the previous findings that cultured fibroblast and vascular smooth muscle cells synthesize TF constitutively (Bevilacqua et al 1985), whereas cultured endothelial cells do not synthesize TF unless the cells are stimulated (Stern et al 1984). When these cells are damaged at trauma sites, TF comes into contact with circulating factor VII to initiate blood coagulation.

The high level of TF-mRNA was observed in human atherosclerosis plaques (Wilcox et al 1989). TF-antigen is localized in the extracellular matrix of the necrotic cores and the macrophage-rich region of the plaques; TF is probably synthesized in the surrounding smooth muscle-like cells adjacent to vessels and trapped in extracellular matrix. The rupture of atherosclerotic plaque may also trigger coagulation, which leads asymptomatic atherosclerosis to become symptomatic.

Interaction of TF with factor VII

When latent TF is exposed to blood, it will bind with factor VII in the presence of Ca^{2+}. TF/factor VII complex exhibits a potent coagulant activity; it activates factor X and factor IX into their active forms to initiate the extrinsic and intrinsic pathways of blood coagulation (Osterud & Rappaport 1977). The binding of cell-associated TF to factor VII was studied using human bladder carcinoma cells (Sakai et al 1989). Factor VII or VIIa specifically bound to TF exposed on the cells in the presence of 5 mM $CaCl_2$. The binding of radiolabelled factor VII or VIIa to the cells was saturable and competitively inhibited by non-labelled factor VII or VIIa. This binding was also completely inhibited by the pretreatment of the cells with anti-TF monoclonal antibody. The binding affinities (K_d) were high − 3.2 ± 0.51 nM for factor VII and 3.25 ± 0.31 nM for factor VIIa. The cells contained 256 000 ± 39 000 binding sites/cell for factor VII and 320 000 ± 31 000 for factor VIIa.

After incubation of factor VII or VIIa with the cells, the cells were washed and examined for the activation of factor X. Cell-bound factor VII and VIIa activated factor X at an equal rate in the presence of Ca^{2+}. Cell-bound factor VII was then dissociated with EDTA and examined for the molecular change on SDS–PAGE. Factor VII (single-chain) was progressively converted into factor VIIa (two-chain) on the cell surface. This conversion was possibly initiated by a trace of factor VIIa and proceeded by an autoactivation manner (Pedersen et al 1989). When cell-bound factor VII was incubated with factor X, it was completely converted into the two-chain form by the resulting factor Xa. Since factor VII was enzymatically inactive (Pedersen et al 1989), the question is how the first molecule of factor VIIa is formed. A trace of factor Xa that may circulate in blood or an unrecognized cellular enzyme, which activates factor VII or factor X, is considered to be a potential enzyme for the generation of the very first molecule of factor VIIa. The above results observed with carcinoma cells are probably similar to the physiological mechanism for the initiation of extrinsic pathway at the sites of trauma or atherosclerosis rupture.

THROMBOMODULIN

Thrombomodulin (TM) was found in endothelium as a cofactor for the thrombin-catalysed activation of a vitamin K-dependent plasma protein, protein C (Esmon & Owen 1981). Activated protein C is the most potent anticoagulant agent inactivating factor Va and factor VIIIa (Suzuki et al 1983, Eaton et al 1986). TM was found to inhibit procoagulant activities of thrombin (Esmon et al 1982a, Esmon et al 1983) and factor Xa (Thompson & Salem 1986). Thus, TM plays a role as an important anticoagulant on vascular walls.

Purification and physicochemical properties of TM

TM has been isolated from lung of various animals and human placenta (Esmon et al 1982b, Salem et al 1984). In all cases, TM was extracted with a non-ionic detergent, Triton X-100, from the cell membrane fraction. Affinity chromatography on DIP–thrombin–agarose was the major step for the purification of TM (DIP–thrombin is the inactivated thrombin formed by treatment with diisopropylfluorophosphate). For the purification of bovine and human lung TM, we (Suzuki et al 1987) used a gel filtration step after DIP–thrombin–agarose chromatography. For the purification of human placenta TM, ion-exchange chromatography on DEAE–Sepharose or DEAE–Trisacryl seemed to be necessary for the successful binding of TM to and subsequent elution from the DIP–thrombin–agarose column (Salem et al 1984). A concanavalin A–Sepharose column was used prior to DIP–thrombin–agarose chromatography for the purification of human placenta TM (Freyssinet et al 1986).

The purified TM preparations have similar physicochemical properties regardless of their sources. TM is a single-chain glycoprotein with estimated molecular weights of 68 000–78 000. It is unusually stable in solutions containing various detergents and resistant to high temperature, alkaline and acidic conditions. Human TM has the amino-terminal sequence of Ala-Pro-Ala-Glu-Pro-Gln-Pro-Gly-Gly-Ser-Gln-Ser- (Suzuki et al 1987) and bovine TM has the sequence of X-Ala-Pro-Pro-Glu-Pro-Glu-Pro-Leu-Gly-Gly-Gln- (Suzuki et al, unpublished).

The structure of human TM and its gene

The primary structure of human TM was deduced from the cDNA sequence by three research groups (Suzuki et al 1987, Jackman et al 1987, Wen et al 1987). The isolated human TM cDNA consisted of a 5'-noncoding region of 153 b.p., an open reading frame of 1725 b.p., a stop codon, a 3'- noncoding region and a poly(A) tail. The deduced amino acid sequence showed that the human TM precursor consisted of a mature protein of 557 amino acid residues and a signal peptide of 18 residues. Five potential *N*-glycosylation and several *O*-glycosylation sites are distributed throughout the molecule. The mature human TM can be divided into five tentative domains (Fig. 3.2). The first domain is located at the extracellular amino-terminal region (1–226 residues), the sequence of which is homologous with animal lectins. The second domain (residues 227–462) contains 36 half-Cys residues and is composed of multiple repeat sequences, which

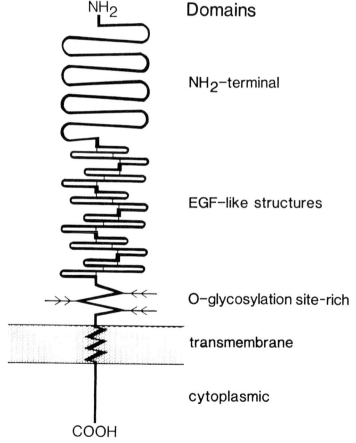

Domains

NH₂-terminal

EGF–like structures

O–glycosylation site-rich

transmembrane

cytoplasmic

Fig. 3.2   Schematic structure of human thrombomodulin. (Reproduced with permission from Suzuki et al 1987.)

are highly homologous (maximum 45% identity) with the mouse epidermal growth factor (EGF) precursor. These EGF-like structures are found in low-density lipoprotein receptors and proteins involved in blood coagulation, fibrinolysis and the complement system, e.g. factor VII, factor IX, factor X, protein C, protein S, protein Z, factor XII, tissue and urinary plasminogen activators. The third domain (residues 463–498) is rich in Ser, Thr and Pro residues and probably contains several O-linked carbohydrate chains. The fourth domain (residues 499–521) is a hydrophobic putative transmembrane domain. The fifth domain (residues 522–557), which is situated at the carboxyl-terminal end of the molecule, is sequestered into the cytoplasmic side of plasma membrane. A Ser residue in this domain of mouse haemangioma TM was found to be phosphorylated in response to phorbol 12-myristate 13-acetate (PMA), which was a stimulant of protein kinase C (Dittman et al 1988).

The human TM gene, 3.7 kb.p. in length (Jackman et al 1987), is located at chromosome 20p12-cen. In the 5′- flanking region a potential TATA box sequence at nucleotide –196 and a CAAT box sequence at nucleotide –279 were identified. The nucleotide sequence of the coding region and that of most of the 3′- non-coding and/or flanking region of the gene were identical to those of TM cDNA, indicating that the human TM gene was free from introns in both the coding and non-coding regions. This is an unusual case in eukaryotic genes; only a few genes without introns have been found, e.g. the genes for mitochondrial proteins, *Drosophila* histon HI, human α- and β-interferon and angiogenine.

Functional properties of TM

TM binds to thrombin with high affinity ($K_d = 5 \times 10^{-10}$ M), and TM/thrombin complex activates protein C in the presence of calcium ions. The kinetic analysis showed that the formation of TM–thrombin complex decreases not only the K_m value of thrombin for protein C, but also increases the catalytic rate of thrombin to activate protein C. The rate of protein C activation by thrombin is increased over 2000-fold on cultured endothelial cells and over 1000-fold in the presence of isolated TM (Esmon et al 1982b).

Phospholipid vesicles composed of phosphatidylcholine and phosphatidylserine appeared to increase the catalytic activity of TM–thrombin complex a few fold (Freyssinet et al 1986, Galvin et al 1987). This effect was not seen in the activation of γ-carboxyglutamic acid (Gla)-domainless protein C. This indicates that Gla-dependent interaction via Ca^{2+} between protein C and phospholipid vesicles is required. Recently, rabbit TM was reported to serve as a cofactor for the protein C activation by factor Xa (Haley et al 1989). This activation required both Ca^{2+} and phospholipids. Like the activation by TM–thrombin complex, Gla-domainless protein C was not activated by TM–factor Xa complex.

The activation of protein C by TM–thrombin complex was inhibited by antithrombin III–heparin, hirudin and inhibitors specific to thrombin such as dansyl-N-(3-ethyl-1,5-pentanedyl)amide (DAPA) and monoclonal antibodies specific to thrombin. The activation by TM–factor Xa complex was also inhibited by antithrombin III–heparin or monoclonal antibody specific to factor Xa (Haley et al 1989).

TM blocks procoagulant activities of thrombin, e.g. fibrinogen clotting, factor V activation (Esmon et al 1982a) and platelet activation (Esmon et al 1983). TM also inhibited prothrombinase by blocking the factor Xa activity (Thompson & Salem 1986).

Structure–function relationship of TM

Thrombin–TM interaction

The alteration of the substrate specificity of thrombin by binding to TM is probably due to a conformational change around the catalytic site of thrombin (Musci et al 1988). Both β-thrombin and γ-thrombin had low activities to activate protein C in the presence of TM (Bezeaud et al 1985), indicating that the site of interaction between TM and thrombin was located on the B-chain of α-thrombin. γ-Thrombin, which is cleaved at Arg_{73} in the B-chain, markedly lost the affinity for TM. A region, Arg_{62}–Arg_{73} of the B-chain, which was probably located in a surface loop relatively distant from the catalytic site of thrombin, was suggested to interact with TM as well as fibrinogen and hirudin (Noé et al 1988).

Monoclonal antibody specific to human thrombin, which inhibited the protein C activating activity of thrombin, was prepared by the authors (K.S.). This antibody blocked the TM–thrombin interaction and also inhibited the fibrinogen clotting activity of thrombin. The epitope was found to locate within the residues Thr_{147}–Asp_{175} in the B-chain. A synthetic peptide, Thr_{147}–Ser_{158}, blocked the thrombin–TM interaction and inhibited the fibrinogen clotting activity of thrombin. This region is thought to localize near the catalytic site of thrombin and also near the region of Arg_{62}–Arg_{73} on the thrombin molecule. The TM binding site on Thr_{147}–Ser_{158} in the B-chain probably shares the binding for fibrinogen (Suzuki et al 1990).

The binding site of thrombin within TM has also been precisely elucidated. An elastase fragment of rabbit TM (Kurosawa et al 1987) and a recombinant human protein that were composed of six EGF-like structures (Suzuki et al 1989) showed the cofactor activity for the protein C activation. Thrombin bound to these proteins with the same affinity ($K_d = 2.1 \times 10^{-10}$ M) as the TM–thrombin interaction. A cyanogen bromide fragment of rabbit TM composed of the fifth and sixth EGF-like structures was capable of binding to thrombin, but the complex of this fragment and thrombin could not activate protein C (Kurosawa et al 1988). The region required for the cofactor activity was narrowed by analysing recombinant proteins composed of several EGF-like structures (Zushi et al 1989, Hayashi et al 1990). The complete cofactor activity was detected in a protein containing three consecutive EGF-like structures from the fourth to the sixth (EGF456), and approximately one-tenth of the activity was detected in the protein composed of the fourth and fifth EGF-like structures (EGF45), but the activity could not be detected in the protein composed of the fifth and sixth EGF-like structures (EGF56). These experiments suggest that the fourth and fifth EGF-like structures are prerequisite for the minimum cofactor activity of TM. All recombinant proteins, EGF456, EGF45 and EGF56, blocked the TM–thrombin interaction, indicating that the binding site of TM to thrombin could be located within the fifth EGF-like structure.

Protein C–TM interaction

The activation of protein C by thrombin–TM complex requires the presence of Ca^{2+}, whereas that by thrombin alone is inhibited by Ca^{2+} (Esmon et al 1982b). Ca^{2+} probably induces a conformational change of the protein C molecule rather than the TM molecule. Beside the Gla-domain, Ca^{2+} possibly binds to EGF-like structures of protein C and/or the activation peptide. Elastase-digested TM also had the cofactor activity, which increased in parallel with Ca^{2+} concentration and the maximum activity was obtained at 250–300 μM. However, this cofactor activity decreased at higher Ca^{2+} concentrations, unlike the Ca^{2+} dependence observed with intact TM (Kurosawa et al 1987). The optimal Ca^{2+} concentration was not seen when Gla-domainless protein C was used. Digestion with elastase would expose a binding site of TM for Gla-residues of protein C. These phenomena were also observed when recombinant human TM proteins, the protein composed of six EGF-like structures, EGF456 and EGF45 were used (Hayashi et al 1990). These findings suggest that the binding site of TM for protein C probably via Ca^{2+} ions is located at the fourth or fifth, or both of these EGF-like structures.

Factor Xa–TM interaction

TM interacts with factor Xa with a high affinity ($K_d = 5.7 \times 10^{-10}$ M), which results in the formation of a 1 : 1 complex and accelerates the protein C activation by factor Xa (Haley et al 1989), and this interaction inhibits prothrombinase activity (Thompson & Salem 1986). TM binds to factor Xa and converts procoagulant factor Xa into an anticoagulant agent by a similar manner as observed in the interaction with thrombin.

Cellular distribution of TM

The distribution of TM antigen is similar both in tissues and organs of human (Maruyama et al 1985) and rabbit (DeBault et al 1986). It has been found on the surface of arterial, venous, lymphatic and capillary endothelium. TM is localized on the outer cell surface and in the Golgi–endoplasmic reticulum complex. Lung has the highest concentration of TM, followed by placenta, spleen, pancreas, liver and heart in that order. TM is also detected to a slight extent on endothelium of kidney and its glomerular capillary loops. The TM antigen is found in rabbit brain, but not in the microcirculation of human brain. This result was confirmed by the observation that the TM-mRNA was not detected in human brain (Wen et al 1987). The TM distribution in syncytiotrophoblasts of placenta may be important to maintain blood fluidity, since this cell is situated at the transportation site for nutrients from maternal blood to embryo. Functionally active TM is also present in platelets. Umbilical endothelial cells contain 30 000–55 000 TM molecules per cell (Maruyama & Majerus 1985).

Imada et al (1990) found that fetomodulin, a cell surface marker protein that was upregulated in murine fibroblast by cyclic AMP, was identical to TM in its amino acid sequence and physicochemical properties. During embryonic development, fetomodulin is localized not only in vasculatures but also at sites of cell-to-cell contact, including lung bud and neural epithelium. This suggests that TM may play a role not only in regulation of blood coagulation but also in embryogenesis.

Cellular dynamics of TM

TM activity decreases after exposure of endothelial cells to endotoxin, interleukin-1, TNF or thrombin, which is known to induce TF in endothelial cells. TNF promotes endocytosis and the degradation of TM, and inhibits transcription of the TM gene (Nawroth et al 1986, Moore et al 1989). In addition, TNF appears to increase the binding sites for factor IXa on endothelium. PMA, which activates protein kinase C, appears to increase the level of TF mRNA and decrease cell surface TM antigen and its activity, though PMA does not change the level of TM-mRNA. This may be associated with phosphorylation and endocytosis of TM (Dittman et al 1988). Thrombin stimulates the synthesis of TF and appears to stimulate endocytosis and recycling of TM in human umbilical vein endothelial cells (Maruyama & Majerus 1985), whereas transcription of TM-mRNA in mouse haemangioma cells is increased by thrombin as well as cyclohexamide (Dittman et al 1989). These phenomena generally imply that the increase in procoagulant activity on endothelial cells is closely related to the decrease in anticoagulant activity.

Plasma-soluble TM

TM is detected not only in endothelium but also in blood and urine (Ishii & Majerus 1985). Plasma-soluble TM is a mixture of proteins with molecular weights 28 000–105 000 observed under reducing conditions. Plasma TM still has the cofactor activity for protein C activation, but its affinity for thrombin is reduced to approximately one-third of that of cellular TM. Plasma TM is likely derived from cells with injury and/or inflammation but not from the release reaction of endothelial cells. In fact, it has been reported that the level of plasma TM is increased in patients with disseminated intravascular coagulation, systemic lupus erythematosus, diabetes mellitus, patients undergoing haemodialysis therapy and in pregnant women, whose vascular walls would be injured. The plasma TM probably becomes a molecular marker to diagnose injury in vascular endothelium.

Recently, mouse TM and recombinant soluble human TM were found to be potent antithrombotic agents for both in vitro and in vivo use.

LIPOCORTINS, Ca^{2+}-DEPENDENT PHOSPHOLIPID BINDING PROTEINS

Lipocortins are the group of proteins that bind acidic phospholipid in the presence of Ca^{2+}. They are ubiquitously distributed in tissues and organs, and discovered by a number of investigators in different fields. Lipocortins were found to be the major protein of which synthesis was stimulated by the antiinflammatory agent glucocorticoid (Flower & Blackwell 1979). The isolated lipocortin was shown to inhibit phospholipase A_2 activity (Davidson et al 1987). The inhibition of phospholipase activity decreases the release of arachidonic acid and hence may diminish the production of prostaglandins, which leads to inflammation. The proteins p35 and p36, found as the substrates of protein tyrosine kinase and serine–threonine kinase, are also members of the lipocortins (Fava & Cohen 1984, Saris et al 1986). These proteins may relate to cell growth or differentiation. Calelectrin and chromobindins were found as the Ca^{2+}-dependent membrane binding proteins and are thought to be involved in exocytosis (Geisow et al 1984). The anticoagulant proteins described below are also members of the lipocortin family.

Placental anticoagulant proteins

Placental anticoagulant protein (PAP), vascular anticoagulant protein (VAC) and calphobindin are the same anticoagulant protein, discovered in placenta and umbilical cord independently by three groups (Funakoshi et al 1987a, Iwasaki et al 1987, Maurer-Fogy et al 1988). These proteins prolong kaolin- or factor Xa-induced clotting time of normal human plasma or platelet-rich plasma. To date at least six anticoagulant proteins that belong to the lipocortin family have been isolated.

The isolation and structure of PAP

Lipocortins are present in a soluble fraction, if tissues are homogenized in the presence of EDTA. It is present in insoluble fraction, however, when tissues are homogenized in the absence of EDTA or the presence of Ca^{2+}. PAP was first found in cultured bovine endothelial cells but the content was not sufficient to be isolated. It was purified from the soluble fraction of placenta homogenate by ammonium sulphate fractionation, DEAE–Sepharose, gel filtration and HPLC (mono S) column chromatography (Funakoshi et al 1987a). The isolated protein was non-glycosylated, with a molecular weight of 32 000. The complete primary structure was deduced from the nucleotide sequence of cDNA (Funakoshi et al 1987b). It was composed of 319 amino acids and the amino group of the amino-terminal alanine was acetylated. The molecule was composed of four internal repeats; each repeat has 70–80 amino acid residues with around 25% identity with each other. The repeats contain two regions that are commonly present in lipocortins; the amino-terminal 17 residues conform to a consensus sequence of Lys-Gly-X-Gly-Thr-Asp-Glu-X-X-h-h-X-h-h-X-Ser-Arg (h represents hydrophobic residues and X non-specialized amino acid residues) and a stretch of six hydrophobic residues at the carboxyl portion of each repeat. These two regions are thought to be directly involved in the binding to phospholipid (Geisow 1986).

Later, three more PAPs, PAP-II, PAP-III and PAP-IV, were isolated from placenta (Tait et al 1988). The sequences of these proteins are homologous with PAP-I. PAP-II, PAP-III and PAP-IV have molecular weights of 33 000, 34 000 and 34 500, respectively.

PAP prolongs factor Xa-induced clotting time of human plasma, indicating that it inhibits prothrombinase, a complex of factor Xa, factor Va, Ca^{2+} and phospholipid. In order to study the inhibition mechanism, effects of PAP on reconstituted prothrombinase were studied. PAP inhibited prothrombinase activity if phospholipid was present in the reaction; but it did not inhibit the prothrombinase activity, when phospholipid was deleted from the reaction. These experiments indicated that PAP inhibited the prothrombinase activity probably by interacting with phospholipid (Funakoshi et al 1987a).

PAP was shown to bind phospholipid vesicles in the presence of Ca^{2+} by a gel filtration technique. The binding affinity of PAP to phospholipid was studied by quenching of fluorescence of PITC–PAP (Tait et al 1989). PAP was labelled with PITC and mono-labelled PITC–PAP was purified. The binding of PITC–PAP to a mixture of phosphatidylcholine and phosphatidylserine (80%/20%) was obtained in the presence of 2 mM Ca^{2+}. Phosphatidylserine was the essential component of phospholipid vesicles and 20% of phosphatidylserine was maximal for the interaction, which gave the maximal clotting activity of reconstituted prothrombinase. The binding constant (K_d) of PAP with acidic phospholipid was found to be less than 0.1 nM.

This interaction was found to be 700 times higher than that of factor Xa and 2400 times higher than that of prothrombin with phospholipid vesicles by competitive binding experiments. Accordingly, PAP inhibits the prothrombinase activity by blocking the phospholipid–factor Xa or phospholipid–prothrombin interaction with its strong affinity to phospholipid. Two other reactions in coagulation cascade, activation of factor X or factor IX by TF–factor VIIa and factor X activation by factor VIIIa–factor IXa, which requires phospholipid, were also inhibited by PAP (Kondo et al 1987). Figure 3.3 shows the comparative binding affinity of coagulation factors with phospholipid. Only the binding of factor Xa to factor Va present on the surface of platelets is comparable to the affinity of PAP.

Possible physiological roles of PAP

PAP is most abundant among other lipocortins and has the highest binding affinity with phospholipid vesicles. PAP-II has 160 times weaker affinity than PAP-I, and PAP-III is 700 times weaker. Thus, these proteins may have different physiological roles. The PAP antigen was also found in platelets and liver. Circulating blood contains a trace of PAP. To date, no significant relation of the blood level of PAP with any specific disease has been found. Although the physiological significance of PAP remains to be elucidated, it may play a role in preventing excessive coagulation at trauma sites, where acidic phospholipid is exposed to circulating blood to trigger coagulation.

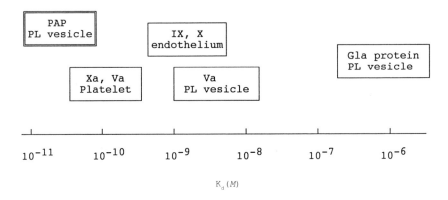

Fig. 3.3 Comparison of the membrane binding affinities of PAP-I and clotting factors. PL represents acidic phospholipid.

REFERENCES

Back R, Konigsberg W H, Nemerson Y 1988 Human tissue factor contains thiolester-linked palmitate and stearate on the cytoplasmic half-cystine. Biochemistry 27: 4227–4231

Bevilacqua M P, Pober J S, Wheeler M E, Cotran R S, Gimbrone M A Jr 1985 Interleukin-1 activation of vascular endothelium: effects on procoagulant activity and leukocyte adhesion. Am J Pathol 121: 394–403

Bezeaud A, Denninger M H, Guillin M H 1985 Interaction of human α-thrombin and γ-thrombin with antithrombin III, protein C and thrombomodulin. Eur J Biochem 153: 491–496

Broze G J, Leykam J E, Schwartz B D, Miletich J P 1985 Purification of human brain tissue factor. J Biol Chem 260: 10917–10920

Davidson F F, Pennis E A, Powell M, Glenny J R Jr 1987 Inhibition of phospholipase A_2 by 'Lipocortins' and calpactins. J Biol Chem 262: 1698–1705

DeBault L E, Esmon N L, Olson J R, Esmon C T 1986 Distribution of the thrombomodulin antigen in the rabbit vasculature. Lab Invest 54: 172–178

Dittman W A, Kumada T, Sadler J E, Majerus P W 1988 The structure and function of mouse thrombomodulin: phorbol myristate acetate stimulates degradation of thrombomodulin without affecting mRNA levels in haemangioma cells. J Biol Chem 263: 15815–15822

Dittman W A, Kumada T, Majerus P W 1989 Transcription of thrombomodulin mRNA in mouse hemangioma cells is increased by cyclohexamide and thrombin. Proc Natl Acad Sci USA 86: 7179–7182

Eaton D, Rodriguez H, Vehar G A 1986 Proteolytic processing of human Factor VIII: correlation of specific cleavages by thrombin, Factor Xa, and activated protein C with activation and inactivation of Factor VIII coagulant activity. Biochemistry 25: 505–512

Esmon C T, Owen W G 1981 Identification of an endothelial cell cofactor for thrombin-catalyzed activation of protein C. Proc Natl Acad Sci 78: 2249–2252

Esmon C T, Esmon N L, Harris K W 1982a Complex formation between thrombin and thrombomodulin inhibits both thrombin-catalyzed fibrin formation and factor V activation. J Biol Chem 257: 7944–7947

Esmon N L, Owen W G, Esmon C T 1982b Isolation of a membrane-bound cofactor for thrombin-catalyzed activation of protein C. J Biol Chem 257: 859–864

Esmon N L, Carroll R C, Esmon C T 1983 Thrombomodulin blocks the ability of thrombin to activate platelets. J Biol Chem 258: 12238–12242

Fava R A, Cohen S 1984 Isolation of a calcium-dependent 35-kilodalton substrate for epidermal growth factor receptor/kinase from A-431 cells. J Biol Chem 259: 2636–2645

Fisher K L, Gorman C M, Vehar G A, O'Brien D P, Lawn R H 1987 Cloning and expression of human tissue factor. Thromb Res 48: 89–99

Flower R J, Blackwell G J 1979 Anti-inflammatory steroids induce biosynthesis of a phospholipase A_2 inhibitor which prevents prostaglandin generation. Nature 278: 456–459

Flower R J, Wood J N, Parente L 1984 Macrocortin and the mechanism of action of the glucocorticoids. Adv Inflamm Res 7: 61–69

Freyssimet J M, Gauchy J, Cazenave J P 1986 The effect of phospholipids on the activation of protein C by the human thrombin–thrombomodulin complex. Biochem J 238: 151–157

Funakoshi T, Heimark R L, Hendrickson L E, McMullen B A, Fujikawa K 1987a Human placental anticoagulant protein: isolation and characterization. Biochemistry 26: 5572–5578

Funakoshi T, Hendrickson L E, McMullem B A, Fujikawa K 1987b Primary structure of human placental anticoagulant protein. Biochemistry 26: 8087–8092

Galvin J B, Kurosawa S, Moore K, Esmon C T, Esmon N L 1987 Reconstitution of rabbit thrombomodulin into phospholipid vesicles. J Biol Chem 262: 2199–2205

Geisow M J 1986 Common domain structure of Ca^{++} and lipid-binding proteins. FEBS Lett 203: 99–103

Geisow M, Childs J, Dash H et al 1984 Cellular distribution of three mammalian Ca^{++}-binding proteins related to *Topeds* calelectrin. EMBO J 3: 2969–2974

Gregory S A, Morrissey J H, Edgington T S 1989 Regulation of tissue factor gene expression in the monocyte. Mol Cell Biol 9: 2752–2755

Guha A, Bach R, Konigsberg W, Nemerson Y 1986 Affinity purification of human tissue factor: interaction of factor VII and tissue factor in detergent micelles. Proc Natl Acad Sci USA 83: 299–302

Haley P E, Doyle M F, Mann K G 1989 The activation of bovine protein C by Factor Xa. J Biol Chem 264: 16303–16310

Hayashi T, Zushi M, Yamamoto S, Suzuki K 1990 Further localization of binding sites for thrombin and protein C in human thrombomodulin. J Biol Chem (in press)

Imada S, Yamaguchi H, Nagumo M, Katayanagi S, Iwasaki H, Imada M 1990 Identification of fetomodulin, a surface marker protein of fetal development, as thrombomodulin by gene cloning and functional assay. Dev Biol 140: 113–122

Ishii H, Majerus P W 1985 Thrombomodulin is present in human plasma and urine. J Clin Invest 76: 2178–2181

Iwasaki T, Suda M, Nakao H et al 1987 Structure and expression of cDNA for an inhibitor of blood coagulation isolated from human placenta: a new lipocortin-like protein. J Biochem (Tokyo) 102: 1261–1273

Jackman R W, Beeler D L, Fritze L, Soff G, Rosenberg R D 1987 Human thrombomodulin gene is intron depleted: nucleic acid sequences of the cDNA and gene predict protein structure and suggest sites of regulatory control. Proc Natl Acad Sci 84: 6425–6429

Kondo S, Noguchi M, Funakoshi T, Fujikawa K, Kisiel W 1987 Inhibition of human factor VIIa-tissue factor activity by placental anticoagulant protein. Thromb Res 48: 449–459

Kurosawa S, Galvin J B, Esmon N L, Esmon C T 1987 Proteolytic formation and properties of functional domains of thrombomodulin. J Biol Chem 262: 2206–2212

Kurosawa S, Stearns D J, Jackson K W, Esmon C T 1988 A 10-kDa cyanogen bromide fragment from the epidermal growth factor homology domain of rabbit thrombomodulin contains the primary thrombin binding site. J Biol Chem 263: 5993–5996

Mackman N, Morrissey J H, Fowler B, Edgington T S 1989 Complete sequence of the human tissue factor gene, a highly regulated cellular receptor that initiates the coagulation protease cascade. Biochemistry 28: 1755–1762

Maruyama I, Majerus P W 1985 The turnover of thrombin–thrombomodulin complex in cultured human umbilical vein endothelial cells and A 549 cancer cells. J Biol Chem 260: 15432–15438

Maruyama I, Bell C E, Majerus P W 1985 Thrombomodulin is found on endothelium of arteries, veins, capillaries, and lymphatics and on syncytiotrophoblast of human placenta. J Cell Biol 101: 363–371

Maurer-Fogy I, Reutelingsperger C P M, Pieters J, Bodo G, Stratowa C, Hauptmann R 1988 Cloning and expression of cDNA for human vascular anticoagulant, a Ca^{++}-dependent phospholipid-binding protein. Eur J Biochem 174: 585–592

Moore K L, Esmon C T, Esmon N L 1989 Tumor necrosis factor leads to the internalization and degradation of thrombomodulin from the surface of bovine aortic endothelial cells in culture. Blood 73: 159–165

Morrissey J H, Fakhrai H, Edgington T S 1987 Molecular cloning of the cDNA for tissue factor, the cellular receptor for the initiation of the coagulation protease cascade. Cell 50: 129–135

Musci G, Berliner L J, Esmon C T 1988 Evidence of multiple conformation changes in the active center of thrombin induced by complex formation with thrombomodulin: an analysis employing nitroxide spin-labels. Biochemistry 27: 769–773

Nawroth P P, Bank I, Handley D, Cassimeris J, Chess L, Stern D 1986 Tumor necrosis factor/cachectin interacts with endothelial cell receptors to induce release of interleukin 1. J Exp Med 163: 1363–1375

Noé G, Hofsteenge J, Rovelli G, Stone S R 1988 The use of sequence-specific antibodies to identify a secondary binding site in thrombin. J Biol Chem 263: 11729–11735

Osterud B, Rappaport S I 1977 Activation of factor IX by the reaction product of tissue factor and factor VII: additional pathway for initiating blood coagulation. Proc Natl Acad Sci USA 74: 5260–5264

Paborsky L R, Tate K M, Harris R J et al 1989 Purification of recombinant human tissue factor. Biochemistry 28: 8072–8077

Pedersen A H, Lund-Hansen T, Bisgaard-Frantzen H, Olsen F, Petersen L C 1989 Autoactivation of human recombinant coagulation factor VII. Biochemistry 28: 9331–9336

Sakai T, Lund-Hansen T, Paborsky L, Pedersen A H, Kisiel W 1989 Binding of human factor VII and VIIa to a human bladder carcinoma cell line (J82). J Biol Chem 264: 9980–9988

Salem H H, Maruyama I, Ishii H, Majerus P W 1984 Isolation and characterization of thrombomodulin from human placenta. J Biol Chem 259: 12246–12251

Saris C J M, Tack B F, Kristensen T, Glenny J R Jr, Hunter T 1986 The cDNA sequence for the protein-tyrosine kinase substrate p36 (calpactin I heavy chain) reveals a multidomain protein with internal repeats. Cell 46: 201–212

Scarpati E M, Wen D, Broze G J et al 1987 Human tissue factor: cDNA sequence and chromosome localization of the gene. Biochemistry 26: 5234–5238

Spicer E K, Horton R, Bloem L et al 1987 Isolation of cDNA clones coding for human tissue factor: primary structure of the protein and cDNA. Proc Natl Acad Sci USA 84: 5148–5152

Stern D M, Drillings M, Kisiel W, Nawroth P, Nossel H L, LaGamma K S 1984 Activation of factor IX bound to cultured bovine aortic endothelial cells. Proc Natl Acad Sci USA 81: 913–917

Suzuki K, Stenflo J, Dahlbäck B, Teodorsson B 1983 Inactivation of human coagulation Factor V by activated protein C. J Biol Chem 258: 1914–1920

Suzuki K, Kusumoto H, Deyashiki Y et al 1987 Structure and expression of human thrombomodulin, a thrombin receptor on endothelium acting as a cofactor for protein C activation. EMBO J 6: 1891–1897

Suzuki K, Hayashi T, Nishioka J, Zushi M, Honda G, Yamamoto S 1989 A domain composed of epidermal growth factor-like structures of human thrombomodulin is essential for thrombin binding and for protein C activation. J Biol Chem 264: 4872–4876

Suzuki K, Nishioka J, Hayashi T 1990 Localization of thrombomodulin-binding site within human thrombin. J Biol Chem 265: 13263–13267

Tait J F, Sakata M, McMullen B A et al 1988 Placental anticoagulant proteins: isolation and comparative characterization of four members of the lipocortin family. Biochemistry 27: 6226–6268

Tait J F, Gibson D, Fujikawa K 1989 Phospholipid binding properties of human placental anticoagulant protein-I, a member of the lipocortin family. J Biol Chem 264: 7944–7949

Thompson E A, Salem H H 1986 Inhibition by human thrombomodulin of factor Xa-mediated cleavage of prothrombin. J Clin Invest 78: 13–17

Wen D, Dittman W A, Ye R D, Deaven LL, Majerus P W, Sadler J E 1987 Human thrombomodulin: complete cDNA sequence and chromosome localization of the gene. Biochemistry 26: 4350–4357

Wilcox J N, Smith K M, Schwartz S M, Gordon D 1989 Localization of tissue factor in the normal vessel wall and in the atherosclerotic plaque. Proc Natl Acad Sci USA 86: 2839–2843

Zushi M, Gomi K, Yamamoto S, Maruyama I, Hayashi T, Suzuki K 1989 The last three consecutive epidermal growth factor-like structures of human thrombomodulin comprise the minimum functional domain for protein C-activating cofactor activity and anticoagulant activity. J Biol Chem 264: 10351–10353

4

Haemostasis and atherosclerosis

O.N. Ulutin

The history of atherosclerosis in general dates from ancient times. Differences in the blood vessels of old and young human beings were observed and noted during the mummification procedures practised in ancient Egypt (Sinzinger & Widhalm 1981).

The terms 'arteriosclerosis' and 'atherosclerosis' were first used by J.F. Lobstein in 1833 and Felix Marchand in 1904 although the vascular changes were presented much earlier in the medical literature (McMillan 1985). These terms are morphological and do not precisely define the pathological process. There are various hypotheses on the pathogenesis of the disease. We will mainly discuss the relationship between the disease and the haemostatic mechanism in this review. Other hypotheses will briefly be mentioned as they may relate to haemostasis. The experiments and discussions that link the disease to haemostasis began 150 years ago. Carl Von Rokitansky postulated in 1841 that the disease is due to the abnormal deposition of blood components including fibrin in the intima (see also Woolf 1987). The theory of tissue response to endothelial injury by Virchow followed this concept in 1856. We will not enter these theories in detail since the historical aspects of this concept have been widely covered in previous reviews. There are many overviews covering the relationship between haemostasis and atherosclerosis (Mehta 1987, Ross 1986, Ulutin 1986a, 1986b, Woolf 1987). We will discuss and summarize the following questions in this short review. What is the nature of clinical and laboratory changes present in the various haemostatic tests in patients with atherosclerosis? Are changes in these parameters present in the young members of families with familial atherosclerosis? Can a haemostasis-related working hypothesis be formulated from these findings?

ENDOTHELIAL CELL

There is increasing evidence that the endothelial cell (EC) is involved in numerous physiological and pathological processes in the vascular system as well as in the haemostatic mechanism. The importance of the EC is being increasingly recognized. The EC has a strong antithrombotic action due to the substances it contains and synthesizes. It has been demonstrated that these functions are reduced in patients with atherosclerosis and there is no doubt that the EC constitutes the most important 'key cell' together with changes in the vascular wall in the development of atherosclerosis. It has been shown in various studies that the EC is the key regulatory cell in vascular homeostasis. The EC performs this by both releasing the substances it has synthesized and by stimulating platelets and leucocytes which are inhibitory. Arachidonic acid (AA) metabolites, surface glycoproteins, chemotactic factors and coagulation factors play roles in the process. It is known that intact human platelets do not adhere to a morphologically and functionally intact normal endothelium. I would also like to mention at this point that there are various types of EC according to the functional type of the vessels and their location.

The internal surface of the EC which faces the circulation is covered by this proteoglycan layer. Many substances are synthesized in the EC. The substances that are produced by the EC for its antithrombotic effect are listed in Table 4.1. Many proteoglycans such as heparan sulphate (HS), dermatan sulphate (DS) and heparin are among the substances synthesized in the EC. The demonstration that heparin is produced in ECs other than in mast cells and basophils and the inhibitory effect of heparin on smooth muscle cell (SMC) hyperplasia have gained considerable importance in relation to the pathogenesis of atherosclerosis (Buonassi 1973, Marcum et al 1986, Marcum & Rosenberg 1985).

Buonassi showed in 1973 that heparan sulphate is synthesized in EC cultures. This finding has been confirmed in both his own and in Marcum & Rosenberg's (1985) studies. It has been demonstrated that HS, which has an anticoagulant effect, is produced in clonal EC cultures of cattle and mice whereas this substance and activity is not present in SMC cultures (Marcum et al 1986, Marcum & Rosenberg 1985). It has also been shown that heparin added to EC cultures adheres to ECs and to their surfaces. As we will discuss later, we consider the relationship between heparin and SMC to be important. Early publications claimed that patients with atherosclerosis had a diminished amount of heparin and these patients show resistance to heparin (Ulutin 1986b).

Tissue plasminogen activator (t-PA) and plasminogen activator inhibitor

Table 4.1 The substances produced by the endothelial cell which have antithrombotic and prothrombotic activity

Antithrombotic	Prothrombotic
t-PA	PAI
Proteoglycans	15-HETE
PGI$_2$	vWF
EDRF (NO)	TT
13-HODE	PAF
Protein S	Endothelin
Thrombomodulin	

(PAI) synthesized in ECs play a prominent role in the regulation of fibrino-lytic activity (Balkuv-Ulutin 1986, Collen & Juhan-Vague 1988). I will try to summarize the knowledge on EC, and the relationship between the fibri-nolytic system and atherosclerosis. It has been known for a long time that t-PA and PAI are produced in the EC and also that fibrinolytic activity is decreased in patients with atherosclerosis due to the altered relationship between these two enzymes. It is known that PAI is also synthesized in cells other than the EC. It has also been demonstrated that lipopolysaccharides and interleukin I (IL-I) increase the level of PAI. When the EC is stimu-lated by the DDAVP and the cuff test, the increase in fibrinolytic activity is less than in normal controls, as shown in Table 4.2. It has been demon-strated using the ELISA technique that there are two types of response in patients with atherosclerosis. A decrease in the production and/or the release of t-PA and an increase in PAI leads to reduced fibrinolytic activity in atherosclerosis. This becomes more significant if one considers that both these substances are synthesized in the EC. It has been shown that an increase in PAI is the most commonly observed cause for the reduced fibrinolytic activity in cases of venous thrombophlebitis (Juhan-Vague et al 1987, Nilsson et al 1985). Huber et al (1988) have observed the changes in cases with unstable coronary artery disease and acute myocardial infarction. They were not able to demonstrate a significant difference between the levels of t-PA in patients and in the control group whereas they found a highly significant difference between the levels of PAI. Sloan & Firkin showed in 1989 that PAI was in excess in 27 of 34 cases of thrombosis with reduced fibrinolytic activity whereas t-PA was deficient in seven cases. According to Norden et al (1989) the response to the venous occlusion test decreases as the atherosclerotic process becomes more widespread. They have also demonstrated that there is a significant increase in the level of fibronectin and in the numbers of peripheral monocytes. The importance of this increase becomes significant when one considers the role of fibronectin in platelet adhesion. As is known, fibronectin is a high-molecular-weight substance which plays a role in cellular adhesion. It has been demonstrated that it is synthesized in various cells including the EC and is present in the α-granules of platelets.

We have shown that t-PA is decreased and PAI is in excess in our patients

Table 4.2 Results of the cuff test (venous stasis test) in normal controls (N=50) and in patients with atherosclerosis (N=50)

		Before	After	Change (%)	Difference
ELT (min)	Normal control	107 ± 23	59 ± 27	44.8	43
	Atherosclerotics	167 ± 27	142 ± 24	8.5	25
Fibrin plate unheated (mm^2)	Normal control	44.4 ± 9.6	86.2 ± 16.4	93.6	41.8
	Atherosclerotics	25.8 ± 9.4	37.6 ± 12.6	45	11.8

with atherosclerosis (coronary sclerosis, cerebrosclerosis and peripheral obliterative vascular diseases (POVD) of atherosclerotic origin) with decreased fibrinolytic activity (Table 4.3).

There were patients among those deficient in t-PA who responded to the cuff test as well as those who did not, whereas increased levels of PAI inhibitor were also present. We can classify patients with atherosclerosis into four groups depending on their levels of t-PA and PAI and their response to the cuff test, but these findings are not consistent and change in both directions with time, in the same person. This classification is therefore artificial.

Type I: low levels of t-PA and normal PAI. These patients do not respond to the cuff test (6 cases).

Type II: normal or slightly elevated t-PA, slightly increased PAI, both parameters increase in the cuff test (14 cases).

Type III: normal t-PA, increased PAI. A slightly increased t-PA whereas marked increased PAI after the cuff test (18 cases).

Type IV: the same results as the control group in fibrinolytic activity, fibrin plate, t-PA and PAI (12 cases).

These variations are positively related to the extent of vascular changes, the stage of the illness and the presence of microthrombi and should be investigated further.

A general evaluation of our series of 50 type IV cases yielded normal results in 12 (24%), 18 (36%) in type III, 14 (28%) in type II and 6 (12%) in type I patients. All of these findings emphasize the importance of the amounts of t-PA and PAI in atherosclerosis and thromboembolism. There have been various studies in the medical literature which have stressed the relationship between the fibrinolytic system and the generation of atherosclerosis (Balkuv-Ulutin 1986, Collen & Juhan-Vague 1988). Atherosclerotic changes in animals treated with inhibitors of the fibrinolytic

Table 4.3 t-PA and PAI levels before and after cuff test in 50 cases of atherosclerosis. Determinations were done using Asserachrom-t-PA and Stachrom PAI kits

	Type I (N=6)		Type II (N=14)		Type III (N=18)		Type IV (N=12)	
	Before	After	Before	After	Before	After	Before	After
t-PA (ng/ml)	3.2±0.6	3.6±0.4	8.6±2.6	13.2±3.4	4.6±2.6	5.6±2.9	5.2±2.4	9.4±2.9
PAI (IU/ml)	3.4±1.4	3.2±1.8	16.4±3.4	24.2±4.2	19.6±3.7	41.7±6.1	3.4±1.2	4.6±2.3

Mean of all types together	Before	After
t-PA (N=50) (ng/ml)	5.6±2.3	8.4±2.7
PAI (N=50) (IU/ml)	12.8±2.7	23.27±4.1

system have been demonstrated in various reports (Deutsch 1965, Hosgör et al 1989, Kwaan 1979, Özer et al 1989). These studies showed that decreased fibrinolytic activity enhances the formation of experimental atherosclerosis and thrombus formation (Fig. 4.1). It has also been shown that activation of the fibrinolytic system in animals prevents smooth muscle

A

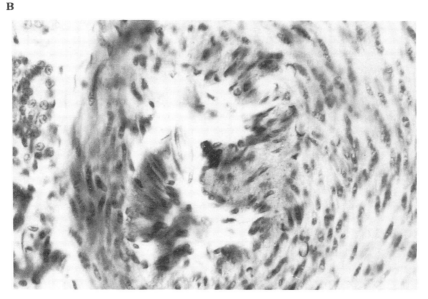

B

Fig. 4.1 A, B Endothelial and smooth muscle cell proliferation and thrombus formation are seen in pulmonary arteries of two different cats given t-AMCA for 3 hours. (From Hosgör et al 1989.)

hyperplasia and the EC alteration caused by experimental thrombosis (Balkuv-Ulutin et al 1981, Ulutin et al 1986).

PGI_2 (prostacyclin) and NO (EDRF)) synthesized by the EC play an important role in the changes related to atherosclerosis. As is known, PGG_2 and PGH_2 are produced in the EC by the interaction of arachidonic acid and cyclooxygenase, and PGH_2 is further converted to PGI_2 with the help of prostacyclin synthetase. PGI_2 is a very potent anti-aggregator and a vasodilator substance (Ulutin 1986b). A decrease in the plasma level of PGI_2 and a decrease or absence in the formation of PGI_2 in the vascular wall of patients with experimental or clinical atherosclerosis have been demonstrated in various studies (Ulutin & Cizmeci 1985a). Our findings have been summarized in Table 4.4.

The highest concentrations of PGI_2 have been found in the EC in measurements performed from the vascular wall. It progressively decreases in the intima and media and disappears in the adventitia. Various substances activate the EC and the cell responds to the stimulus by increasing the generation of PGI_2 and endothelial derivative relaxing factor (EDRF). EDRF is a vasodilator that relaxes smooth muscle. It also inhibits aggregation and adhesion of platelets (Radomski et al 1988). It has been demonstrated in recent studies that it is nitric oxide (NO) in structure. It has been shown that the relaxation due to EC is impaired in hypercholesterolaemic rabbits and monkeys as well as in atherosclerotic human beings (Föstermann et al 1988).

13-Hydroxyoctadecadienoic (13-HODE) is synthesized as a lipo-oxygenase metabolite in the cytosol of the EC. 13-HODE has an anti-adhesive effect (Botting & Vane 1989, Buchanan et al 1985). 13-HODE, which is produced and released from the EC as linoleic acid metabolism, prevents the adhesion of platelets. It has been demonstrated experimentally that platelets become adhesive when the production of 13-HODE decreases.

15-Hydroxyeicosatetraenoic (15-HETE), on the other hand, which is synthesized by the action of 12-lipo-oxygenase on AA, is required for platelet adhesion and platelet adhesion is impaired in the case of lipo-oxygenase deficiency (Buchanan 1988).

Thrombomodulin, which is present in the EC membrane, plays a role in the activation of protein C. It has also been demonstrated that part of protein S is produced in the EC. The EC plays a role in this way, in the activation of natural inhibitors.

Table 4.4 The plasma levels of 6 keto-$PGF_{1\alpha}$ in 22 normal control subjects and 22 patients with atherosclerosis in the same age group determined using radioimmunoassay (values are pg/ml)

Normal control (N=22)	92.6 ± 22
Atherosclerosis (N=22)	35.4 ± 27 $P<0.001$

Other than having an antithrombotic effect, the EC synthesizes substances that are procoagulants and vasoconstrictors. The antithrombotic and procoagulant effects of the EC may concomitantly take place in a balanced fashion (Teitel et al 1982). Such components include tissue thromboplastin (TT), PAI, von Willebrand factor (vWF) and endothelin.

It has been demonstrated that PAI increases and therefore fibrinolytic activity decreases in some patients with thrombophlebitis and atherosclerosis.

There are various observations that vWF is increased in cases with atherosclerosis. We have also demonstrated in our laboratories that VIIIAg (vWF), VIII Ricof and VIIIC increase together with fibrinogen in such cases.

Yanagisawa et al showed in 1988 that a polypeptide consisting of 21 amino acids is a potent vasoconstrictor. It is called endothelin and is present in the EC. The status of this substance, which is ten times more potent then angiotensin II in pathological states is open to further studies and discussion.

It has been demonstrated that a stimulated EC increases the level of platelet-activating factor (PAF; Walsh et al 1975). It is well known that in very small concentrations PAF activates platelets and causes aggregation and also stimulates neutrophils. The production and release of PAF in the EC increase as a result of the stimulation of the EC by thrombin, histamine, bradykinin and leukotrienes. PAF stimulates platelets and facilitates the adherence of neutrophils to the EC by stimulating them. What is of interest is that some of the activators listed above also stimulate the production and release of PGI_2. With the effect of IL-I, TT appeared on the surface of EC.

Thrombin formation also takes place on the cell surface as a result of the effect of XIa, Va and Xa.

SMOOTH MUSCLE CELL

The first morphological signs in cases with atherosclerosis consist of hypertrophy and hyperplasia of smooth muscle cells (SMCs) and the migration of SMCs from the media to the intima. As we have mentioned above, heparin inhibits smooth muscle hyperplasia (Tiozzo et al 1989). Smooth muscle proliferating factor (SMPF — growth hormone) which is released from platelet α-granules causes smooth muscle hyperplasia and a chemotactic substance leads to the migration of smooth muscle cells to the intima.

These stimulated SMCs synthesize collagen, elastic fibrils and various proteoglycans. These substances are important in the pathogenesis of atherosclerosis. Collagen types IV and V are synthesized in the EC. They are released under the EC towards the basement membrane side and only cause platelet adhesion. vWF and specific platelet glycoproteins such as GPI_b and $GPII_b/IIIa$ play a role in this adhesion. If the injury is deep and if platelets contact with collagen type I and type III synthesized by the SMC, adhesion and 'release reaction' take place. Type I and III cause adhesion, aggregation and secretion. It has also been demonstrated that SMPF (platelet derivative growth factor — PDGF) increases the synthesis of cholesterol and phospholipid in smooth muscle.

While the EC synthesizes heparan sulphate, SMC produces dermatan sulphate (DS) and chondroitin sulphate. DS activates mainly heparin cofactor II and in this way inactivates thrombin (Pangrazzi & Gianase 1987).

SMCs which have undergone hyperplasia and which have migrated to the intima and have synthesized connective tissue (collagen, elastin, connective tissue matrix) also produce a chemotactic substance which leads to the migration of monocytes to the intima (Schwartz et al 1986). In 1977 Cloves & Karnovsky demonstrated in mice that SMC hyperplasia takes place after the arterial EC is stimulated and this hyperplasia is inhibited by the infusion of heparin. This finding was also confirmed by in vivo and in vitro studies. It was also demonstrated that this particular effect of heparin was not related to its anticoagulant action (Castellot et al 1987, Guyton et al 1980, Hoover et al 1980, Karnovsky et al 1989, Tiozzo et al 1989). In in vitro concentrations of 5 μg/ml, heparin inhibits SMC proliferation and significantly decreases [^{3}H]thymidine uptake. It has also been shown on the other hand that chondroitin sulphate, dermatan sulphate, protamine sulphate and high-molecular-weight dextrose do not produce such an effect. As we have mentioned previously the importance of these findings in the pathogenesis of atherosclerosis becomes clearer if published findings, e.g. the shorter duration of action of heparin, the resistance to heparin and the low levels of heparin in these cases, are taken into account (Engelberg 1988, Ulutin 1986b).

COAGULATION FACTORS

The most frequently observed finding in these patients is an increase in fibrinogen and in the VIIIc/VIIIAg ratio. The alterations in the other coagulation factors yield discrepant results in various studies. A decrease in the half-lives of fibrinogen and platelets is another finding reported in these cases (Berkarda et al 1968). A laboratory picture of chronic disseminated intravascular coagulation (DIC) in atherosclerotic patients is another aspect (Ulutin & Ulutin 1975).

In the prethrombotic stage of atherosclerotic patients there is not only a significant increase in the level of fibrinogen but also an increase in the fibrin polymerization curve (Fig. 4.2). Fibrinogen is more responsive to thrombin compared with normal control subjects. It has also been reported that ristocetin cofactor activity is increased (Rak et al 1986). These authors have shown in their studies that compared to normal there is a difference in the electrophoretic mobility of vWF Ag. Many researchers accept that the changes in fibrinogen and high levels of fibrinogen are important findings concerning atherosclerosis and the prethrombotic stage.

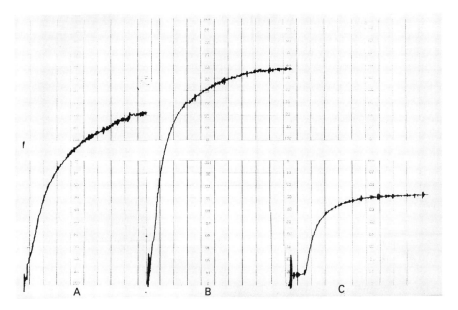

Fig. 4.2   Fibrin polymerization curves in **A** atherosclerosis with hypercoagulability, **B** prothrombotic stage and **C** normal control subject.

NATURAL INHIBITORS

Heparin, AT-III (heparin cofactor I), heparin cofactor II, protein C and protein S are among the natural inhibitors. Extensive experiments have been done concerning their relation to atherosclerosis. Various reports have described resistance to heparin in atherosclerotic patients, shorter action of heparin compared to normal subjects, that therapy with intermittent low-dose heparin has a beneficial effect and also that it prevents thrombosis if administered preoperatively. We have summarized the general literature and our own findings elsewhere (Ulutin 1986b). Various experiments are currently being performed that examine the effects of low-molecular-weight heparin, pentasaccharides and hirudin rather than unfractionated (UF) heparin on animals and the relationship of these effects to those mentioned above (Cloves & Karnovsky 1977).

There is no consensus on the state of AT-III in patients with atherosclerosis. The level of AT-III may show secondary changes depending on the clinical state. It has been demonstrated in cases of diabetes mellitus with vascular complications that levels of thrombin–antithrombin III complexes (TAT) and plasmin–α_2-antiplasmin complexes increase and are indicators of continuous activation of coagulation and fibrinolysis (Takahashi et al 1989). We have found in our own atherosclerotic patients that the levels of protein C and S are at the lower side of the normal range and are decreased significantly compared to normal (Table 4.5). Protein S has been shown to be produced in endothelial cell cultures (Fair et al 1986) and also is present in the EC (Stern et al 1986). The presence of two of the main factors of the protein C system, thrombomodulin and protein S, in the EC shows that it is also a key cell in the regulation of natural inhibitors. The presence of a low-grade chronic DIC-like mechanism in atherosclerosis is being considered. We think at this point that the fluctuations in the levels of AT-III, protein C and S are usually secondary in that they are affected by the extent of the disease, by the presence and absence of thrombosis and that they cannot be related quantitatively to the pathogenic process.

FIBRINOLYTIC SYSTEM

Changes in the fibrinolytic system play an important role in atherosclerosis. The decrease in fibrinolytic activity in atherosclerosis and the production of vascular changes and thromboembolism by experimental inhibition of the fibrinolytic system in animals have caused alterations of the fibrinolytic system to be of more significance in this disease (Balkuv-Ulutin et al 1989, Deutsch 1965, Hoşgör et al 1989, Kwaan 1979, Özer et al 1989). To summarize the findings we can state that synthesis and release of t-PA is decreased and/or synthesis and release of PAI is increased in the EC of atherosclerotic cases and a decrease in global fibrinolytic activity ensues as a result. On the other hand, antiplasmin activity of plasma increases. Our findings have been summarized in Table 4.3. An increase in PAI rather then a decrease in t-PA has been demonstrated in most of the cases in recent experiments (Balkuv-Ulutin 1986, Collen & Juhan-Vague 1988, Huber et al 1988, Juhan-Vague et al 1984). The increase of inhibitors (PAI and α_2-antiplasmin) is considered more important although the activity of the fibrinolytic system is found to be decreased in tests such as the euglobulin lysis time (ELT) and fibrin plate. The excess of inhibitors changes the direction of the system in various experiments although the synthesis of activator is increased (Takahashi et al 1989). The vascular wall and the liver play a regulatory role in the fibrinolytic system. The balance between the production of activator and inhibitor and inactivation controls fibrinolysis in both systems (Balkuv-Ulutin 1978, Juhan-Vague et al 1984, Sprengers &

Table 4.5 Protein C and protein S levels in normal subjects (N=24) and in patients with atherosclerosis (N=24). Determinations were done using Asserachrom protein C and Stachrom protein S kits

	Protein C	Protein S
Normal control (N=24)	109.24 ± 11.7	110.42 ± 13.1
Atherosclerosis (N=24)	88.91 ± 14.6 $p<0.01$	89.64 ± 14.8 $p<0.05$

Kluft 1987). The liver controls the increased fibrinolytic activity by inactivating t-PA and by increasing the release of antiplasmin and PAI.

A progressive decrease in fibrinolytic activity and a related increase in thrombotic tendency is observed in atherosclerotic cases. The latest experiments reveal that an increase in PAI is more frequently observed here compared to a decrease in t-PA and this constitutes one of the reasons for thromboembolism in these patients.

LEUCOCYTES

The leucocytes of the circulation enter extravascular tissues by initially adhering to the EC and then reaching the subendothelium by passing through the endothelium by diapedesis. A close relationship is established between the leucocytes and endothelial cell in this way, even in physiological circumstances, they can lead to endothelial injury in pathological conditions. The presence of certain substances in leucocytes affects the EC metabolism, and also leucocytes have procoagulants causing a prethrombotic stage when they are destroyed.

The degradation of heparin sulphate by the heparinase found in leucocytes, the presence of proteases that lead to vascular injury and cause lysis of the basal membrane, the presence of TT especially in monocytes and the increase in EC and neutrophil adhesion by LTB_4 may be cited as examples (Harlan 1987, Jonasson et al 1986, Matzner et al 1985). It has also been demonstrated that IL-1 derived from monocytes increases the adhesion of segmented neutrophils to the EC. Some authors assume that the adhesion of segmented leucocytes to the EC represents acute inflammation and together with the adhesion of monocytes are signs of an atherosclerotic lesion.

It can be demonstrated that monocytes migrate towards the intima, and are transformed into phagocytic tissue histiocytes and into foam cells as a result of the chemotactic substance that is released during smooth muscle hypertrophy. The whole process has a role in atherogenesis (Gerrity 1981, Harlan 1985, Jauchem et al 1982, Jonasson et al 1986, Schwartz et al 1986). Monocytes are transformed into phagocytic macrophages in the intima. If plasma levels of triglycerides, very-low-density lipoproteins (VLDLs) and cholesterol are high, monocytes phagocytose them and these are transformed to foam cells (Gianturco & Bradley 1988). It has also been demonstrated that VLDLs are toxic to the EC.

PLATELETS

The most extensive changes in haemostasis in atherosclerotic cases take place in platelets and platelet function. Platelets have three main functions: adhesion, aggregation and secretion (Castellot et al 1987, Takahashi et al 1989). Platelet functions and the alterations in their biochemistry are summarized in Table 4.6. It has been demonstrated by various methods that platelet adhesion and aggregation increase in atherosclerotic subjects (Ulutin 1976). The increase in the platelet adhesiveness and aggregation were more pronounced in the prethrombotic stage and during transient ischaemic attacks. It is also known that factors such as vWF and fibrinogen which play a role in platelet adhesion are increased compared to normal. Significant changes in the differential count and in the formation of islands on foreign surfaces have also been observed in addition to the adhesion of platelets to these surfaces (Rebuck et al 1961, Vague et al 1987, Walsh et al 1975). We found that platelets change into more active forms and produce bigger aggregates in atherosclerotic patients when we performed differential platelet counts on formvar with the Rebuck method (Table 4.7). They are more prominent in the prethrombotic stage and in transient ischaemic attacks. We have also demonstrated in our studies that anti-aggregating drugs and defibrotide reverse these patterns towards normal

Table 4.6 Functional and biochemical alterations of platelets in the patients with atherosclerosis

Increase of platelet adhesion
Alteration of surface activation
Hyperaggregation with aggregating agents
Occasionally spontaneous aggregation
Hypersecretion
Increase level of platelet markers in plasma
Increase of platelet α_2-antiplasmin
Decrease of platelet AT-III
Decrease of γ-glutamyl transferase in platelets
Low levels of cyclic AMP in intact platelets
Alteration of membrane phospholipids
Increase of $PGF_{2\alpha}$, PGE, MDA and TXA_2 formation in platelets
Defective [^{14}C]glucose membrane transport due to decrease or alteration of glucose binding membrane protein
Increase of galactose incorporation into platelets
Alterations of platelet membrane glucoprotein distribution
Shortened half-life of platelets

Table 4.7 Differential platelet counts on formvar surfaces in normal subjects and atherosclerotic patients in the same age group using shadow-casting technique of EM of Rebuck et al (1961)

	R	D	I	S	Aggregates per 100 single platelets	
					Small	Gross
Normal control (N=22)	3.2 ± 1.6	66.4 ± 8.1	20.3 ± 5.6	10.2 ± 2.4	4.5 ± 2.4	–
Atherosclerosis (N=32)	2.1 ± 0.7 $p<0.01$	24.6 ± 9.2 $p<0.001$	25.1 ± 8.2 n.s.	47.4 ± 9.2 $p<0.001$	12.6 ± 6	5.2 ± 3 $p<0.001$

R, round; D, dendritic; I, intermediates; S, spread.

(Ulutin et al 1975). Spread forms and aggregate formation decrease especially with defibrotide (Ulutin 1988, 1989). Increased adhesion and increased aggregation are findings frequently observed in these cases. Tschopp et al (1979), on the other hand, did not demonstrate any difference between normal subjects and atherosclerotic cases with the method of subendothelial adhesion of Baumgartner. Platelets respond to a greater degree and with lower concentrations of thrombin, ADP and adrenaline compared with normal subjects. We have observed in our cases that an excessive response to all aggregating agents is present in most of the subjects whereas some of them respond excessively only to ADP or adrenaline. In some patients, spontaneous aggregates occur in the circulation, causing transient ischaemic attacks as well as release reactions during circulation.

Stimulated platelets secretes the substances in their dense bodies, α_1 and α_2 granules, in the order mentioned above by a mechanism that we will discuss later (Ulutin 1976). Increased secretion as well as increased adhesion and increased aggregation have also been demonstrated in platelets of patients with atherosclerosis. We have demonstrated this excessive secretion in our laboratories by measuring ADP, PF4, βTG, platelet fibrinogen and platelet α_2-antiplasmin (Ulutin 1976).

'Molecular markers' have recently been utilized to measure platelet activity, degradation and secretion (Fareed et al 1986) (Table 4.8).

One of our recent studies (Yardimci et al 1990) demonstrated that γ-glutamyl transferase (γ-GT) activity was 50.78 ± 3.37 u/10^8 platelets for normal control subjects whereas in platelets obtained from atherosclerotic subjects γ-GT activity values decreased to 24.78 ± 3.98 u/10^8 platelets. This difference was highly significant. On the other hand glutathione levels were found to be 12.24 ± 1.28 μg/10^9 platelets and 11.94 ± 1.8 μg/10^9 platelets for normal and atherosclerotic subjects. The difference was not significant. These findings need further study and interpretation.

As observed in the tables, increased adhesion, increased aggregation and increased secretion constitute the main alterations in platelets of atherosclerotic patients. As we will discuss further this increase in activity shows that platelets play a very important role in the pathogenesis and progression of atherosclerosis and in the formation of thrombosis. Some of the substances stored in the granules of platelets play a direct role in these

Table 4.8 The plasma levels of molecular markers of platelets in plasma in normal controls and in atherosclerosis with hypercoagulability. Determinations were done using Asserochrom-B-TG and PF-4 kits (results in IU/ml)

	Normal Control	Atherosclerosis	Significance
B-TG (N=20)	16.4 ± 9.1	82.6 ± 21.4	$p<0.001$
PF-4 (N=20)	4.2 ± 2.2	19.9 ± 8.6	$p<0.001$

pathological alterations. The laboratory finding of platelet-acquired storage pool disease observed in chronic DIC may also be seen in atherosclerosis. We had defined this condition as 'acquired storage pool deficiency' stating that a release reaction ensues in the circulation (Ulutin & Ulutin 1975).

Some alterations in the substances stored in the granules of platelets have also been observed in these cases. It has been shown that the level of AT-III, which is stored in platelets and is secreted when the platelets are stimulated, is lower in cases with atherosclerosis (Aktulga & Ulutin 1977a, Ulutin & Gürsoy 1983). This might be one of the reasons for the increased aggregation with small amounts of thrombin. We have also demonstrated in our laboratory that α_2-antiplasmin, which is a releasable substance stored in the α-granules of the platelet, is significantly increased compared to normal (Balkuv-Ulutin & Latallo 1980). The demonstration of PAI in platelets has opened a new dimension in this subject. Increased levels of this substance is one reason that the clot in atherosclerotic patients is resistant to lysis.

It is known that the level of cyclic AMP decreases when the platelets are stimulated. We have demonstrated that there is a decrease in intact circulating platelets (Yardimci et al 1979). This is evidence in support of the fact that platelets circulate in the active form.

There are various alterations in the prostanoid metabolism in the platelets of atherosclerotic patients. A number of studies have revealed that the distribution and the amount of phospholipids in the platelet membrane vary (Aktulga & Ulutin 1977b, 1979, Hoak 1988). In our own study the amount of total membrane phospholipids was found to be increased, but each phospholipid was increased at a different rate. After induction of release by ADP and collagen, the order of phospholipids available was also altered in atherosclerosis. Discrepant results were obtained with different release inducers (Aktulga & Ulutin 1977b, 1979). New experiments are needed to explain these findings.

It has been demonstrated that the synthesis of $PGF_{2\alpha}$, PGE_2, malondialdehyde (MDA) and TXA_2 is a significantly increased compared to normal after induction with collagen and ADP (Ulutin 1986b, Ulutin & Cizmeci 1985a) (Table 4.9). As we have mentioned above, this increase is

Table 4.9 The effect of collagen induction on $PGF_{2\alpha}$, PGE, MDA and TX-B$_2$ formation in platelets obtained from normal control subjects and from the cases of atherosclerosis with hypercoagulability

	TX-B$_2$ (pmol/ml)	MDA (n mol/3 × 10^8 platelets)	$PGF_{2\alpha}$ (pg/10^9 platelets)	PGE (pg/ml)
Control				
Before	1.20 ± 0.40	5.6	240.77 ± 16.1	2400 ± 600
After	1.35 ± 0.55	9.4	559.16 ± 89	5800 ± 950
Atherosclerosis				
Before	2.6 ± 1.6	12.6	355.1 ± 24	6300 ± 1200
After	5.9 ± 2.4	28.4	2764.39 ± 239	9200 ± 1800

seen together with a decrease in platelet cyclic AMP levels. It should be mentioned at this point that the platelet prostanoid metabolism is active in atherosclerotic cases and this has an important role in atherosclerosis and thromboembolism.

The importance of the roles of eicosanoid metabolism in atherosclerosis and thrombosis is becoming more important as the effect of eicosonoid metabolism on the EC and on platelets is recognized (Aktulga & Ulutin 1977b, 1979, Brook & Aviram 1988, Buchanan et al 1985, Sinzinger 1986, Stam et al 1989, Ulutin 1986b, Ulutin & Çizmeci 1985b, Willis & Smith 1989, Yardimci et al 1979).

The AA metabolites that are synthesized in platelets, TXA_2 and others, are pro-atherosclerotic and prethrombotic whereas the AA metabolite prostacyclin, which is synthesized in the EC, is not. Linoleate metabolites dihomo-γ-linoleic acid and eicosapentanoic acid, on the other hand, have opposite effects. The demonstration of increased amounts of AA metabolites after stimulation of platelets compared to normal subjects is important in relation to the atherosclerotic process as well as promoting the formation of thrombi.

Various studies have shown that an increase in plasma lipids and cholesterol results in an increase in platelet activity (Brook & Aviram 1988). An increase in platelet adhesion, aggregation and release, an increase in the plasma levels of PF-4 and βTG and especially an increase in the availability of PF3 are among the findings that are reported in such cases. Observations showed that lowering the level of plasma lipoprotein is concomitant with a decrease in platelet activity. It has been shown in in vitro studies that LDL and VLDL increase whereas HDL decreases platelet activity (Stam et al 1989, Willis & Smith 1989). The role of lipid peroxidation in atherogenesis is progressively gaining recognition. It has been demonstrated in aortic EC and SMC cultures that lipid peroxides inhibit EC proliferation whereas they stimulate SMC proliferation, a phenomenon that ultimately is atherogenic. Lipid peroxides, which are produced as a result of the peroxidation of unsaturated fatty acids, have been found in the wall of the aorta and have been found to be in a higher concentration in atherosclerotic cases. The lipid peroxides which are found in high concentrations in cases with ischaemic heart disease and POVD are progressively gaining importance. The subject is open to further study.

It was possible to observe additional changes in platelets of patients with atherosclerosis. Some alterations in the membrane transport systems of the platelets of atherosclerotic patients have been shown. The transport of [^{14}C]glucose through the platelet membrane has been found to be defective in atherosclerotic cases as depicted in the tables and figures. Depending on the severity and duration of the illness, it has been demonstrated that time-dependent and concentration-dependent transport is either decreased or blocked, although the degree of the impairment varies (Tables 4.10 and 4.11) (Ulutin 1986a, Yardimci 1980a, 1980b, Yardimci & Ulutin 1986). A defect in the transport of amino acids and galactose, in contrast, has not

Table 4.10   The timing of accumulation of [^{14}C]glucose by platelets of normals, atherosclerotic patients, adult type diabetes mellitus (DM) (type II) and juvenile diabetes mellitus (type I). Mean ± s.e.; N=case no.; results are expressed as nmol glucose/10^9 platelets)

	1 min	2 min	5 min	10 min	15 min	20 min
Normal (37°C) (N=22)	2.36±0.19	3.02±0.21	4.07±0.26	5.08±0.34	5.78±0.42	6.24±0.46
Normal (4°C) (N=10)	1.09±0.12	–	–	–	–	1.31±0.26
Atherosclerosis (37°C and 4°C) (N=26)	0.43±0.09	0.60±0.09	0.94±0.11	1.16±0.16	1.31±0.17	1.43±0.23
Adult type DM (37°C and 4°C) (N=12)	0.66±0.13	0.73±0.18	1.18±0.24	1.38±0.26	1.45±0.27	1.50±0.28
Juvenile DM (37°C) (N=4)	1.94±0.5	2.79±0.48	4.2±0.55	5.47±0.29	6.51±0.41	7.33±0.61

Table 4.11   The concentration dependence of [^{14}C]glucose transport in platelets of normals, atherosclerotic cases, adult type diabetes mellitus (DM) (type II) and juvenile diabetes mellitus (type I) cases. (mean ± s.e.; N=case no.; each case represents the average of three determinations; results are expressed as nmol/10^9 platelets/30 s)

	1×10^{-5} M glucose	2×10^{-5} M glucose	5×10^{-5} M glucose	10×10^{-5} M glucose	K_M 10^{-5} M	V_{max} nmol/10^9 platelets/30 s
37°C	3.71±0.42	5.61±0.54	9.33±0.85	13.36±1.27	–	–
4°C (N=8)	0.68±0.11	1.33±0.17	2.99±0.96	5.83±0.78	–	–
Normal net transport (active transport)	3.01±0.37	4.29±0.48	6.35±0.81	7.54±1.16	2.15±0.28	9.11±1.49
1/V (1/nmol/10^9 platelets/30 s) (37°C, 4°C)	0.38±0.08	0.26±0.05	0.18±0.03	0.15±0.023	–	–
Atherosclerosis (N=10) (37°C, 4°C)	0.36±0.09	0.67±0.16	1.43±0.29	2.72±0.59	–	–
Adult type DM (N=4)	0.47±0.10	0.98±0.21	2.27±0.48	4.68±0.91	–	–
37°C	5.0	6.2	9.3	11.5		
4°C	0.2	0.4	1.0	2.0	–	–
Juvenile DM net transport (active transport)	4.8	5.8	8.3	9.5	1.54	10.87
1/V 1/nmol/10^9 platelets/30 s	0.21	0.17	0.12	0.11	–	–

been observed (Emekli 1982, Emekli & Ulutin 1980, Yardimci 1980b). [^{14}C]Glucose normally binds to the protein peak when osmotic shock is produced and the supernatant is fractionated by chromatography, but it does not bind to a protein and stays as free glucose in atherosclerotic cases with impaired transport (Yardimci & Ulutin 1986). The absence of a binding protein (glucoprotein) for glucose, a molecular alteration and a plasmatic aetiology can be discussed at this point. We have obtained some data in one of our ongoing studies that favour a plasmatic origin for the defect (Göker et al 1988). The relationship of this blockage to plasma lipid alterations may be discussed.

The transport of [^{14}C]galactose to platelets has been found to be normal (Emekli 1982, Emekli & Ulutin 1980, Ulutin 1986b). The incorporation of galactose to protein, on the other hand, is significantly increased and some alterations on the membrane glucoprotein pattern have taken place compared to normal. Increases in GPIb and GPIIa have been demonstrated. These may explain at least partially the hyperaggregation observed in these cases.

In our laboratory, however, it has been shown in some of the in vitro studies that platelets obtained from atherosclerotic patients produce more lactate (Avanoğlu 1986) (Fig. 4.3) and that platelets of atherosclerotic patients contain less glycogen (Ünlüer et al 1986) (Fig. 4.4). The increase in glycogenolysis and glyconeogenesis in this case is open to discussion.

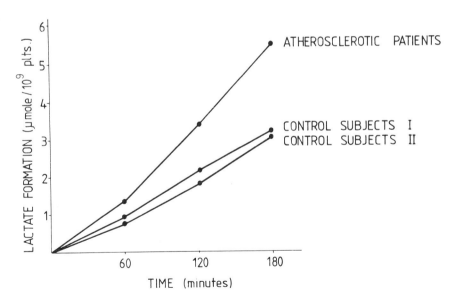

Fig. 4.3 Lactate formation in the resting platelets of normal and atherosclerotic subjects at 37°C. Lactate formation was time dependently increased in platelets of normal and atherosclerotic subjects. Lactate formation in resting platelets of atherosclerotic patients was more than that in resting platelets of control groups. The difference was statistically significant ($P<0.001$) (Avanoğlu 1986).

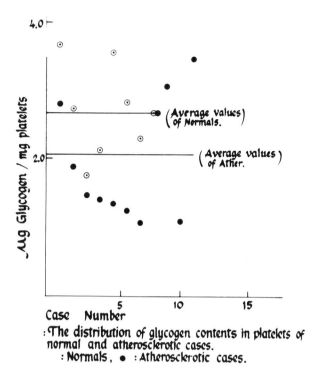

Fig. 4.4   The distribution of glycogen contents in platelets of normal and atherosclerotic cases. ⊙ Normal, ● Atherosclerotic cases.

Young familial members

It is an interesting finding that some of the defects presented above are present in some of the young members of atherosclerotic families although no clinical and classical laboratory alterations were found in these young cases . No specific clinical findings were observed; fundoscopic examinations and serum lipid levels and distribution were within normal limits.

Findings such as reduced EC functions and an increase in platelet activity were observed and they varied from subject to subject. These are most commonly seen in mothers and fathers whose families have complications of atherosclerosis and thromboembolism. Marriages within families are frequently observed in some areas of Turkey and the findings mentioned above are seen in some of the young members of these families. We will publish the results of this ongoing study in the future. Further studies are required to evaluate this ongoing study and to delineate the character of the genetic defect. The preliminary studies suggest that the primary marker is impairment of function of the EC in these young members.

CONCLUSIONS

Our studies and previous published findings suggest that the phenomenon is a modern combination of the hypothesis of Rokitansky and Virchow. I would wish to exclude from this debate lipid alterations as these have been extensively studied in published work.

The concept proposed by Von Rokitansky in 1841 that atherosclerosis is caused by the incorporation of mural thrombi into the vascular wall was reinforced in 1946 by the findings of Duguid that supported further those of Rokitansky. The further demonstration of fibrin and platelet products in the vascular wall and the progression of mural thrombi into atherosclerotic plaques have reinforced these concepts (Woolf 1987).

The relationship between the EC, platelet, SMC and monocyte/histiocyte revealed by experimental EC injury, supports Virchow's tissue response theory. Recent studies provide added support for the EC injury theory. As we will discuss below, new findings embrace both Rokitansky's and Virchow's point of view, and support the role of EC injury.

In order to discuss a working hypothesis we will summarize the development of atherosclerosis as follows. The primary defect in the first stage is EC dysfunction. EC shows defective resistance to endothelial injury because of a genetic defect. Sensitivity of endothelial cells to injury could be the primary alteration in this disease of the vessel wall. Genetic factors may lower the resistance of EC to injury or, as we have mentioned above, EC hypo-dysfunction may be the basis for this sensitivity. The genetic defect should be defined at the molecular level. This genetically sensitive EC may be injured by risk factors such as high fat intake, hypertension, smoking, toxins, viraemia, immunological causes, mechanical causes, activated leucocytes, etc.: events in which the EC lining is very easily injured.

Independent of genetics as a primary origin of the sensitivity to injury of ECs, the primary event is a progressive decrease in the amounts of various substances synthesized by the EC. The main event is a decrease in the production of t-PA and an increase in PAI, and a state of unresponsiveness or diminished response to stimuli that eventually leads to reduced fibrinolysis. The synthesis of proteoglycans decreases and the proteoglycan layer that is situated in the inner side is not able to maintain its continuity.

Prostacyclin synthesis progressively decreases. This in turn leads to the disappearance of the antiplatelet action of EC. Platelets begin to activate. There are new findings that state that the amount of PDRF (NO, nitric oxide), which is a substance that has a vasodilator and antiplatelet effect, decreases in atherosclerotic patients. Platelets eventually adhere to the surface of the EC which shows hypo-dysfunction. Some ECs become denuded and in some areas the subendothelium contacts the circulation.

Thirdly, platelets activate and adhere to the subendothelium and blood is exposed to the denuded area.

The activated prostanoid metabolism, increased synthesis of AA metabolites and increased formation of TXA_2 with a concomitant decrease in cyclic AMP increase the process of secretion in this case from the granules of platelets. Among the secreted substances fibronectin facilitates adhesion, PF-4 has an antiheparin effect, PDGF (SMPF) stimulates smooth muscle hyperplasia/hypertrophy and chemotactic factor stimulates the migration of smooth muscle to the intima.

Fourthly, SMGF (PDGE) which is released from the granules of platelets causes proliferation of SMC, which have a diminished inhibition because of decrease of heparin, and migration towards the intima ensues following the effect of a chemotactic substance derived from platelets. A haemostatic substance that is released by SMC that migrate towards the intima causes the migration of monocytes to the intima. The monocytes that reach the intima are transformed into tissue histiocytes which have phagocytic activity and into foam cells. The hypertrophied SMC form the connective tissue matrix and synthesize collagen and elastin fibres. In the hypoxic area fatty degeneration occurs. Calcium precipitates and plaques of atheroma are formed. Patchy lipid deposition into hypertrophied SMCs and into newly formed connective tissue takes place which is further followed by the formation of atheroma.

Fifthly, a monolayer EC is not present in the region of atheroma and platelets adhere to this surface. Platelets which circulate in the hyperactive state in these cases easily produce the mural platelet thrombosis. The slightest additional activation leads to thrombosis in these cases who have already reached the prethrombotic stage because of hypercoagulability, reduced fibrinolytic activity and decreased activity of natural anticoagulants. We believe that smoking, hypertension, diabetes mellitus, increase in cholesterol and lipids, abnormal lipoprotein metabolism, viral agents, immunological agents, etc., are risk factors rather than causative factors and that they extend EC injury and accelerate and extend the disease process.

THERAPEUTIC PRINCIPLES

Numerous experiments are being performed and published on the classical aspects of the treatment of atherosclerosis, which include lowering the high lipid concentrations by drugs and/or diet, discouraging smoking, controlling hypertension and lowering the other risk factors. The therapy that we discuss relates to the haemostatic mechanism and can be divided into four categories.

1. Oral anticoagulant treatment does not have a role in this disease except for thromboembolic complications. On the other hand, heparin therapy has gained importance after it was demonstrated that heparin prevents smooth muscle hyperplasia (Cloves & Karnovsky 1977). Low-molecular-weight heparin produces

fibrinolytic activity by increasing t-PA and decreasing PAI (Balkuv-Ulutin et al 1989).

2. The importance of antiplatelet therapy becomes more prominent when the role of the substances that are secreted from the platelets on the formation of atherosclerosis and on thromboembolism are taken into account. Platelets have a stimulating effect in atherosclerosis and thromboembolism because of their increased adhesion, aggregation and especially secretion. Secreted substances such as antiheparin factor (PF-4), SMPF (mitogen growth factor), chemotactic factor against smooth muscle, etc., are substances that have a pathogenic effect in atherosclerosis. The role of these drugs may be beneficial even from a hypothetical point of view because secretion, adhesion and aggregation are inhibited and the platelet surface reaction is modified (Buchanan 1988, Harker 1986, Ulutin et al 1975).

3. Fibrinolytic therapy: this therapeutic regimen has become conventional in treating thrombosis but should be evaluated further because fibrinolytic activity decreases in atherosclerotic patients, and it has been shown that the decrease of fibrinolytic activity causes vascular wall injury in animal experiments (Balkuv-Ulutin et al 1981, Deutsch 1965, Hosgör et al 1989, Kwaan 1979).

4. Endothelium modulating and supporting treatment: therapy which improves the function of the EC has begun to gain acceptance. This group of substances, which increase the level of proteoglycans, increase t-PA, decrease PAI, increase the synthesis and release of PGI_2 and decrease EC injury and re-endothelialization, are promising (Balkuv-Ulutin et al 1989, Ulutin et al 1986). Metformine and defibrotide are included in this category (Ulutin 1988, Ulutin et al 1986).

SUMMARY

In this short review the findings concerning the haemostatic mechanism observed in atherosclerotic patients are summarized. We stress that fact that some of these changes are observed in young members of atherosclerosis families. We discuss a working hypothesis that is derived from these observations and state that the EC dysfunction seen in the earliest stages and the possible genetic defect are factors that are related to this stage. We briefly discuss therapeutic principles derived from the alterations of the haemostatic system and the EC.

REFERENCES

Aktulga A Z, Ulutin O N 1977a Platelet antithrombin III in atherosclerosis. Thromb Haemostasis 38: 275

Aktulga A Z, Ulutin O N 1977b Platelet phospholipid changes in atherosclerosis. Thromb Haemostasis 38: 32

Aktulga A Z, Ulutin O N 1979 Platelet phospholipids in atherosclerotics and in normals before and after release. In: Neri Serneri G G, Prentice C R M (eds) Haemostasis and thrombosis. Academic Press, London, pp 677–683

Avanoglu Y 1986 The alteration of glucose utilization and lactate formation of platelets in cases of atherosclerosis. In: Ulutin O N, Vinazzer H (eds) Thrombosis and haemorrhagic diseases. Gözlem, Istanbul, pp 417–424

Balkuv-Ulutin S 1986 Fibrinolytic system in atherosclerosis. Semin Thromb Haemostasis 12: 91–101

Balkuv-Ulutin S 1978 Physiological response to enhanced fibrinolytic activity. In: Gaffney P J, Balkuv-Ulutin S (eds) Fibrinolysis: current fundamental and clinical concepts. Academic Press, London, pp 27–36

Balkuv-Ulutin S, Latallo S Z 1980 Determination of the platelets antiplasmin with chromogenic substrate (S-2251) and comparison of the values obtained from atherosclerotics and from normals (Abst. 382). VIth Internat. Congr. Thrombosis, Monte-Carlo.

Balkuv-Ulutin S Girisken G, Tunali H, Uruluer S, Yigitbasi Ö, Toulemond F 1981 Fibrinolytic treatment of experimental thrombosis with and without plasminogen prior to vasoactive agents. In: Ulutin O, Berkarda B (eds) Proc. 1981 International Symposia on Haematology, New Istanbul Contrib Clin Sci 13(suppl. 2): 109–121

Balkuv-Ulutin S, Ulutin T, Özsoy Y, Toulemond F, Ulutin O N 1989 The effect of LMW (CY 222) and unfractionated heparins on the fibrinolytic activity and on platelet functions. VIth Meeting of Danubian League against Thrombosis and Haemorrhagic Disorders, May 31–June 3, Vienna, p 28

Berkarda B, Akogan G, Urgancioglu I 1968 A comparative study on the fibrinogen and thrombocyte. Haseki Tip Bull (Istanbul) 6: 135–141

Bizzozero J 1882 Über einen neuen Formbestandtheil des Blutes und dessen Rolle bei der Thrombose und der Blutgerinnung. Virchow's Arch Pathol Anat Physiol Klin Med 90: 261–332

Botting R, Vane J R 1989 The receipt and dispatch of chemical messengers by endothelial cells. In: Schrör K, Sinzinger H (eds) Prostaglandins in clinical research: cardiovascular system. Liss, New York pp 1–11

Brook J G, Aviram M 1988 Platelet lipoprotein interactions. Semin Thromb Haemostasis 14: 258–265

Buchanan M B 1988 Mechanism of pathogenesis of arterial thrombosis: potential sites of inhibition by therapeutic compounds. Semin Thromb Haemostasis 14: 33–40

Buchanan M R, Butt R W, Magas Z, Van Ryn J, Hirsh J, Nazir D 1985 Endothelial cells produce a lipoxygenase-derived chemorepellent which influences platelet endothelial cell interactions: aspirin and salicylate. Thromb Haemostasis 53: 306–311

Buonassi V 1973 Sulfated mucopolysaccharides synthesis and secretion in endothelial cell culture. Exp Cell Res 76: 363–388

Castellot J J Jr, Wright T C, Karnovsky M J 1987 Regulation of vascular smooth muscle cell growth by heparin and heparan sulfates. Semin Thromb Haemostasis 13: 489–503

Cloves A W, Karnovsky M J 1977 Suppression by heparin of smooth muscle cell proliferation in injured arteries. Nature 265: 625–626

Collen D, Juhan-Vague I 1988 Fibrinolysis and atherosclerosis. Semin Thromb Haemostasis 14: 180–183

Dembinska-Kieć A, Gryglewski R J 1986 Contribution of arachidonic acid metabolites to atherosclerosis. Wienes Klin Wochenschr 98: 198–206

Deutsch E 1965 Discussion on atherosclerosis. In: Garan R, Ulutin O N (eds) Thrombosis and anticoagulants, Sermet Matbaasi, Istanbul, p 128

Duguid J B 1946 Thrombosis as a factor in the pathogenesis of coronary atherosclerosis. J Pathol Bacteriol 58: 207

Emekli N B 1982 Galactose transport and glycoprotein changes in the platelets of atherosclerotics. In: Ulutin O N, Berkarda B (eds) Proceedings of the 1981 Symposium on Haematology. Sermet Matbaasi, Vize-Kirklareli, pp 89–101

Emekli N B, Ulutin O N 1980 ^{14}C-galactose transport in human platelets. VI Internat Congr on Thrombosis of Mediterranean League Against Thromboembolic Diseases, Monaco (Abs. 270)

Engelberg H 1988 Update on the relationship of heparin to atherosclerosis and its thrombotic complications. Semin Thromb Haemostasis 14: 88–105

Fair D S, Marlar R A, Levin E G 1986 Human endothelial cells synthesize protein S. Blood 67: 1168–1171

Fareed J, Walenga J M, Baker W H, Hayes A, Hoppenstendt D A 1986 Molecular markers of haemostatic activation in atherosclerosis: a new concept in diagnostic profiling of endogeneous pathophysiologic transition. Semin Thromb Haemostasis 12: 102–109

Föstermann U, Mugge A, Alheid U, Haverich A, Frolich J C 1988 Selective attenuation of endothelium-mediated vasodilation in atherosclerotic human coronary arteries. Circ Res 62: 185–190

Gerrity R G 1981 The role of the monocyte in atherogenesis. I. Transition of blood-borne monocytes into foam cells in fatty lesions. Am J Pathol 103: 181–190

Gianturco S H, Bradley W A 1988 Lipoprotein-mediated cellular mechanisms for atherogenesis in hypertriglyceridemia. Semin Thromb Haemostasis 14: 165–169

Göker B, Yardimci T, Ulutin O N 1988 Defibrotide' in trombositlerin ^{14}C-glucose transportuna etkisi. XX. Ulusal Haematol Kongresi, Ankara University Press, Ankara, p 56

Goodnight S H Jr 1988 Effects of dietary fish oil and omega-3 fatty acids on platelets and blood vessels. Semin Thromb Haemostasis 14: 285–289

Guyton J R, Rosenberg R D, Cloves A W, Karnovsky M J 1980 Inhibition of rat arterial smooth muscle cell proliferation by heparin. I. In vivo studies with anticoagulant. Circ Res 46: 625–634

Harker L A 1986 Antiplatelet drugs in the management of patients with thrombotic disorders. Semin Thromb Haemostasis 12: 134–155

Harlan J M 1985 Leucocyte–endothelial interactions. Blood 65: 513–525

Harlan J M 1987 Consequences of leucocyte–vessel wall interactions in inflammatory and immune reactions. Semin Thromb Haemostasis 13: 434–444

Hoak J C 1988 Platelets and atherosclerosis. Semin Thromb Haemostasis 14: 202–205

Hoover R L, Rosenberg R D, Haernig W, Karnowsky M J 1980 Inhibition of rat arterial smooth muscle cell proliferation by heparin. II. In vitro studies. Circ Res 47: 578–583

Hosgör I, Yilmazer S, Girisken G, Satiroglu G, Karadayi N, Balkuv-Ulutin S 1989 The morphological alteration of myocardial coronary vessels after the application of tranexamic acid in cats. Proc VIth Meeting Danubian League against Thrombosis and Haemorrhagic Disorders, May 31–June 3, 1989 Vienna

Huber K, Rose D, Resch I et al 1988 Circadian fluctuation of plasminogen activator inhibitor and tissue plasminogen activator levels in plasma of patients with unstable coronary artery disease and acute myocardial infarction. Thromb Haemostasis 60: 372–376

Jauchem J R, Lopez M, Sprague E A, Schwartz C I 1982 Mononuclear cell chemoattractant activity from cultured arterial smooth muscle cells. Exp Mol Pathol 37: 166–174

Jonasson L, Holm J, Skalli O, Bandjers G, Hansson G K 1986 Regional accumulations of T cells, macrophages, and smooth muscle cells in the human atherosclerotic plaque. Arteriosclerosis 6: 131–138

Juhan-Vague I, Moerman B, De Cock F, Aillaud M F, Collen D 1984 Plasma levels of a specific inhibitor of tissue-type plasminogen activator (and urokinase) in normal and pathological conditions. Thromb Res 33: 523–530

Juhan-Vague I, Valadier J, Alessi M J et al 1987 Deficient t-PA release and elevated PA inhibitor levels in patients with spontaneous or recurrent deep venous thrombosis. Thromb Haemostasis 57: 67–72

Karnovsky M J, Wright T C Jr, Castellot J J Jr, Choay J, Lormeau J C, Petitou M 1989 Heparin, heparan sulfate, smooth muscle cells and atherosclerosis. Ann N Y Acad Sci 556: 268–281

Kwaan H C 1979 Physiologic and pharmacologic implications of fibrinolysis. Artery 5: 285–291

Lucchesi B R 1987 Role of neutrophils in ischemic heart disease, pathophysiologic role in myocardial ischemia and coronary artery reperfusions. In: Mehta J L (ed) Thrombosis and platelets in myocardial ischaemia. Davis, Philadelphia, pp 35–48

Marcum J A, Rosenberg D A 1985 Heparin-like molecules with anticoagulant activity are synthesized by cultured endothelial cell. Biochem Biophys Res Commun 126: 365–372

Marcum J A, Atha D H, Fritze D S M, Nawroth P, Stern D, Rosenberg R D 1986 Cloned bovine aortic endothelial cells synthesize anticoagulant active heparan sulfate proteoglycan. J Biol Chem 261: 7507–7517

Matzner Y, Bar-Ner N, Yahalom J, Ishai-Michaeli R, Fuks Z, Vladavsky I 1985 Degradation of heparan sulfate in the subendothelial extracellular matrix by a readily released heparanase from human neutrophils. J Clin Invest 76: 1306–1313

McMillan G C 1985 Nature and definitions of atherosclerosis. Ann N Y Acad Sci 454: 1–4

Mehta J L 1987 Thrombosis and platelets in myocardial ischemia. Davis, Philadelphia

Nievelstein P F E M, Houdijk W P M, Sakariassen K S, DeGroot P G, Sixma J J 1985 The role of fibronectin for platelet deposition on purified vessel wall component. Thromb Haemostasis 54: 230

Nilsson I M, Ljugner H, Tengborn L 1985 Two different mechanisms in patients with venous thrombosis and defective fibrinolysis: low concentration of plasminogen activator or increased concentration of plasminogen activator inhibitor. Br Med J 290: 1453–1459

Norden C, Jermolin G A, Reimann H et al 1989 Impaired fibrinolysis characterizes the state of thrombophilia on extent of arteriosclerotic lesion. Thromb Haemostasis 62: 228 (Abst 706)

Özer A F, Pamir M N, Erbengi T, Iplikcoioğlu A 1989 Inhibited fibrinolytic activity and cerebral arterial vasospasm: an experimental electronmicroscopic study. 9th Internat Congr Neurological Surgery, Oct 8–13, New Delhi (Abst 203048)

Pangrazzi J, Gianase F 1987 Dermatan sulfate as a potential antithrombotic drug. Haematologica 75: 459–464

Radomski M W, Palmer R M J, Moncada S 1988 Endogenous nitric acid inhibits human platelet adhesion to vascular endothelium. Lancet 2: 1057–1058

Rak K, Hàrsfalvi J, Tornai I, Boda Z 1986 Increased plasmatic level of Willebrand factor protein: its clinical significance. In: Ulutin O N, Vinazzer H (eds) Thrombosis and hemorrhagic diseases. Gözlem, Istanbul, pp 74–82

Rebuck J W, Riddle J M, Brown M G, Johnson S A, Monto R W 1961 Volumetric and ultrastructural studies of abnormal platelets. In: Johnson S A, Monto R W, Rebuck J W, Horn R C (eds) Blood platelets. Little, Brown & Co, Boston, pp 533–552

Ross R 1986 The pathogenesis of atherosclerosis: an update. N Engl J Med 314: 488–500

Schwartz C J, Valente A J, Sprague E A et al 1986 Monocyte–macrophage participation in atherogenesis: inflammatory component of pathogenesis. Semin Thromb Haemostasis 12: 79–86

Schwartz C J, Valente A J, Kelley J L, Sprague E A 1988 Thrombosis and the development of atherosclerosis: Rokitansky revisited. Semin Thromb Haemostasis 14: 189–195

Sinzinger H 1986 Role of platelets in atherosclerosis. Semin Thromb Haemostasis 12: 124–133

Sinzinger H, Widhalm K 1981 Atherosclerose seit der zeit der Pharaonen. Österreich Arztezeitung 20: 1

Sloan I G, Firkin B C 1989 Impaired fibrinolysis in patients with thrombotic or hemostatic defects. Thromb Res 55: 559–567

Sprengers E D, Kluft C 1987 Plasminogen activator inhibitors. Blood 69: 381–387

Stam H, Hülsmann W C, Jangkind J F, van der Kraaig A M M, Koster J F 1989 Endothelial lesions, dietary: composition and lipid peroxidation. Eucosanoid 3: 1–14

Stern D M, Brett J, Harris K, Nawroth P P 1986 Participation of endothelial cells in the protein C and S anticoagulant pathway: synthesis and release of protein S. J Cell Biol 102: 1971–1978

Stringer M D, Görog P G, Freeman A, Kakkar V V 1989a Lipid peroxides in atherosclerosis (Abst 1568). Thromb Haemostasis 62: 500

Stringer M D, Görög P G, Kakkar V V 1989b Atherogenic effects of lipid peroxides on cultured aortic endothelial and smooth muscle cells (Abst 421). Thromb Haemostasis 62: 132

Takahashi H, Tsuda A, Tatewaki W, Wada K, Niwano H, Shibata A 1989 Activation of blood coagulation and fibrinolysis in diabetes mellitus: evaluation by plasma levels of thrombin–antithrombin III. Complex and plasmin alpha 2–plasmin inhibitor complex. Thromb Res 55: 727–735

Teitel J M, Bayer K A, Lau H K, Rosenberg R D 1982 Studies of the prothrombin activation pathway utilizing radioimmunoassay for the F_1/F_{1+2} fragment and thrombin–antithrombin complex. Blood 59: 1348–1352

Tiozzo R, Cingi M R, Pietrangelo A, Albertazzi L, Calandra S, Milani M R 1989 Effect of heparin like compounds on the in vitro proliferation and protein synthesis of various cell types. Arzneim-Forsch/Drug Res 39: 15–20

Tschopp T B, Baumgartner H R, Silberbauer K, Sinzinger H 1979 Platelet adhesion and platelet thrombus formation on subendothelium of human arteries and veins exposed to following blood in vitro: a comparison with rabbit aorta. Haemostasis 8: 19–29

Ulutin O N 1976 The platelets: fundamentals and clinical applications. Kaḡit ve Basim Isleri AS, Istanbul

Ulutin O N 1986a Introductory historical remarks on atherosclerosis and haemostasis. Semin Thromb Haemostasis 12: 77–78

Ulutin O N 1986b Atherosclerosis and haemostasis. Semin Thromb Hemostasis 12: 156–174

Ulutin O N 1988 Clinical effectiveness of defibrotide in vaso-occlusive disorders and its mode of actions. Semin Thromb Hemostasis 14: 58–63

Ulutin O N 1989 The clinical and pharmacological results during defibrotide treatment of peripheric obliterative vascular diseases. In: Strano A, Novo S (eds) Advances in vascular pathology 1989, Vol 3. Excerpta Medica, Amsterdam pp 9–13

Ulutin S B, Ulutin O N 1969 A study on the platelet antiplasmin activity in atherosclerotics and normal people. Vth Congr Asian-Pacific Soc Haematology, Istanbul (Abst 162)

Ulutin O N, Ulutin S B 1975 Acquired storage pool deficiency in chronic disseminated intravascular coagulation. In: Ulutin O N (ed) Platelets: recent advances in basic research and clinical aspects. Excerpta Medica, Amsterdam pp 329–333

Ulutin O N, Gürsoy A 1983 Platelet antithrombin III in normal persons and in atherosclerotics. Ann Univ Sarav Med (suppl 3): 149–150

Ulutin O N, Cizmeci G 1985a Alteration of prostanoids in atherosclerosis. Semin Thromb Hemostasis 11: 362–368

Ulutin O N, Cizmeci G 1985b Alteration of prostanoids in atherosclerosis. Semin Thromb Hemostasis 11: 362–366

Ulutin O N, Tunali H, Uḡur M S, Ayti S, Erbengi T, Balkuv-Ulutin S 1986 Effect of defibrotide in electrically induced thrombosis in dogs. Haemostasis 16(suppl 1): 9–12

Ulutin S B, Aktulga A, Aktuḡlu G et al 1975 Observations on the effects of antiaggregating drugs on platelet function. In: Ulutin O N (ed) Platelets: recent advances in basic research and clinical aspects. Excerpta Medica, Amsterdam pp 282–291

Ünlüer A, Avanoḡlu Y, Erdaḡ A, Yardimci T 1986 Glycogen levels in the platelets of normal and atherosclerotic cases. In: Ulutin O N, Vinazzer H (eds) Thrombosis and Hemorrhagic Diseases. Gözlem, Istanbul pp 425–428

Vague P, Juhan-Vague I, Alessi M C et al 1987 Metformin decreases the elevated levels of plasminogen activator inhibitor, plasma insulin and tryglyceride in non-diabetic obese subjects. Thromb Haemostasis 57: 326

Virchow R 1856 Phlogose und Thrombose in Gefässystem. Gesammelte Abhandlungen zur Wissenschaftlichen Medizin, Meidinger, Frankfurt/Main, pp 458–463

Von Rokitansky K 1841 Handbuch der Pathologischen: Anatomie. Braunmuller & Seidel, Berlin

Walsh R T, Bauer R B, Barnhart M I 1975 Platelet function in transient ischaemia and cerebrovascular disease: effect of aspirin and contrast media. In: Ulutin O N (ed) Platelets: recent advances in basic research and clinical aspects. Excerpta Medica, Amsterdam pp 367–377

Whatley R E, Zimmerman G A, McIntyre T M, Taylor R, Prescott S M 1987 Productions of platelet-activating factor by endothelial cells. Semin Thromb Hemostasis 13: 445–453

Willis A L, Smith D L 1989 Eicosanoid aspects of atherosclerosis. In: Schrör K, Sinzinger H (eds) Prostaglandins in clinical research. Liss, New York, pp 73–84

Woolf N 1987 Thrombosis and atherosclerosis. In: Bloom A L, Thomas D P (eds) Haemostasis and thrombosis, 2nd edn. Churchill Livingstone, Edinburgh pp 651–678

Yanagisawa M, Kurihara H, Kimura S et al 1988 A novel potent vasoconstrictor peptide produced by vascular endothelial cells. Nature 332: 411–415

Yardimci T U 1980a Membrane transport systems in human platelets. Haematologica 65: 498–508

Yardimci T U 1980b The effect of osmotic shock on platelet membrane transport. Haematologica 65: 516–522

Yardimci, T U, Ulutin O N 1986 Alteration of platelet glucose transport system in atherosclerosis. Wiener Klin Wochenschr 98: 221–224

Yardimci T, Emekli N, Uğur M S, Ulutin O N 1979 c-AMP and c-GMP levels in the platelets of atherosclerosis and normal controls. IVth Meeting of the Asian-Pacific Division of ISH, Seoul, Korea

Yardimci T, Yaman A, Ulutin O N 1990 γ-Glutamyl transferase and glutathione levels in the platelets of normal and atherosclerotic subjects. 11th Internat Congr Thromb L jubljana, Yugoslavia, June 24–28

5

Molecular biology in blood coagulation

J.H. McVey   J.K. Pattinson   E.G.D. Tuddenham

The development of molecular biological techniques over the past two decades has made an enormous impact on medical research. In the field of blood coagulation it has allowed the molecular cloning and the sequencing of the genes encoding all the components of the intrinsic pathways of blood coagulation. The deduced primary structure of these proteins has aided our understanding of their cleavage and activation although a full understanding of the tertiary structure and function of these molecules is some way off (for review see Tuddenham 1989). Equally important, the cloning of these genes has provided us with probes to analyse the genetic defect(s) in patients with bleeding disorders. These gene-specific probes and polymorphic probes tightly linked to the disease locus have allowed us to offer carrier diagnosis to families at risk of having an affected baby (Gitschier et al 1985c, Antonarakis et al 1985b). However, because of the technical difficulties involved many laboratories have avoided the use of DNA analysis and it still remains a very specialized area.

The recent development of the polymerase chain reaction (PCR) (Saiki et al 1985, 1986, 1988, Scharf et al 1986, Mullis & Falcona 1987, Erlich et al 1988), although not as fundamentally important as the techniques for cloning and sequencing DNA, is clearly one of the most substantial advances in molecular genetics in the past decade. The procedure allows the amplification of a defined segment of DNA more than a million-fold in only a few hours from relatively impure DNA. This ability to amplify allows the analysis of DNA in fixed pathological specimens (Shibata et al 1988a, 1988b, Ipraim et al 1987), buccal cells from mouthwashes (Lench et al 1988), human hairs (Lench et al 1988, Higuchi et al 1988), and even single cells from various sources (viz. lymphoid, Crescenzi et al 1988, Jeffreys et al 1988; tissue culture, Li et al 1988; human embryo, Handyside et al 1989; oocyte, Coutelle et al 1989; or sperm, Li et al 1988) which would have been impossible using standard DNA cloning methods.

The polymerase chain reaction method is based on the repetitive cycling of three simple reactions differing only in their incubation temperature. All three reactions occur in the same tube and the repetitive cycling can therefore be fully automated. In addition to the target DNA to be amplified, the necessary reagents are simply the following: two single-stranded synthetic oligonucleotides (primers) complementary to the boundaries of the target sequence, an excess of the four deoxynucleotide triphosphates, and a thermostable DNA polymerase isolated from the thermophilic bacterium *Thermus aquaticus*.

The first step in the procedure (Fig. 5.1) is the heat denaturation of native double-stranded DNA. The resultant single-stranded DNA can then anneal to the excess of single-stranded primers in those regions containing complementary sequences. One of the advantages of the PCR technique is that the target DNA does not need to be particularly pure or plentiful; it can be a minor species in a complex mixture of other DNA species.

The second step in the procedure is the annealing of the primers to the denatured DNA; this occurs at a lower temperature. The primers define the two ends of the DNA segment to be amplified and represent sequences on opposite strands of the DNA. The specificity of the PCR method is defined by the precision of this annealing step.

The third step in the procedure is the synthesis of a complementary strand of DNA extending from the 3'- end of the oligonucleotide primers. A new strand of DNA is synthesized from each annealed primer and each newly synthesized strand of DNA can serve as a template in the next round of the cycle. The result is the logarithmic amplification of new DNA products.

After extension of the primers the cycle is repeated, firstly raising the temperature to denature all the double stranded DNA, secondly lowering the temperature to allow the primers to anneal and thirdly allowing the extension of the newly annealed primers. After the completion of n cycles the defined segment of DNA would theoretically have been amplified by 2^n, and will be so abundant that it will appear to be the only detectable DNA in the reaction mixture. Typically the reaction undergoes 30 cycles which are completed in only a few hours. If necessary, the amplified segment of DNA can then be further analysed by more conventional molecular biology techniques, although in some cases the presence or absence of an amplified segment is sufficient.

The power of the PCR technique lies in its extraordinary sensitivity, its ability to amplify segments from crude samples, its suitability for automation, and its speed. The sensitivity of the technique also eliminates the need in most cases to use radiolabelling for detection.

However, the extraordinary sensitivity of the technique is also one of its greatest problems. False positive amplifications from carry-over of previously amplified DNA or from cloned DNA, which may be present in the laboratory in milligram quantities, do occur. Laboratories must therefore take particular care to avoid these artefacts by the use of positive and negative controls, physical separation of the PCR preparation and amplification from the analysis of the PCR and from all cloned DNAs and the use of positive displacement pipettes to reduce cross-contamination (Kwok & Higuchi 1989).

Reagents

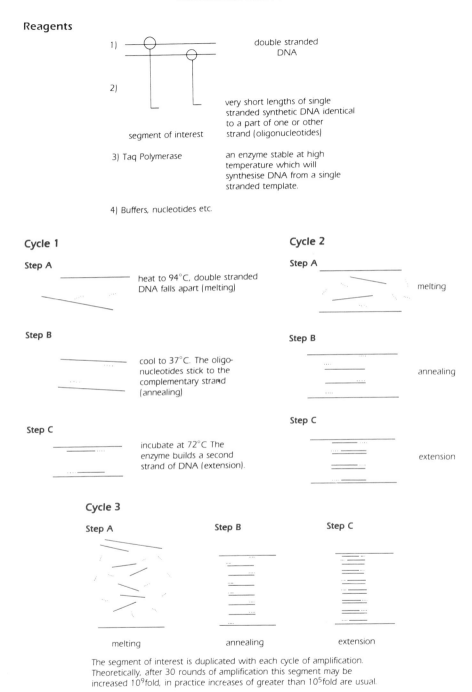

1)   double stranded
                                            DNA

2)

                                            very short lengths of single
                                            stranded synthetic DNA identical
                                            to a part of one or other
segment of interest   strand (oligonucleotides)

3) Taq Polymerase   an enzyme stable at high
                                            temperature which will
                                            synthesise DNA from a single
                                            stranded template.

4) Buffers, nucleotides etc.

Cycle 1   **Cycle 2**

Step A   **Step A**

            heat to 94°C, double stranded   melting
            DNA falls apart (melting)

Step B   **Step B**

            cool to 37°C. The oligo-   annealing
            nucleotides stick to the
            complementary strand
            (annealing)

                                            Step C

Step C

            incubate at 72°C The   extension
            enzyme builds a second
            strand of DNA (extension).

Cycle 3

Step A   **Step B**   **Step C**

        melting   annealing   extension

The segment of interest is duplicated with each cycle of amplification.
Theoretically, after 30 rounds of amplification this segment may be
increased 10^9fold, in practice increases of greater than 10^5fold are usual.

Fig. 5.1 A schematic representation of the polymerase chain reaction.

The technique of PCR is potentially useful in any situation that requires DNA analysis. However, its principal application in medicine will be mostly as a diagnostic tool, to answer the question: does a given sequence of DNA exist in a given clinical specimen? (for review see Eisenstein 1990).

We will illustrate the power of the PCR technique in the field of blood coagulation by describing how it has been used in the study of haemophilia A. We will also outline some of the exciting prospects which this technique holds for the future.

CARRIER DIAGNOSIS

Currently carrier diagnosis of haemophilia A is performed by using intragenic polymorphic DNA sequences. These polymorphisms involve recognition sites for the restriction enzymes BclI (Gitschier et al 1985b), BglI (Antonarakis et al 1985a) and XbaI (Wion et al 1986); the presence or absence of the sites provides a haplotype for the haemophilia mutation in a pedigree analysis. This analysis relies on radioactive Southern blot technology which is costly, time consuming and technically demanding. By contrast PCR offers a rapid, non-radioactive technique for screening large numbers of samples for DNA polymorphisms. Using appropriately selected primers it is possible to amplify specifically the segment of DNA containing the restriction enzyme polymorphisms and then to score the amplified DNA for the absence or presence of the restriction enzyme cut site in much the same way as with Southern bolt analysis (Kogan et al 1987). However, because the target polymorphic DNA segment has been amplified the analysis can be carried out by visualizing the DNA fragments on a standard agarose gel system.

The example shown in Figure 5.2 illustrates how the technique works. DNA extracted from peripheral blood was amplified in a PCR reaction using primers which flank the polymorphic BclI restriction site; following amplification the samples were restricted with the enzyme BclI and the digests analysed on a 2% agarose gel. The agarose gel separates the fragments according to size. In the absence of the cut site the DNA migrates as a fragment of 142 base pairs (band A, Fig. 5.2), and in the presence of the cut site there are two bands of 99 and 43 base pairs (bands B and C, Fig. 5.2). Analysis of the pedigree shows that the presence of the cut site tracks with the disease phenotype. In this family I.1 is an affected individual who is hemizygous for the BclI cut site. His sister I.3 is heterozygous for the BclI site, and may be a carrier but is uninformative since neither of the haplotypes of the parents is known, although it can be inferred that her mother was an obligate carrier. The other brother I.4 was affected but although deceased his BclI haplotype can be inferred, his daughter II.2 is heterozygous and being an obligate carrier is fully informative. As seen in her sons (III.1 and III.2), any male child must either have the BclI cut site and be affected or not have the cut site and be unaffected. However, her grand-daughter IV.1

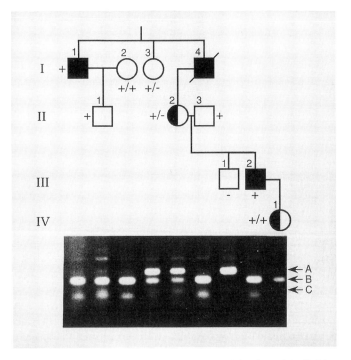

Fig. 5.2 A haemophilia A pedigree analysed by PCR amplification of the Bcl I polymorphism in the factor VIII gene. DNA extracted from peripheral blood of the family members was amplified using the oligonucleotides:

5′ T A A A G C T T T A A A T G G T C T A G G C 3′
5′ T T C G A A T T C T G A A A T T A T C T T G T T C 3′

as primers. The amplified material was digested with the restriction enzyme Bcl I and the digests analysed on a 2% agarose gel (A– 142 b.p., B– 99 b.p., C 43 b.p.). Individuals were scored + or – for either the presence or absence of the restriction enzyme cleavage site.

is homozygous for the presence of the cut site and although an obligate carrier is uninformative.

The above example illustrates both the success and the limitations of using the available restriction length polymorphisms for carrier detection in haemophilia A, restrictions which arise when individuals are homozygous, or a new mutation is involved. This can be overcome if the actual mutation in the patient is known. At present this is a rare occurrence; however, as we will discuss below PCR offers the prospect of rapid identification of the mutation in an affected individual. If the mutation is known and is a point mutation there are two alternative stratagems for screening: either to use the more generally applicable technique of allele specific oligonucleotide hybridization, or in some cases to take advantage of the fortuitous creation or destruction of a restriction enzyme site by the point mutation, the presence or absence of which can be scored in a similar fashion to the standard restriction fragment length polymorphism (RFLP) analysis described above (Gitschier et al 1988). The results shown in Figure 5.3 illustrate the use of allele-specific oligonucleotide hybridization. A segment of DNA spanning the mutation site is amplified using PCR. This DNA is next applied to a membrane which is then hybridized with a synthetic oligonucleotide representing either the wild-type sequence or the mutant sequence. The filter is then washed under conditions which allow only the totally homologous hybrid to remain bound. It is therefore possible to definitively score potential carriers for the mutation. In the example shown there are three individuals whose amplified DNA binds only the oligonucleotide with the C→T mutation and does not bind the wild-type oligonucleotide. These individuals are therefore hemizygous for the point mutation which results in premature termination of the primary translation product.

The use of a linked RFLP is a more generally applicable method of screening carriers; however, as discussed above in the case of the factor VIII gene a very limited number of RFLPs have been identified and these are only informative in about 75% of cases. The human genome contains a class of dispersed repeat elements each of which consist of a number of tandemly repeated sequences. In many cases, the number of tandem repeats at a particular locus is highly variable, so that multiple alleles are detectable simply as length polymorphisms (Bell et al 1982, Capon et al 1983, Jeffreys et al 1985). This high degree of allelic variability makes these informative genetic markers useful for pedigree analysis. In general these hypervariable repeats are scattered throughout the genome. Hypervariable repeats have been reported near a number of structural genes implicated in human disease such as apoB (Knott et al 1986, Huang & Breslow 1987), insulin (Bell et al 1982), α-globins and the Hras oncogene (Capon et al 1983). Using primers complementary to unique sequences flanking a hypervariable repeat locus it is possible to amplify the region by PCR and to analyse the length of the products by gel electrophoresis (Jeffreys et al 1988). This method should be directly applicable to other loci such as the factor VIII gene.

PRE-IMPLANTATION DIAGNOSIS

In the above section we have discussed the practical problems of offering carrier diagnosis and how we predict that PCR will improve the ability to detect carriers. Currently prenatal diagnosis is carried out using RFLP on DNA samples extracted from chorionic villus biopsied at about ten weeks of gestation (Gitschier et al 1985c, Antonarakis et al 1985b). The parents are then faced with the dilemma of whether or not to abort an affected fetus. The sex of the fetus is determined so that in certain X-linked inherited disorders for which a specific diagnosis is not yet available the parents can terminate all male pregnancies, although half of these are

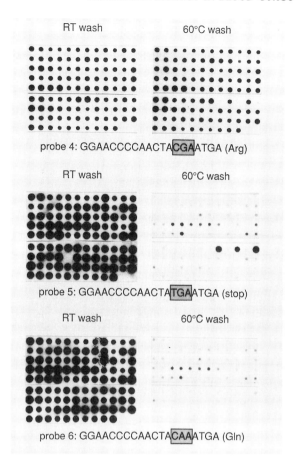

probe 4: GGAACCCCAACTACGAATGA (Arg)

probe 5: GGAACCCCAACTATGAATGA (stop)

probe 6: GGAACCCCAACTACAAATGA (Gln)

Fig. 5.3 Identification of mutations in the factor VIII gene by discriminant oligonucleotide hybridization to amplified DNA. DNA extracted from peripheral blood of haemophiliac patients was amplified using the oligonucleotides:
5′ A T G G C A T G G A A G C T T A T G T C A A 3′
5′ C A A C A G T G T G T C T C C A A C T T C 3′
as primers. The amplified material was denatured before applying to a nylon membrane (Genescreen) in triplicate. Each filter was then hybridized with a [32]P 5′-labelled oligonucleotide corresponding to either the wild-type sequence (probe 4) or the sequence with a C→T transition (probe 5) or the sequence with a G→A transition (probe 6). The blots were then washed at room temperature, autoradiographed and further washed at 60°C before autoradiography.

unaffected. The detection of inherited diseases or sex determination in very early preimplantation embryos would allow the selection and transfer of only healthy zygotes to the uterus. Although preimplantation sexing would not allow the birth of a healthy boy, it would prevent unnecessary termination of an established pregnancy. Thus couples could embark on a pregnancy knowing that it was free from a specific serious inherited disorder.

Such a diagnosis would have to be made on embryonic cells taken at an early stage of development, and preferably be quick enough to allow the pre-embryo to be transferred in utero without cryopreservation. Previously this was impossible because the techniques available were not rapid or sensitive enough to analyse single copy sequences and thus to genotype a single cell. However, using PCR it is now possible to detect sequences amplified from a single cell.

Recently we were able to demonstrate that it is possible to remove a single cell from a human embryo after in vitro fertilization and to determine the sex of the embryo using PCR (Handyside et al 1989). We increased the sensitivity of the technique by amplifying a repeated sequence unique to the Y-chromosome (Nakahori et al 1986). Figure 5.4 shows typical results obtained when a single cell was removed from each of eight embryos (A to H) at the 6–10 cell stage. The cells were incubated at 94°C for 30 minutes to ensure complete lysis, and the Y-specific segment was amplified. It was unnecessary to purify the DNA from the cell; similarly it is possible to amplify sequences from blood and chorionic villus samples without prior extraction of the DNA (Kogan et al 1987). The samples are simply treated with a combination of detergent and boiling to release the genomic DNA. Four of the embryos (D, F, G and H) are positive for Y chromosome material as shown by the dense band at 152 base pairs (b.p.) and are therefore male, three (A, C and E) are negative and are therefore female. Each of these determinations was independently corroborated by karyotype analysis of the respective embryo. However, in one other amplified sample (B) there is a faint but detectable band migrating at the expected position for the Y-specific material. This is a minor product when compared to the positives (D, F, G and H). This embryo proved to be female and therefore

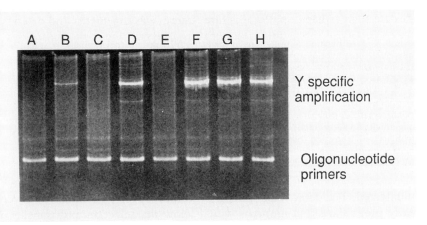

Fig. 5.4 Sexing of single cells biopsied from human preimplantation embryos by DNA amplification. Single cells were removed from human preimplantation embryos at the 6–10 cell stage. Immediately before amplification the cells were incubated at 94°C for 30 min in reaction buffer to ensure complete lysis. The DNA was amplified using oligonucleotides encompassing 152 b.p. of a 3.4-kb repeat sequence on the Y-chromosome (Nakahori et al 1986). After amplification the products were analysed on a 12% polyacrylamide gel.

this amplification most probably represents contamination of the PCR reaction by fragments of genomic DNA from the skin surfaces of the male operator. False positive amplifications are a major problem when amplifying sequences which are present at low copy number in the sample. It is essential to take precautions to eliminate the principal sources of contamination. The PCR preparation and amplification should be performed in a physically separated area from the post-PCR and cloning manipulations. Additionally, ultraviolet irradiation has been used to eliminate DNA contamination from the PCR buffers; the amplification reactions can be set up in a class II exhaust protected cabinet to reduce contamination from the operator's skin surfaces and it may be necessary to wear appropriate protective clothing (Kwok & Higuchi 1989, Kitchin et al 1990).

The biopsy and PCR sexing described above was achieved within about 8 hours, thus selected female embryos could have been transferred to the uterine environment on the day of diagnosis. Indeed, several such sexed embryos have now been implanted in mothers carrying severe X-linked disorders (Handyside et al 1990). It has also been shown that it is possible to genotype single human oocytes for markers closely linked to cystic fibrosis (Coutelle et al 1989, Lench et al 1988) and Duchenne muscular dystrophy (Coutelle et al 1989). Although it is possible at present to investigate by these means only a small proportion of the large number of inherited diseases, the availability of closely linked hypervariable repeat loci should widen the range in the near future.

MUTATION SCREENING

Identification of the mutation in a particular individual affected by a genetic disease such as haemophilia A is rare. Large rearrangements and deletions within a gene can usually be identified by classical Southern blot analysis, comparing the pattern obtained with the affected sample with the normal (Antonarakis et al 1985a, Gitschier et al 1985a, Youssoufian et al 1987), but account for less than 5% of cases. However, identification of point mutations and small deletions or rearrangements in the case of the human factor VIII gene has been hampered by its large size and its complex structure (Gitschier et al 1984). Using classical molecular biological techniques it would be necessary to clone and sequence the entire gene of the affected individual, a far from trivial task. PCR, however, offers alternative, more rapid methods of mutation screening. Initially we and others have successfully used a directed-search strategy (Gitschier et al 1988, Pattinson et al 1990a, 1990b). By amplifying specific segments of the factor VIII gene and screening for mutations by allele-specific oligonucleotide hybridization, it is possible to screen large numbers of samples for mutations at these sites. We chose to target sequences thought to be essential for biological activity and also sequences we predicted would be hypermutable. The dinucleotide CpG is thought to be hypermutable because it is the preferred site for cytosine methylation in higher eukaryotes and 5-methylcytosine is prone to mutate to thymidine by deamination (Duncan & Miller 1980). There are 70 CpG dinucleotides in the human factor VIII gene, of which 12 occur in arginine codons (CGA) which a C to T transition would convert to a TGA termination codon. Five of these arginine codons form part of the recognition site of the restriction endonuclease TaqI. Mutations in these codons can therefore be detected using either Southern blot analysis or PCR amplification across the restriction site and digestion of the amplified material with the restriction enzyme to test for the presence or absence of the cut site (Gitschier et al 1985a, 1985b, 1985c, Antonarakis et al 1985a, 1985b, Youssoufian et al 1986, Gitschier et al 1986). We have studied the remaining eight arginine codons, namely: the cleavage sites for either activated protein C or thrombin at the following codons, 336, 372 and 1689, and the 5 CpG dinucleotides within codons −5, 427, 583, 795 and 1696 using PCR and discriminant oligonucleotide hybridization (Table 5.1). Oligonucleotide primers were synthesized that flank the CpG dinucleotides and these were used to amplify DNA isolated from peripheral blood of 793 unrelated haemophilia A patients. The amplified samples were subsequently applied to a membrane and hybridized to oligonucleotides corresponding to the wild-type sequence or containing a C to T or a G to A transition (G to A transition would result from deamination of the C residue on the anti-sense strand) (see Fig. 5.3). Point mutations were identified in 16 patients. This methodology has allowed us to carry out an extensive survey of a large number of haemophilic samples for mutations at these selected sites (Pattinson et al 1990a).

However, since this approach has only identified 2% of the mutations in this population, more generalized schemes must be developed to allow us to identify the remaining mutations. Because of the size and complexity of the factor VIII gene, rapid screening methods are needed as a first step to roughly localize mutations. Sequencing of isolated cloned DNA or direct sequencing of DNA amplified by PCR will be necessary as a final step to identify the exact base changes. Attempts have been made to improve the efficiency of mutation detection by using methods which will allow detection of a single base pair mismatch in a heteroduplex formed between variant DNA and wild-type DNA. Segments of the patient's gene are amplified using PCR and these are then hybridized with radiolabelled DNA and RNA which is complementary to the wild-type sequence. The heteroduplexes formed between the wild-type and variant DNAs have been treated in various ways to detect single base pair mismatches. Thus the single-strand specific S1 nuclease has been used to cleave the DNA at a point of mismatch (Shenk et al 1975). Chemicals such as osmium tetroxide and hydroxylamine have been used to cleave at single base pair mismatches (Cotton et al 1988). RNase A has been used to cleave RNA.DNA heteroduplexes at points of mismatch (Myers et al 1985a). After cleavage the fragments are analysed by electrophoresis on denaturing polyacrylamide

Table 5.1 Predicted mutation 'hotspots' in the factor VIII gene

Codon			Normal			Expected effect
Number	DNA	Amino acid	function	Probable mutations		of mutation*
−5	CGA	Arg	?Propeptide cleavage	TGA	Term.	Severe haem. A. CRM⁻
				CAA	Gln	?Neutral
336	CGA	Arg	Inactivation	TGA	Term.	Severe haem. A. CRM⁻
				CAA	Gln	Thrombophilia
372	CGC	Arg	Activation	TGC	Cys	Moderate or severe
				CAC	His	Haem. A. CRM⁺
427	CGA	Arg	?	TGA	Term.	Severe haem. A. CRM⁻
				CAA	Gln	?Neutral
583	CGA	Arg	?	TGA	Term.	Severe haem. A. CRM⁻
				CAA	Gln	?Neutral
795	CGA	Arg	B domain release	TGA	Term.	Severe haem. A.? CRM±
				CAA	Gln	?Neutral or mild haem. A
1689	CGC	Arg	Activation and release from vWF	TGC	Cys	Severe or moderate haem. A. CRM⁺
				CAC	His	Severe or moderate haem. A. CRM⁺
1696	CGC	Arg	?	TGA	Term.	Severe haem. A. ? CRM±
				CAA	Gln	? Neutral

* Severe haem. A – haemophilia A, factor VIII 0%. Moderate haem. A – haemophilia A, factor VIII 1–5%.
CRM⁺ᵒʳ⁻: non-circulating hypofunctional factor VIII present⁺ or absent⁻.

gels. The length of the cleaved fragment is the distance from the radiolabelled nucleotide to the mismatched base pair. Levinson et al (1987) have successfully used the method of RNase A cleavage to identify a missense mutation in the factor VIII gene at position 2116 (Arg to Pro).

Alternatively, it is possible to identify mutations in a segment of DNA using the technique of denaturing gradient gel electrophoresis. In this method heteroduplexes formed between wild-type and mutant DNA molecules are separated by gel electrophoresis in polyacrylamide gels containing a gradient of denaturant. Duplex DNA fragments move through these gels with a constant mobility determined by molecular weight until they migrate into a region of the gel containing a denaturant concentration sufficient to melt the DNA. When the DNA undergoes melting, its electrophoretic mobility abruptly decreases. Thus, the final position of a DNA fragment in the gel is determined by its melting temperature (Fischer & Lerman 1983, Myers et al 1985b, 1985c, 1985d). The difference in melting temperature between two fragments that differ by a single base change is sufficient to allow their separation on the denaturing gradient gel.

These methods are being further developed and refined and offer the prospect of rapid identification of the causative mutation in any individual patient.

SUMMARY

The recent development of the polymerase chain reaction provides a readily accessible, automated, rapid, non-radioactive method for analysing a large number of DNA samples. The technique is immediately applicable in the clinical context for haplotype analysis and for carrier detection. In the future it offers the prospect of identification of the particular mutation giving rise to the disease in any individual where a gene map of the disease locus is available and of preimplantation diagnosis of genetic disease.

REFERENCES

Antonarakis S E, Waber P G, Smith M S et al 1985a Haemophilia A: detection of molecular defects and of carriers by DNA analysis. N Engl J Med 313: 842–848
Antonarakis S E, Copeland K L, Carpenter R J et al 1985b Prenatal diagnosis of haemophilia A by factor VIII gene analysis. Lancet 1: 1407–1409
Bell G I, Selby M J, Rutter W J 1982 The highly polymorphic region near the human insulin gene is composed of simple tandem repeating sequences. Nature 295: 31–35
Capon D J, Chen E Y, Levinson A D et al 1983 Complete nucleotide sequences of the T24 human bladder oncogene and its normal homologue. Nature 302: 33–37
Cotton R G H, Rodrigues N R, Campbell R D 1988 Reactivity of cytosine and thymine in single base pair mismatches with hydroxylamine and osmium tetroxide and its application to the study of mutations. Proc Natl Acad Sci USA 85: 4397–4401
Coutelle C, Williams C, Handyside A et al 1989 Genetic analysis of DNA from single human oocytes: a model for preimplantation diagnosis of cystic fibrosis. Br Med J 299: 22–24
Crescenzi M, Seto M, Herzig G P et al 1988 Thermostable DNA polymerase chain amplification of t(14, 18) chromosome breakpoints and detection of minimal residual disease. Proc Natl Acad Sci USA 85: 4869–4873
Duncan B K, Miller J H 1980 Mutagenic deamination of cytosine residues in DNA. Nature 287: 560–561
Eisenstein B I 1990 The polymerase chain reaction: a new method of using molecular genetics for medical diagnosis. N Engl J Med 322: 178–183
Erlich H A, Gelfand D H, Saiki R K 1988 Specific DNA amplification. Nature 331: 461–462
Fischer S G, Lerman L S 1983 DNA fragments differing by single base-pair substitutions are separated in denaturing gradient gels: correspondence with melting theory. Proc Natl Acad Sci USA 80: 1579–1583
Gitschier J, Wood W I, Goralka T M et al 1984 Characterization of the human factor VIII gene. Nature 312: 326–330
Gitschier J, Wood W I, Tuddenham E G D et al 1985a Detection and sequence of mutations in the factor VIII gene of haemophiliacs. Nature 315: 427–430
Gitschier J, Drayna D, Tuddenham E G D et al 1985b Genetic mapping and diagnosis of

haemophilia A achieved through a Bcl polymorphism in the factor VIII gene. Nature 314: 738–740

Gitschier J, Lawn R M, Rotblat F et al 1985c Antenatal diagnosis and carrier detection of haemophilia A using factor VIII gene probe. Lancet 1: 1093–1094

Gitschier J, Wood W I, Shuman M A, Lawn R M 1986 Identification of a missense mutation in the factor VIII gene of a mild hemophiliac. Science 232: 1415–1416

Gitschier J, Kogan S, Levinson B, Tuddenham E G D 1988 Mutations of factor VIII cleavage sites in hemophilia A. Blood 72: 1022–1028

Goodbourn S E Y, Higgs D R, Clegg J B, Weatherall D J 1983 Molecular basis of length polymorphism in the human globin gene complex. Proc Natl Acad Sci USA 80: 5022–5026

Handyside A H, Pattinson J K, Penketh R J A et al 1989 Biopsy of human preimplantation embryos and sexing by DNA amplification. Lancet 1: 347–349

Handyside A H, Kontogianni E H, Hardy K, Winston R M L 1990 Pregnancies from biopsied human preimplantation embryos sexed by Y-specific DNA amplification. Nature 344: 768–770

Higuchi R, von Beroldingen C H, Sensabaugh C F, Erlich H A 1988 DNA typing from single hairs. Nature 332: 543–546

Huang L-S, Breslow J L 1987 A unique AT rich hypervariable minisatellite 3' to the Apo B gene defines a high information restriction fragment length polymorphism. J Biol Chem 262: 8952–8955

Ipraim C C, Saiki A K, Erlich H A et al 1987 Analysis of DNA extracted from formalin-fixed, paraffin-embedded tissues by enzymatic amplification and hybridization with sequence-specific oligonucleotides. Biochem Biophys Res Commun 142: 710–716

Jarman A P, Nicholls R D, Weatherall D J et al 1986 Molecular characterisation of a hypervariable region downstream of the human α-globin gene cluster. EMBO J 5: 1857–1863

Jeffreys A J, Wilson V, Thein S L 1985 Hypervariable 'minisatellite' regions in human DNA. Nature 314: 67–73

Jeffreys A J, Wilson V, Newmann R, Keyte J 1988 Amplification of human minisatellites by the polymerase chain reaction: towards DNA fingerprinting of single cells. Nucleic Acids Res 16: 10953–10971

Kitchin P A, Szotyori Z, Fromholc C, Almond N 1990 Avoidance of false positives. Nature 344: 201

Knott T J, Wallis S C, Pease R J et al 1986 A hypervariable region 3' to the human apolipoprotein B gene. Nucleic Acids Res 14: 9215–9216

Kogan S C, Doherty M, Gitschier J 1987 An improved method for prenatal diagnosis and carrier detection of genetic diseases by analysis of specifically amplified polymorphic sequences: application to haemophilia A. N Engl J Med 317: 985–990

Kwok S, Higuchi R 1989 Avoiding false positives with PCR. Nature 339: 237–238

Lench N, Stanier P, Williamson R 1988 Simple non-invasive method to obtain DNA for gene analysis. Lancet 1: 1356–1358

Levinson B, Janco R, Phillips III J, Gitschier J 1987 A novel missense mutation in the factor VIII gene identified by analysis of amplified haemophilia DNA sequences. Nucleic Acids Res 15: 9797–9805

Li H, Gryllensten U B, Cui X et al 1988 Amplification and analysis of DNA sequences in single human sperm and diploid cells. Nature 335: 414–417

Mullis K B, Falcona F A 1987 Specific synthesis of DNA in vitro via a polymerase-catalyzed chain reaction. Methods enzymol 155: 335–350

Myers R M, Larin Z, Maniatis T 1985a Detection of single base substitutions by ribonuclease cleavage at mismatches in RNA:DNA duplexes. Science 230: 1242–1246

Myers R M, Lumelsky N, Lerman L S, Maniatis T 1985b Detection of single base substitutions in total genomic DNA. Nature 313: 495–498

Myers R M, Fischer S G, Maniatis T, Lerman L S 1985c Modification of the melting properties of duplex DNA by attachment of a GC rich DNA sequence as determined by denaturing gel electrophoresis. Nucleic Acids Res 13: 3111–3129

Myers R M, Fischer S G, Lerman L S, Maniatis T 1985d Nearly all single base substitutions in DNA fragments joined to a G–C clamp can be detected by denaturing gradient gel electrophoresis. Nucleic Acids Res 13: 3131–3145

Nakahori Y, Mitani K, Yamada M, Nakagome Y 1986 A human Y-chromosome specific repeated DNA family (DYZ 1) consists of tandem assay of pentanucleotides. Nucleic Acids Res 14: 7569–7580

Pattinson J K, Millar D S, McVey J H et al 1990a The molecular genetic analysis of haemophilia A: a directed search strategy for the detection of point mutations in the human factor VIII gene. Blood (in press)

Pattinson J K, McVey J H, Boon M, Ajani A, Tuddenham E G D 1990b CRM⁺ haemophilia A due to a missense mutation (372→Cys) at the internal heavy chain thrombin cleavage site. Br J Haematol 75: 73–77

Saiki R K, Scharf S, Falcona F et al 1985 Enzymatic amplification of β-globin genomic sequences and restriction site analysis for diagnosis of sickle cell anemia. Science 230: 1350–1354

Saiki R K, Bugawan T L, Horn G T et al 1986 Analysis of enzymatically amplified β-globin and HLA-DQα DNA with allele-specific oligonucleotide probes. Nature 324: 163–166

Saiki R K, Gelfand D H, Stoffel S et al 1988 Primer-directed enzymatic amplification of DNA with a thermostable DNA polymerase. Science 239: 487–491

Scharf S J, Horn G T, Erlich H A 1986 Direct cloning and sequence analysis of enzymatically amplified genomic sequences. Science 233: 1076–1078

Shenk T E, Rhodes C, Rigby P W J, Berg P 1975 Biochemical method for mapping mutational alterations in DNA with S1 nuclease: the location of deletions and temperature sensitive mutations in Simian virus 40. Proc Natl Acad Sci USA 72: 989–993

Shibata D, Martin W J, Arnheim N 1988a Analysis of DNA sequences in forty year old paraffin embedded thin-tissue sections: a bridge between molecular biology and classical histology. Cancer Res 48: 4564–4566

Shibata D K, Arnheim N, Martin W J 1988b Detection of human papilloma virus in paraffin embedded tissue using the polymerase chain reaction. J Exp Med 167: 225–230

Tuddenham E G D (ed) 1989 The molecular biology of coagulation. Baillière's Clinical Haematology 2 (4)

Wion K L, Tuddenham E G D, Lawn R M 1986 A new polymorphism in factor VIII gene for prenatal diagnosis of haemophilic A. Nucleic Acids Res 14: 4535–4542

Youssoufian H, Kazazian H H, Philips D G et al 1986 Recurrent mutations in haemophilia A give evidence for CpG mutation hotspots. Nature 324: 380–382

Youssoufian H, Antonarakis S E, Aronis S et al 1987 Characterization of five partial deletions of the factor VIII gene. Proc Natl Acad Sci USA 84: 3772–3776

6

Warfarin and the metabolism and function of vitamin K

J.A. Sadowski   E.G. Bovill   K.G. Mann

Evidence for the existence of a dietary factor responsible for the maintenance of haemostasis was obtained over sixty years ago when Heinrich Dam (1929) first observed that chicks fed a diet low in fat for cholesterol-balance studies, developed haemorrhages and that blood obtained from these chicks clotted slowly. After studying the distribution of this antihaemorrhagic factor in vegetable and animal tissues, establishing its solubility in fat solvents and the inability of vitamins A, D and E to replace it, Dam (1935) defined the factor as vitamin K. K was the first letter in the alphabet not to be occupied by existing or hypothetical vitamins and happened to be the first letter in the word 'Koagulation' according to the German and Scandinavian spelling.

The relation of vitamin K to the clotting process was explained on the basis of the classical theory of blood coagulation (Eagle 1937). This theory presumed that in the presence of calcium ions, thromboplastin derived from the fluid of wounded tissues or from ruptured blood platelets, activates a plasma proenzyme, prothrombin, into an enzyme, thrombin, which then converts the fibrinogen of the plasma into the insoluble fibrin clot. In 1935 Schonheyder was able to trace the vitamin K-dependent coagulation defect to a lack of prothrombin by demonstrating that blood from normal chicks accelerated the clotting of plasma from vitamin K-deficient chicks. Since thromboplastin, calcium and fibrinogen were not lower in the plasmas of vitamin K-deficient chicks, he concluded that the only factor contributing to the acceleration of the clotting time was prothrombin. Subsequently, Dam et al (1936) demonstrated that a precipitate from normal plasma which contained prothrombin could restore normal coagulability when added to plasmas obtained from vitamin K-deficient chicks. The corresponding precipitates from vitamin K-deficient chicks were inactive. The concept that the bleeding associated with vitamin K deficiency was simply due to a lack of prothrombin became commonly accepted. Recognition of the fact that several factors other than prothrombin depend on vitamin K came slowly. Today, it is known that at least five other vitamin K-dependent proteins are actively involved in normal haemostasis. These are: Factor VII (stable factor, proconvertin), factor IX (Christmas factor, plasma thromboplastin component), factor X (Stuart-Prower factor), protein C and protein S. Their functional roles in haemostasis are shown in Figure 6.1. Two other plasma proteins, proteins Z and M, are also vitamin K dependent. These proteins may also play a role in haemostasis. The biochemical characteristics of the vitamin K-dependent coagulation proteins are summarized in Table 6.1.

Immediately after the discovery of vitamin K, its chemical properties were studied by many groups of workers in an effort to isolate and characterize the active material. Physical and chemical properties of a number of crude extracts and concentrates from various plant and animal sources high in vitamin K activity filled the literature. In 1939 McKee, Doisy and coworkers reported the isolation of two pure substances possessing vitamin K activity (McKee et al 1939). One substance, a light yellow oil isolated from alfalfa, was called vitamin K_1 (phylloquinone). The other material was a light yellow crystalline compound isolated from putrefied sardine meal and designated vitamin K_2 (menaquinone). The oxidized (yellow) form of each compound absorbed one mole of hydrogen to form a colourless compound.

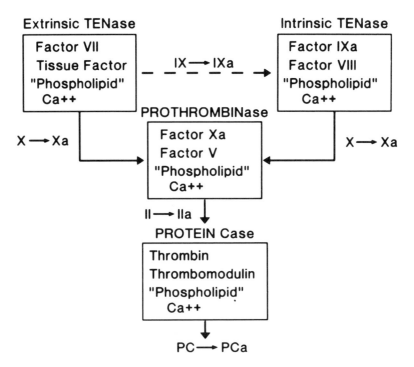

Fig. 6.1 Vitamin K-dependent complex enzymes of blood coagulation, each represented by a box naming the appropriate constituents. The first component is a serine protease which catalyses the respective bond cleavages; the second is the cofactor protein required. All the reactions require a membrane surface which may be replaced by purified phospholipid preparations. The assembly of all catalysts requires calcium ions. The arrows between the complex enzymes represent the proteolytic transformations catalysed by the respective catalysts. (From Mann et al 1984a, with permission.)

Table 6.1 Biochemical characteristics of the vitamin K-dependent haemostatic proteins

	Molecular weight	Approximate Plasma concentration (μg/ml)	Number Gla residues/ molecule	Half-life (h)	References
Prothrombin	72 000	100	10	60	Magnusson et al (1974), Mann (1976)
Factor VII	46 000	0.5	10	6	Kisiel & Davie (1975), Bajaj et al (1981), McMullen et al (1983)
Factor IX	55 000	4	12	24	Discipio et al (1977), Osterud et al (1978), McMullen et al (1983), Thompson (1986)
Factor X	59 000	10	11	30	Roberts et al (1965), Fujikawa et al (1972), Discipio et al (1977), McMullen et al (1983)
Protein C	62 000	3	9	6	Kisiel & Davie (1981), Howard et al (1988), Haley et al (1989)
Protein S	69 000	15 (total)	10	42	Discipio & Davie (1979), Dahlback (1983), Bovill et al (1987), D'Angelo et al (1988)
Protein Z	55 000	2.6	13	2–3	Prowse & Esnouf (1977), Broze & Miletich (1984), Miletich & Broze (1987)

A quinone structure was indicated from the absorption spectra, reduction behaviour, and lability toward light and alkali.

The chemical structure for vitamin K_1 was determined by Binkley and coworkers in Doisy's laboratory using degradative methods (Binkley et al 1939). Confirmation of the structural formula for vitamin K_1 as 2-methyl-3-phytyl-1,4-naphthoquinone was obtained through synthesis from phytyl bromide and 2-methyl-1,4-naphthohydroquinone. These results were simultaneously reported by Fieser (1939). In 1940 vitamin K_2 was found to contain the same aromatic nucleus as vitamin K_1 but a longer and more unsaturated side chain consisting of six isoprene units (Binkley et al 1940). The chemical structures for vitamins K_1 and K_2 are shown in Figure 6.2.

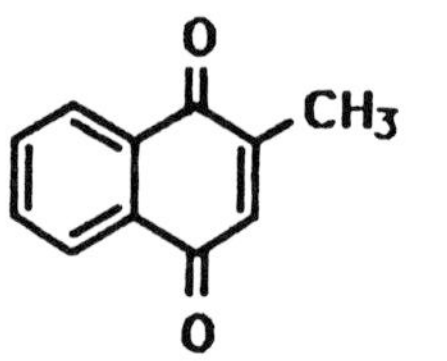

Menadione (Vitamin K$_3$)

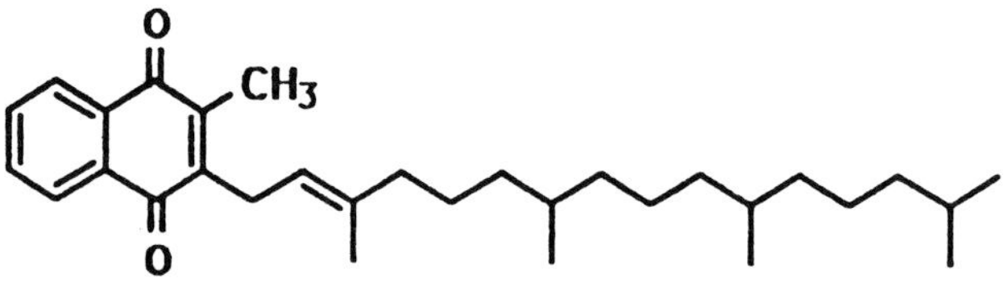

Phylloquinone (Vitamin K$_1$)

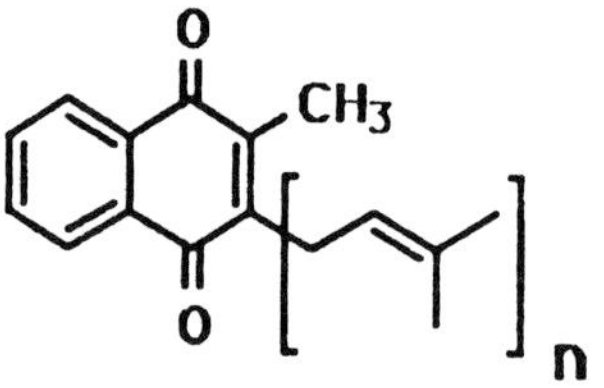

For example, if n = 7, MK-7

Menaquinone(s) (Vitamin K$_2$)

Fig. 6.2   Chemical structures of compounds with vitamin K. activity

The menaquinones of the vitamin K$_2$ family have been found to occur in nature with side chains ranging from 20 carbon atoms with four isoprene units to 65 carbons with 13 isoprene units. Vitamin K$_1$ has only been found in nature as the phytyl derivative. The isolation of two naturally occurring forms of vitamin K having different numbers of carbon atoms and different degrees of unsaturation in the side chain led Isler and coworkers to carry out a systematic investigation on members of the vitamin K$_1$ and K$_2$ series with different numbers of isoprenoid units in the side chain. By 1959 many synthetic isoprenologues of vitamin K$_1$ and K$_2$ had been synthesized and tested for their relative biological activities (Isler & Wiss 1959). A clear dependence on chain length was shown when these compounds were injected intramuscularly into vitamin K-deficient chicks and their abilities to restore the prothrombin time to normal were compared. In the K$_1$ series the form found in nature with a side chain of 20 carbon atoms had maximum effectiveness and in the K$_2$ series the isoprenologue with a 25-carbon side chain was most effective.

EARLY THEORIES REGARDING THE MODE OF ACTION OF VITAMIN K

Attempts to elucidate the mechanism of action of vitamin K in the synthesis of prothrombin were begun even before the vitamin had been isolated in the pure state. Dam and coworkers (1936) observed that when crude vitamin K_1 concentrates from alfalfa extracts were added to blood from vitamin K-deficient chicks in vitro there was no observable improvement in the prothrombin content even if the extract remained in contact with the blood for hours at body temperature. They also observed that if the concentrate was injected intravenously to vitamin K deficient chicks, the prothrombin content of the blood did not rise immediately but required several hours before it reached normal levels. These results soon led to the realization that vitamin K was probably not identical with prothrombin.

Another early hypothesis centred around the idea that vitamin K might enter the prothrombin molecule as a prosthetic group. However, this hypothesis was abandoned when it was observed that large quantities of the prothrombin fraction of normal chicken blood fed to vitamin K-deficient chicks failed to restore normal coagulation (Dam et al 1936). Dried beef blood was also inactive when fed to deficient chicks at 10% of the diet (Dam 1942). These results were not taken as absolute proof since vitamin K could have remained in prothrombin in some bound and biologically inactive form. Solvonuk et al (1952), using radioactive menadione (2-^{14}C-methyl-1,4-napthoquinone), showed that there was no radioactivity associated with prothrombin after administration of the labelled vitamin to mice and dogs. Ray et al (1962) showed that a preparation of prothrombin, satisfying the usual criteria of purity, failed to show the presence of vitamin K chemically or biologically.

Demonstration that the liver is the site of prothrombin synthesis came from several lines of evidence. Andrus et al (1939) removed livers from normal dogs and found that prothrombin decreased regardless of whether vitamin K was supplied. Brinkhouse & Warner (1940) observed that ingestion of chloroform produced hypoprothrombinaemia that could not be prevented or cured by vitamin K. Direct proof that the liver is the site of prothrombin synthesis came when Anderson & Barnhart (1962) demonstrated that the liver cells of dicumarol-treated dogs with low plasma prothrombin were devoid of prothrombin as measured by immunofluorescence. However, when vitamin K was given there was a rapid appearance of antigenic material in the endoplasmic reticulum of the liver cells.

ELUCIDATION OF THE MOLECULAR BASIS OF VITAMIN K ACTION

Significant advances in the understanding of the molecular biology of protein synthesis and maintenance provided a new basis for studying the role of vitamin K in the synthesis of prothrombin and factors VII, IX, and X during the 1960s. A premise gradually developed that the vitamin could theoretically function at any one of a number of steps from transcription of the prothrombin gene to degradation of the gene product (Jacob & Monod 1961). A number of hypotheses based on this premise were tested and argued, sometimes rather heatedly; they are listed in Table 6.2.

Eventually it became apparent that in the absence or chemical antagonism of vitamin K, abnormal prothrombin molecules were synthesized that shared many similarities with prothrombin but were not capable of forming thrombin under physiological conditions. Some of these properties are listed in Table 6.3. In 1973 Nelsestuen & Suttie isolated a peptide from a tryptic digest of normal prothrombin by adsorption to and elution from barium citrate. Using the identical procedure, no similar peptide was isolated from abnormal prothrombin. They reasoned that this peptide contained the vitamin K-dependent portion of prothrombin. The peptide was capable of binding calcium ions, had an apparent molecular weight based on gel filtration and dry weight analysis which was far in excess of that anticipated from the

Table 6.2   Proposals regarding the mechanism of action for vitamin K

1. As prothrombin
2. As a part of prothrombin
3. As a component of the electron transport system for the production of ATP
4. As an effector molecule regulating the synthesis of prothrombin:
   A.   At the level of DNA transcription
   B.   At the level of RNA translation
5. As a regulator in the degradation of prothrombin
6. As a modulator for the secretion of prothrombin
7. As an active agent in the post-translational modification of a precursor to prothrombin:
   A.   Folding the molecule into the proper configuration
   B.   Adding carbohydrate residues
   C.   Introducing calcium binding sites:
      i.   By addition of an unknown prosthetic group
      ii.   By modification of some amino acid

Table 6.3   Properties of abnormal prothrombin

Property	Comparison with prothrombin
Molecular weight	Indistinguishable
Amino acid composition	Apparently identical
End-terminal residues	Apparently identical
Carbohydrate composition	Apparently identical
Immunochemical determinants	Originally identical
Electrophoretic mobility	Similar at most pHs
Hydrodynamic properties	Indistinguishable
Circular dichroism spectra	Indistinguishable
Adsorption to barium salts	Very low
Calcium binding	Very low
Biological activity	Lacking or very low
Activation by trypsin	Apparently identical
Activation by snake venoms	Apparently identical

known amino acid content, was unusually resistant to further proteolysis by several other proteases, and was located in the N-terminal lipid binding region of prothrombin. Due to the preponderance of glutamic acid residues in the peptide they suggested the existence of a covalently attached non-carbohydrate prosthetic group through the γ-carboxyls of glutamic acid. Further analysis of the peptide by titration revealed that it contained a large excess of carboxyl groups over that predicted by amino acid analysis (Howard & Nelsestuen 1974).

Stenflo (1974), using a combination of enzymatic and chemical techniques, was able to isolate two peptides from the amino terminal activation fragment of prothrombin which differed from the corresponding peptides obtained from abnormal prothrombin. One peptide, consisting of residues 4–10, had too high an anodal electrophoretic mobility to be consistent with its composition. However, the corresponding peptide from the abnormal prothrombin had a mobility expected from its amino acid composition. The other peptide from normal prothrombin, residues 12–44, had an arginine residue which was not attacked by trypsin. The same peptide from the abnormal prothrombin, however, was replaced by smaller peptides.

Stenflo further treated the heptapeptide, residues 4–10, of abnormal and normal prothrombin with aminopeptidase M and carboxypeptidase B to obtain a tetrapeptide of the sequence Leu-Glx-Glx-Val. The mass spectrum of the peptide from normal prothrombin revealed the presence of a new amino acid, γ-carboxyglutamic acid (Gla) (Stenflo et al 1974). Nelsestuen et al (1974), using similar methods, independently reported the presence of γ-carboxyglutamic acid in another region of prothrombin. Magnusson et al (1974) subsequently demonstrated that all ten of the glutamic acid residues in the first 33 residues of prothrombin were modified in the same way.

During the same period while the abnormal prothrombins were being characterized, efforts were made to develop in vitro systems that synthesized active prothrombin molecules in response to the addition of vitamin K. Soon after the presence of γ-carboxyglutamic acid residues in prothrombin was reported, a rat liver microsomal activity that fixed ^{14}C-bicarbonate into glutamic acid residues of endogenous precursor proteins to form ^{14}C-γ-carboxyglutamic acid residues in prothrombin after the addition of vitamin K was described (Esmon et al 1975).

It is now generally understood that vitamin K functions in the maintenance of haemostasis through its action as a cofactor in the post-translational carboxylation of glutamic acid residues in the vitamin K-dependent haemostatic factors to form γ-carboxyglutamic acid residues. These residues are responsible for the calcium ion-mediated interaction of these proteins with negatively charged phospholipid surfaces.

ANTAGONISTS OF VITAMIN K ACTION

Research into the mode of action of vitamin K has been greatly aided through the use of vitamin K antagonists to produce hypoprothrombinaemia. It is tempting to suggest that γ-carboxyglutamic acid might still not be identified as a product of vitamin K action had it not been for the discovery of coumarin anticoagulants and their use in medicine.

At approximately the same time that Dam noticed the haemorrhagic disease in chicks fed low-fat diets which led to the discovery of vitamin K, a new mysterious haemorrhagic disease was observed in cattle feeding on spoiled sweet clover hay on the prairies of North Dakota in the United States and in Alberta, Canada. It was soon recognized that the disease was reversible and could be controlled by substituting good hay for spoiled hay and by transfusion of blood drawn from healthy cattle. Roderick (1931) ascertained that the deficiency was due to a lack of prothrombin synthesis and concluded that the spoiled hay contained some substance which causes a depletion in the prothrombin level. Subsequently, Campbell & Link (1941) isolated the haemorrhagic agent in 1941 and identified it as a 3,3'-methylenebis-(4-hydroxycoumarin) which later became known as dicumarol (Fig. 6.3). With the publication of the structure of vitamin K in 1939, attention was paid to the structural similarity of the anti-haemorrhagic vitamin K and the haemorrhagic dicumarol. Butt et al (1941) treated the first patient with dicumarol in 1941. By 1942 a reversible antagonism between dicumarol and vitamin K was shown by Overman et al (1942) in experiments with animals and by Lehmann (1942) in man.

Since the discovery of dicumarol, several hundreds of derivatives of coumarin and other structural analogues of vitamin K possessing antivitamin K activity have been synthesized. The chemical structures of some of these compounds are shown in Fig. 6.3. The most popular of the coumarin-based anticoagulants used has been warfarin, 3-(a-acetonylbenzyl)-4-hydroxycoumarin. This compound was found to have more potent anticoagulant activity in rats than dicumarol and was first introduced as a rodenticide in 1948. Its application in humans came about when it was observed through accidental poisoning and a suicide attempt that, except for its depression of the clotting factors, warfarin had no other significant effects in humans. Warfarin was introduced into anticoagulant therapy in 1953 (Shapiro 1953). Because of the ease with which warfarin may be administered (water-soluble sodium salt) and its even depression of the clotting factors, it has since found wide clinical use. Early on, the general assumption was made that coumarin anticoagulants compete directly with vitamin K for a receptor protein or proteins, at the site where vitamin K exerts its biological activity. The overall antagonism was presumed to result from the relative affinities of the coumarin drug and vitamin K for the active site and upon the amount of coumarin drug and vitamin K available. Direct competition between the vitamin and coumarin anticoagulants was first postulated as early as 1942 by Collentine & Quick (1942), who studied the antagonism in dogs. They observed that dogs made hypoprothrombinaemic through cholecystonephrostomy returned to normal after injection of vitamin

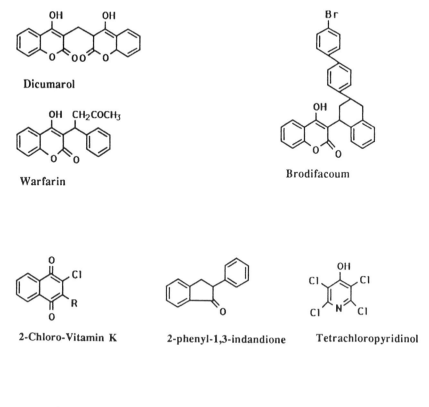

Fig. 6.3   Chemical structures of compounds which act as vitamin K antagonists.

K in 4 hours, but that simultaneous injection of dicumarol blocked the action of the vitamin for up to 96 hours. Since 10 mg of vitamin K_1 was found to counteract 100 mg of dicumarol, they suggested greater affinity on the part of the vitamin for the active site than the anticoagulant.

In 1956 Babson et al presented evidence that the antagonism was not a simple classical competition between two antagonists. They observed that when constant doses of vitamin K_1 and dicumarol in the same ratio were fed to rats over various periods of time, the hypoprothrombinaemia produced by low doses disappeared as the doses increased if the ratio of the drugs was kept the same. In competitive inhibition, increasing the doses but keeping the ratio of the agonist and antagonist constant should not affect the response. However, Babson's hypothesis was criticized because of the possibility that at high doses given over a period of time the ratio of vitamin K to dicumarol might change because of preferential storage of the vitamin and differences in their metabolism.

Lowenthal & Macfarlane (1964) reinvestigated Babson's original hypothesis. They observed that both in vivo and in vitro warfarin inhibited the ability of vitamin K to stimulate the synthesis of factor VII at low doses of vitamin and anticoagulant, but the inhibition was reversed at higher doses. Thus, under entirely different experimental procedures (injected doses and short time intervals) they were able to confirm the earlier findings of Babson. On the basis of these and additional experiments (Lowenthal 1970, Lowenthal & Chowdry 1970) Lowenthal & Macfarlane proposed that the coumarin anticoagulant's action depends upon the irreversible inhibition of normal vitamin K transport to its site of action, and that at higher concentrations of vitamin K the inhibition is overcome by vitamin K entering the cell by an alternate route which is not coumarin sensitive.

In 1969, Olson proposed that the antagonism between vitamin K and the coumarin anticoagulants could best be explained by an allosteric interaction (Olson et al 1969). In the model, vitamin K and coumarin anticoagulants would vie for different sites on the same regulatory protein. The binding of the anticoagulant would render the active site of the vitamin inaccessible, or change the configuration of the protein so that the regulatory protein would be rendered non-functional.

Strains of wild rats have been discovered that are resistant to warfarin and other coumarin anticoagulants (Boyle 1960). The resistance has been shown to be heritable by an autosomal dominant gene (Pool et al 1968, Greaves & Agres 1967). Hermodson et al (1969) demonstrated that rats which are homozygous for warfarin resistance have vitamin K requirements 20 times greater than normal and are from 50 to 500 times less susceptible to warfarin. On the basis of whole body distribution, subcellular distribution and rate of depletion of ^{14}C-vitamin K_1 in the livers of normal and resistant rats, Thierry et al (1970) concluded that it was improbable that the vitamin was metabolized more rapidly or distributed differently in the warfarin-resistant rats. Evidence was also obtained that ribosomes prepared from controls and incubated with radioactive warfarin contained two to three times as much warfarin as the ribosomes from resistant rats (Lorusso & Suttie 1972). On the basis of these results it was proposed that the warfarin binding protein is the protein which when combined with vitamin K allows for the synthesis of prothrombin.

Hereditary resistance to oral anticoagulants has also been described in man. From clinical studies on these warfarin-resistant families, it was proposed that a genetic mutation of the vitamin K-anticoagulant receptor site, transmitted by an autosomal dominant gene, was responsible for the resistance.

All of these theories regarding the nature of the antagonism between warfarin and vitamin K and the nature of the resistance in rats and humans have a common denominator: vitamin K and coumarin drugs compete for an active site or sites on the same regulatory protein(s). Insight into the probable nature of these receptors and their function advanced with the discovery of a new metabolite of vitamin K_1 by Matschiner et al (1970). Bell & Matschiner (1969) originally raised the possibility that the coumarin drugs may inhibit the hepatic uptake of vitamin K_1. They found that in warfarin-treated rats the amount of radioactivity in the liver 30 minutes after the injection of radioactive vitamin K_1 did not differ significantly from the control group. However, subsequent experiments, in which liver radioactivity was examined 8 hours after administration of the vitamin, showed that warfarin caused an increase in the amount of radioactivity present in the liver. This observation led to a study of the effect of the anticoagulant on the metabolism of vitamin K. Chromatographic analysis of these liver extracts revealed the presence of a radioactive metabolite which was more non-polar than the vitamin. The metabolite was identified by mass spectroscopy as vitamin K_1-2,3-epoxide. The epoxide was shown to be present in small amounts in the livers and hearts of normal animals fed diets containing tritiated vitamin K_1 and in elevated amounts in animals who received warfarin. The identification of vitamin K_1-2,3-epoxide in normal rats and in increased levels in warfarin-treated rats suggested that the epoxide might be involved in the mechanism of action of the vitamin and/or warfarin.

Subsequent studies by Bell & Matschiner (1972) showed that vitamin K_1-epoxide had approximately the same activity as vitamin K_1 in vitamin K-deficient rats. However, in rats treated 24 hours previously with warfarin, the epoxide failed to produce any response in prothrombin synthesis. These results indicated that the epoxide is rapidly converted to the vitamin in the deficient rats but that in warfarin-treated rats this reaction was inhibited. The hypothesis was further supported by the observation that when the epoxide was administered a few minutes before the anticoagulant protection against warfarin was as great as that obtained by administration of the vitamin before warfarin. Bell & Matschiner raised the possibility that the epoxide was an inhibitor of vitamin K; however, subsequent experiments did not support this theory (Sadowski & Suttie 1974). However, the discovery of vitamin K epoxide and the influence of warfarin on the metabolism of vitamin K suggested that the interconversion between these two forms of the vitamin might in some way be related to the biochemical function of the vitamin.

Willingham & Matschiner (1974), using homogenates and subcellular fractions obtained from control and vitamin K-deficient rats, were first to recognize the enzymatic conversion of vitamin K to its 2,3-epoxide in a reaction requiring molecular oxygen. Based on their observation that vitamin K epoxidase activity increased under conditions where precursors to prothrombin accumulated in the liver, they hypothesized that the epoxidation of vitamin K was involved in the conversion of precursor prothrombin (abnormal prothrombin) to biologically active prothrombin. The relationship between the in vitro epoxidation of vitamin K and the synthesis of biologically active prothrombin was extensively studied by Sadowski et al (1977). These studies demonstrated that the requirements for the in vitro synthesis of prothrombin and for the vitamin K-dependent carboxylation of glutamyl residues in microsomal prothrombin precursors were similar to the requirements for vitamin K expoxidation. Under a variety of experimental conditions, carboxylation or prothrombin synthesis was never observed without simultaneous epoxidation of vitamin K. In addition, stimulation or inhibition of the carboxylase resulted in a similar effect on epoxidation. They specifically demonstrated that both the epoxidation of vitamin K and the carboxylase required a reduced form of pyridine nucleotide that could be substituted for by reduced vitamin K hydroquinone.

Furthermore, both the carboxylation and epoxidation reactions required molecular oxygen. Surprisingly, both the epoxidation of vitamin K and the carboxylation of glutamyl residues in prothrombin precursors were not inhibited by warfarin, a potent in vivo antagonist of vitamin K in the synthesis of γ-carboxyglutamic acid residues in prothrombin. The in vitro refractoriness to warfarin inhibition was later understood to occur as a result of the pharmacologically high concentration of vitamin K_1 used to study the epoxidation and carboxylation reactions (Whitlon et al 1978).

The formation of vitamin K-2,3-epoxide during the carboxylation of vitamin K-dependent proteins results in the requirement for the enzymatic conversion of the epoxide back to the quinone or hydroquinone of vitamin K if the vitamin is to be used catalytically. The enzymatic conversion of vitamin K-2,3-epoxide to vitamin K was first described by Matschiner (Matschiner et al 1974, Zimmerman & Matschiner 1974), and is referred to as the vitamin K epoxide reductase. The epoxide reductase does not utilize reduced pyridine nucleotides as cofactors but instead requires the presence of some cytosolic component that can be replaced by the addition of a non-physiological reducing agent (dithiothreitol). Other investigators also observed a significant stimulation of vitamin K carboxylase activity in the presence of dithiothreitol and were able to demonstrate that lower concentrations of vitamin K were required for the carboxylation when dithiothreitol was present in the incubation mixtures (Friedman & Shia 1976).

ELUCIDATION OF THE VITAMIN K CYCLE

Whitlon et al were able to demonstrate that vitamin K and vitamin K-2,3-epoxide were metabolically interconverted in liver microsomes during the carboxylation and proposed the metabolic pathway shown in Figure 6.4. Based upon their observations, this model proposes that the quinone form of vitamin K is converted to its active cofactor form, vitamin K hydroquinone,

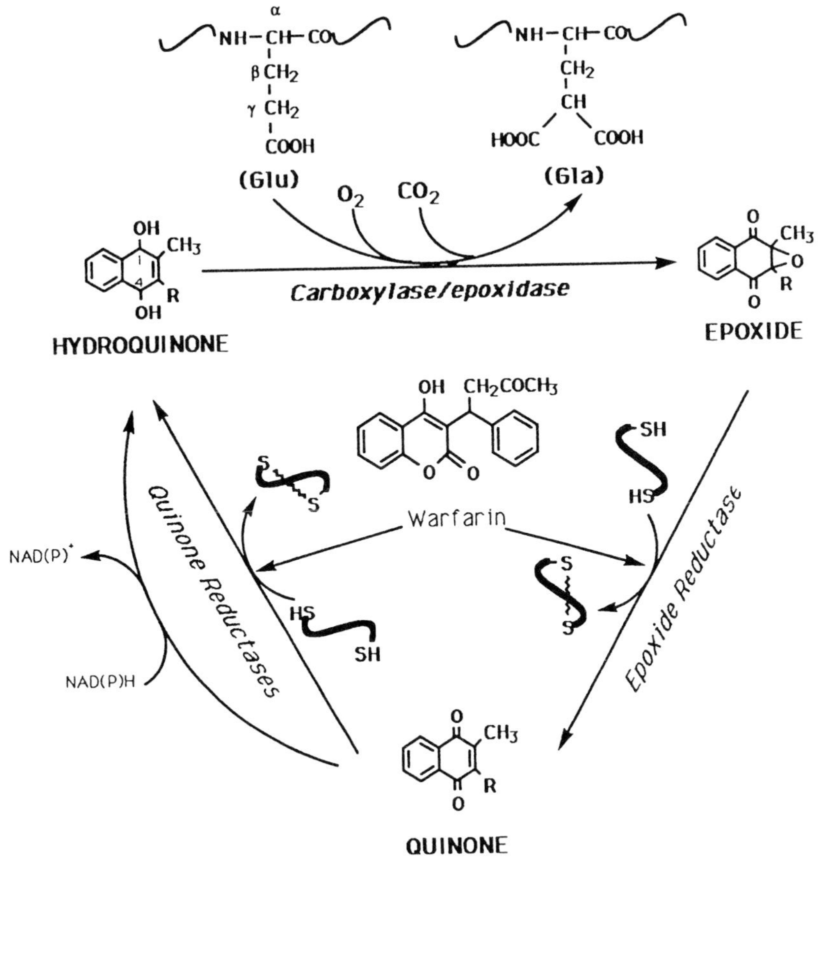

Fig. 6.4 A schematic representation of the vitamin K cycle.

by two different quinone reductases. One quinone reductase requires reduced pyridine nucleotides as cofactors while the other reductase requires some unknown reductant present in the cytosol that can be replaced by dithiothreitol in in vitro experiments. The vitamin K-2,3-epoxide formed during the carboxylation reaction is then converted back into vitamin K quinone by vitamin K epoxide reductase in another reaction requiring reducing equivalents from the unknown cytosolic factor(s) but supported by dithiothreitol in vitro. Both dithiothreitol-dependent enzymatic activities (vitamin K quinone reductase and vitamin K epoxide reductase) were also shown to be strongly inhibited by warfarin, whereas the pyridine nucleotide-dependent quinone reductase was not susceptible to warfarin inhibition at the concentrations of warfarin studied but required higher concentrations of the vitamin to support carboxylation.

The above model provides a simplified explanation for the antagonism of clotting factor biosynthesis by warfarin and other 4-hydroxycoumarin anti-coagulants. This model proposes that under normal physiological and dietary conditions the cyclic interconversion of vitamin K to its hydroquinone and vitamin K-2,3-epoxide is disrupted in the presence of pharmacologically effective doses of warfarin. This metabolic disruption of the cycle results in the decreased availability of the active cofactor form of vitamin K, vitamin K hydroquinone, resulting in a decreased synthesis of γ-carboxyglutamic acid residues in the vitamin K-dependent blood clotting factors. Pharmacological doses of vitamin K or dietary intake of foods containing high concentrations of the vitamin can overcome this inhibition by generating the active hydroquinone cofactor through the warfarin-insensitive pyridine nucleotide-dependent pathway. However, any vitamin K epoxide formed from hydroquinone generated by the pyridine nucleotide-dependent quinone reductase is not recycled due to the warfarin block of the epoxide reductase. Thus, continued antagonism of warfarin by vitamin K results in stoichiometric consumption of the vitamin in contrast to catalytic recycling. Further proof for the existence of these enzymes and their function in the metabolic conversion of vitamin K and its role in the carboxylation of vitamin K-dependent proteins has been provided by other investigators. Despite the extensive investigation into the nature of the vitamin K cycle, purification and characterization of the enzymes responsible for these interconversions has been unsuccessful; thus, no detailed biochemical explanation for the mechanism of warfarin inhibition at the molecular level is generally accepted.

Strains of wild rats have been developed that are resistant to the pharmacological effects of warfarin on the metabolism of vitamin K. Studies from these animals indicate that both the dithiothreitol-dependent reductases (quinone and epoxide reductases) are much less sensitive to the antagonistic effects of warfarin. However, a structurally related compound (brodifacoum) has been shown to be equally effective in warfarin-resistant rats. These 'super warfarin' anticoagulants, in addition to being more potent inhibitors of the metabolism of vitamin K, are slowly metabolized and exert their biological effects for a significantly longer time. Persons exposed to these second-generation anticoagulant rodenticides require daily doses of vitamin K that far exceed the daily vitamin K requirement in the absence of coumarin antagonism. The estimated daily requirement of vitamin K has been suggested to be approximately 0.5 to 1.0 μg/kg of body weight in humans. In the presence of brodifacoum, the requirement is increased approximately 1000-fold, and because of the long half-life of brodifacoum this therapy must be continued for long periods of time (months). Patients who present with bleeding problems of an undiagnosed nature and are refractory to traditional vitamin K therapy should be examined for possible exposure to one of these anticoagulants.

PHYSIOLOGY OF VITAMIN K-DEPENDENT HAEMOSTATIC MECHANISMS IN THE PRESENCE OF NORMAL AND ALTERED VITAMIN K METABOLISM

This section will review the effects of normal and altered vitamin K metabolism on vitamin K-dependent haemostatic mechanisms. The role of the vitamin K-dependent proteins in coagulation can be modelled as a series of linked, multiple component enzyme complexes (Fig. 6.1) (Mann & Fass 1983). A vitamin K-dependent protease is combined with a protein cofactor on a phospholipid membrane surface in the presence of calcium ions in each successive linked reaction. The reactions are linked by the conversion of Gla-containing zymogens to serine proteases incorporated into succeeding reactions leading finally to the conversion of fibrinogen to fibrin by thrombin. Both procoagulant and anticoagulant pathways incorporate vitamin K-dependent proteins. The intrinsic and extrinsic factor X activating complexes and the prothrombinase complex are procoagulant, whereas thrombin bound to thrombomodulin activates protein C (Esmon & Owen 1981). Activated protein C together with the vitamin K-dependent cofactor protein S inhibit the procoagulant pathways by inactivating factors Va and VIIIa (Fulcher et al 1983, Suzuki et al 1983).

The vitamin K-dependent coagulation proteins share a dependence on divalent metal ion binding in the NH_2^- terminal Gla domain for the assumption of their functionally active conformation. Two and potentially three metal ion dependent transitions have been observed in completely carboxylated prothrombin which are necessary for expression of physiological activity. The first transition has been associated with a variety of metal ions by fluorescence techniques and circular dichroism (Bjork & Stenflo 1973, Prendergast & Mann 1977, Bloom & Mann 1978). Antibodies specific for the calcium-stabilized conformation of prothrombin have been utilized to observe a second, calcium-specific conformer of prothrombin and fragment 1 (Furie & Furie 1979, Madar et al 1981, 1982). Phospholipid binding and fragment 1 self-association appear to require this second transition (Nelsestuen 1976, Prendergast & Mann 1977). Five to six metal ion binding sites are provided by the ten Gla residues in prothrombin. These binding sites can be divided into high- and low-affinity classes with the high-affinity sites required for lipid binding (Bajaj et al 1976, Furie et al 1976, 1979, Robertson et al 1978, Borowski et al 1985). Studies of other vitamin K-dependent proteins are limited but they appear to share similar Gla-dependent metal ion binding characteristics. Gla-mediated lipid binding may be explained by either binding site exposure following Ca^{2+}-induced conformational changes (Madar et al 1982) or through Ca^{2+}-mediated cations binding between anionic protein and lipid surfaces (Dombrose et al 1979) or, most likely, by some combination of both mechanisms.

The protein cofactors required by the procoagulant vitamin K-dependent proteins include tissue factor, factor VIIIa and factor Va, which bind factors VIIa, IXa and Xa respectively. Protein S, itself a vitamin K-dependent protein, and thrombomodulin are the anticoagulant protein cofactors, binding thrombin and activated protein C respectively. Thrombomodulin and tissue factor are integral membrane proteins and thus differ from protein S, factor V and factor VIII which associate with acidic lipid membranes which may be made available following membrane perturbation or activation. Furthermore, factors Va and VIIIa require proteolytic activation by thrombin or factor Xa to produce the active cofactors, factor Va and factor VIIIa. Tissue factor and thrombomodulin do not require proteolytic activation to express their binding function.

The prothrombinase complex has been the most thoroughly studied of the multi-component enzyme systems depicted in Figure 6.1 and has been used as a prototype model for these complex systems. This model (Fig. 6.5) was developed from evaluation of discrete binding and ternary interactions amongst the enzyme components (Mann et al 1981). Factor Va embedded in the curved surface of the phospholipid bilayer binds in a 1 : 1 stoichiometric complex with factor Xa. Factor Va appears to bind the lipid membrane through its light chain (Higgins & Mann 1983). Factor Xa binds the light chain of factor Va and interacts with the lipid surface through its Gla domain. Subsequent data have shown that the heavy chain also participates in this interaction. Prothrombin appears to bind to the heavy chain of factor Va and exhibits a Gla-dependent lipid interaction. The model also illustrates prothrombin self-association mediated by Ca^{2+} binding in the Gla domain. A recurrent theme is emphasized by the model and Figure 6.1: vitamin K-dependent enzyme complexes consist of an active vitamin K-dependent serine protease and its zymogen substrate bound together with a protein cofactor to a lipid surface in the presence of Ca^{2+}.

The striking rate enhancement mediated by these multi-component complexes is illustrated in Table 6.4. The intact prothrombinase complex generates thrombin from prothrombin at a rate of 300 000-fold greater than Xa alone. Conversely, the table demonstrates a dramatic rate reduction with the absence of even one of the components of the complex since the integrity of the complex requires the presence of all its constituent parts. The rate enhancement has been attributed to increased local concentrations of reactants (Nesheim et al 1981a) and to changes in the active site of Xa induced by complex formation (Nesheim et al 1981b, Higgins et al 1985).

Although significant differences exist amongst these complexes, their similarities allow consideration of their physiological function under the following general categories: localization, amplification and modulation. Following damage or perturbation of vascular surface the binding of plasma coagulation proteins locally amplifies the haemostatic response by increasing

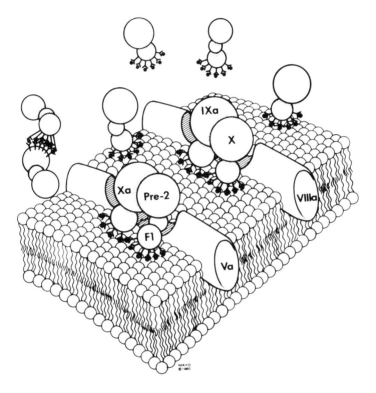

Fig. 6.5 The prothrombinase and intrinsic factor Xase complexes. Structural and functional similarities between the constituents of both complexes suggest that they assemble in a similar manner on a membrane lipid bilayer. In this model, which is based almost exclusively on data pertaining to assembly of the prothrombinase complex, the cofactors, factor Va and factor VIIIa, are shown intimately associated with the lipid bilayer. Factors Va and VIIIa essentially serve as receptors for their respective enzymes (factor Xa and factor IXa) and substrate (prothrombin and factor X). Prothrombin is illustrated as a multidomain molecule composed of fragment 1 (F1), fragment 2 (F2) and prethrombin 2 (Pre-2). Factor Va binds to membrane by virtue of its COOH terminal-derived light chain. Prothrombin, factor X/Xa, and factor IX also possess membrane binding properties which are dependent upon their γ-carboxyglutamic acid (Gla)-containing regions. Calcium ions (small dots) mediate the solution phase dimerization of prothrombin and also contribute to Gla-dependent membrane binding events. The Va–Xa interaction is also mediated by calcium ions. (From Mann et al 1981, with permission.)

Table 6.4 Rates of prothrombin activation in the presence of various combinations of the prothrombinase complex

Components present[a]	Rate[b]
Xa	0.0044
Xa, Ca^{2+}	0.010
Xa, Ca^{2+}, phospholipid	0.092
Xa, Ca^{2+}, Va	1.55
Xa, Ca^{2+}, phospholipid, Va	1210

[a]Proteins are present at potential physiological concentration: prothrombin, ~10^{-6} M; factor Va, ~10^{-3} M; factor Xa, ~10^{-9} M. Phospholipid is present at a concentration adequate to saturate the reaction.
[b]Rates expressed as moles of thrombin per minute per mole of factor Xa. (From Mann 1984b, with permission.)

local reactant concentrations and increasing the catalytic efficiency of the active protease. The dramatic rate enhancement observed with the complete complex implies that the number of complexes formed then modulates a proportionate response to injury. As constituents of the assembled complex, factors Va and Xa are protected from the inhibitory activity of activated protein C and antithrombin III, respectively (Walker & Esmon 1979, Nesheim et al 1982). Dissolution of the complexes leads to both a decrease in catalytic rate and susceptibility to physiological inhibitors. Hereditary deficiency states such as the haemophilias and acquired abnormalities like oral anticoagulant therapy or vitamin K deficiency inhibit vitamin K-dependent haemostasis by decreasing the number of competent complexes formed in response to stimulation of the haemostatic system.

Oral anticoagulant therapy presented a unique opportunity to study vitamin K-dependent haemostatic mechanisms. Early studies demonstrated abnormal forms of prothrombin and the other vitamin K-dependent procoagulant proteins (Hemker & Muller 1968, Prydz & Gladhaug 1971, Veltkamp 1971, Brozovic & Howarth 1974). These early studies found that Gla-deficient prothrombin had only about 3% activity in a two-stage clotting assay compared to normal prothrombin (Nelsestuen & Suttie 1972, Stenflo & Ganrot 1972, Cesbron et al 1973). Subsequent work has demonstrated a spectrum of undercarboxylated isomers of prothrombin in warfarin-treated patients ranging from 0 to 10 mol of Gla per mole of prothrombin (Malhotra 1981, 1989, 1990). These undercarboxylated isoforms appear to have a range of activity disproportionate to the extent of carboxylation (Malhotra 1989, 1990) in functional assays when compared to fully carboxylated prothrombin (9-Gla 78%, 8-Gla 20%, 7-Gla 7% and = <6-Gla 2%). These observed decreases in clotting activity have been elucidated by Ca^{2+} and lipid binding studies of the undercarboxylated isomers. It appears that the loss of as few as three Gla residues severely impairs calcium and lipid binding (Malhotra et al 1985), thus leading to decreased complex formation and inhibition of the haemostatic response. More recently, recombinant vitamin K-dependent proteins with varying degrees of carboxylation have been shown to express functional activity which appears decreased in the undercarboxylated isomers (Walls et al 1989).

The relative position of the Gla residues in the Gla domain also appears to play a role in function. Selected residues appear to be preferentially conserved following warfarin therapy (Bovill et al 1986, Liska & Suttie 1988). Borowski et al (1986) have shown that the Gla residue at position 16 appears to play an important role in the high-affinity metal ion binding required for membrane binding. The other vitamin K-dependent proteins appear to share the metal ion binding properties of prothrombin (Nelsestuen et al 1976, Nesheim et al 1981a, Church et al 1988, 1989). The Gla domains of the other vitamin K-dependent proteins share a high degree of structural homology and will most likely show similar structural and functional changes following oral anticoagulant therapy.

IMPLICATIONS OF LOWER WARFARIN DOSES ON LABORATORY MONITORING STRATEGIES

Pharmacological alteration of vitamin K metabolism by coumarin-related compounds has a well-established role in anticoagulant therapy. However, serious haemorrhagic and thrombotic complications have been reported in association with oral anticoagulant therapy. Haemorrhagic complications occur primarily in individuals with prothrombin clotting times in excess of the therapeutic range (Coon & Willis 1974, Landefeld et al 1989). The present trend toward the use of lower doses of warfarin may decrease the incidence of haemorrhagic complications. The occurrence of thrombotic complications, primarily coumarin-induced skin necrosis, is rare but may have devastating clinical consequences. Although the cause of this seemingly paradoxical response to anticoagulant therapy is unknown, a significant proportion of cases have been associated with heterozygous protein C deficiency. In response to this observation the hypothesis has been put forward that the plasma concentration of the short half-life inhibitory protein, protein C, drops more rapidly than some of the longer half-life procoagulants leading to an increased propensity to clot formation (Broekmans et al 1983). The effect of lower doses of warfarin on the occurrence of skin necrosis is unknown.

Both haemorrhagic complications and skin necrosis appear to be associated with profound alterations of vitamin K-dependent haemostatic mechanisms. However, clinical practice is changing in response to the demonstration of the efficacy of lower doses of warfarin (Hull et al 1982, Hirsh et al 1986). The drop in dosage has been especially dramatic in the regimens referred to as 'mini' or 'very low' dose therapy with the use of as little as 1 mg of warfarin per day (Poller et al 1987, Bern et al 1990). At this lower end of the dosage range there is little effect on the traditional monitoring assays. Consequently, we must reassess our monitoring strategies. Three promising approaches are: (1) measurement of normal and functionally distinct des-carboxy isomers of vitamin K-dependent zymogens (Furie et al 1984, 1988, Church et al 1989, Bovill et al 1988); (2) measurement of the inhibition of the ongoing level of activation of the haemostatic system (Bauer & Rosenberg 1987); and (3) measurement of vitamin K metabolites. The first two alternative monitoring strategies have been reviewed elsewhere (Bovill et al 1990). The evaluation of vitamin K metabolites is a novel idea which would directly measure the effect of warfarin on vitamin K metabolism. If mini-dose warfarin exerts its beneficial effects through subtle reductions in the γ-carboxyglutamic acid content of vitamin K-dependent clotting factors, then subtle effects on the normal distribution of vitamin K and vitamin K epoxide levels should be observed as a result of decreased activity of the vitamin K cycle. This latter strategy is presently under investigation in our laboratory.

Regardless of the monitoring strategy used, the lower dosage regimens will likely be far more sensitive to dietary intake of vitamin K. Vitamin K_1

Table 6.5   The vitamin K content of some common foods and beverages

<1.0 μg/100 g	1–10 μg/100 g	10–50 μg/100 g	50–100 μg/100 g	>100 μg/100 g
Canned pears	Peanut oil	Sunflower oil	Olive oil	Soya bean oil
Banana	Corn oil	Sesame oil	Liver (beef)	Rape seed oil
Orange	Safflower oil	'Vegetable' oil	Cauliflower	Broccoli
Apple (no peel)	Apple (with peel)	Pumpkin	Asparagus	Cabbage
Potatoes	Blueberries	Mustard	Watercress	Spinach
Onions	Cranberries	Cheese		Lettuce
Black tea	Tomatoes	Butter		Brussels sprouts
Orange juice	Sweet potatoes	Liver (pork,		Turnip greens
Apple juice	Squash	chicken)		Kale
Grapefruit juice	Whole wheat	Eggs		Chewing
Cranberry juice	flour	Green beans		tobacco
Lemonade	Milk	Peas		
Ginger ale	Corn	Oats		
Cola	Carrots			
Vinegar	Peaches			
Lemon extract	Corn flakes			
Vanilla extract	cereal			
Almond extract	Rice Krispies			
Brewed coffee	cereal			
Honey				
Salt				
Sugar				
Peanut butter				
Graham crackers				
White flour				
Egg white				
White rice				
Brown rice				
White pasta				
Chicken breast				
Lean pork				
Lean ground beef				

is rapidly absorbed from the diet (Sadowski et al 1988) and therefore only fasting levels of vitamin K_1 truly reflect nutritional status (Sadowski et al 1989). Non-fasting samples of blood only reflect the vitamin K_1 content of the foods most recently consumed (<16 hours). The data in Table 6.5 provide a list of the vitamin K_1 content of common foods and beverages. These data have been obtained in our laboratory (J.A.S.) and others as recently compiled and reviewed by Suttie (1985). The lack of a solid database for the vitamin K_1 content of various foods and beverages is a serious limitation for developing effective strategies for low-dose warfarin therapy. Future clinical practice probably will include dietary counselling for patients taking warfarin at the lower end of the dose range. We are currently addressing this problem and developing a large database for the vitamin K_1 content of common foods, beverages and condiments. There is clearly a need for careful studies of the interaction between diet and lower doses of warfarin. Such studies should address effects on the distribution of vitamin K metabolites and their relationship to changes in the haemostatic system.

REFERENCES

Anderson G F, Barnhart M I 1962 Prothrombin synthesis in the dog. Am J Physiol 206: 929–938
Andrus W, Lord J W, Moore R A 1939 Effect of hepatectomy on the plasma prothrombin and utilization of vitamin K. Surgery 6: 899–900
Babson A I, Malament S, Mangum G H et al 1956 The effect of simultaneous administration of vitamin K and dicoumarol on prothrombin in rat plasma. Clin Chem 2: 243–244
Bajaj S P, Nowak T, Castellino F J 1976 Interaction of manganese with bovine prothrombin and its thrombin-medicated cleavage products. J Biol Chem 251: 6294–6299
Bajaj P S, Rapaport S I, Brown S F 1981 Isolation and characterization of human factor VII. J Biol Chem 256: 253–259
Bauer K A, Rosenberg R D 1987 The pathophysiology of the prethrombotic state in humans: insights gained from studies using markers of haemostatic system activation. Blood 70: 343–350
Bell R G, Matschiner J T 1969 Vitamin K activity of phylloquinone oxide. Arch Biochem Biophys 135: 152–159
Bell R G, Matschiner J T 1972 Warfarin and the inhibition of vitamin K activity by an oxide metabolite. Nature 237: 32–33
Bern M, Lokich J J, Wallach S R et al 1990 Very low doses of warfarin can prevent thrombosis in central venous catheters: a randomized prospective trial. Ann Int Med 112: 423–428
Binkley S B, Chenney L C, Holcomb W F 1939 The constitution and synthesis of vitamin K. J Am Chem Soc 61: 2558–2559
Binkley S B, McKee R W, Thayer S A et al 1940 The constitution of vitamin K2. J Biol Chem 133: 721–729
Bjork I, Stenflo J 1973 A conformational study of normal and dicoumarol-induced prothrombin. FEBS Lett 32: 343–346
Bloom J W, Mann K G 1978 Metal ion-induced conformational transition of prothrombin and prothrombin fragment 1. Biochemistry 17: 4430–4438
Borowski M, Furie B C, Goldsmith G H et al 1985 Metal and phospholipid binding properties of partially carboxylated human prothrombin variants. J Biol Chem 260: 9258–9264

Borowski M, Furie B C, Furie B 1986 Distribution of γ-carboxyglutamic acid residues in partially carboxylated human prothrombins. J Biol Chem 261: 1624–1628

Bovill E G, Malhotra O P, Nesheim M E et al 1986 Future directions in the monitoring of oral anticoagulant therapy. In: Triplett D (ed) Advances in coagulation testing: interpretation and application. College of American Pathologists, Skokie, IL, p 397

Bovill E, Landesman M, Mann K et al 1987 A monoclonal antibody solid phase competitive RIA which measures all forms of protein S in plasma. Thromb Haemostasis 58: 1836

Bovill E, Bhushan F, Mann K G et al 1988 Measurement of abnormal prothrombin and protein C in normal and warfarin-treated individuals. Blood 72: 1362

Bovill E G, Malhotra O P, Mann K G 1990 Mechanisms of vitamin K antagonism. In: Hirsh J (ed) Baillière's clinical haematology vol 3 no 3. Baillière Tindall, London, p 555

Boyle C M 1960 Case of apparent resistance of Rattus norvegicus Berkenhout to anticoagulant poisons. Nature 188: 517

Brinkhouse K M, Warner E D 1940 Effect of vitamin K on hypoprothrombinemia of experimental liver injury. Proc Soc Exp Biol Med 44: 609–610

Broekmans A W, Bertina R M, Coeliger E A et al 1983 Protein C and the development of skin necrosis during anticoagulant therapy. Thromb Haemostasis 49: 244–248

Broze G J 1982 Binding of human factor VII and VIIa to monocytes. J Clin Invest 70: 526–535

Brozovic M, Howarth D J 1974 Demonstration of PIVKA-VII. Boerhave course on synthesis of prothrombin and related coagulation factors. Leiden, Netherlands

Broze G J, Miletich J P 1984 Human protein Z. J Clin Invest 73: 933–938

Butt H R, Allen E V, Billman J L 1941 A preparation of spoiled sweet clover. 3,3' methylenebis (4 OH coumarin) which prolongs coagulation and prothrombin time of the blood: preliminary report of experimental and clinical studies. Proceedings of the staff meetings of the Mayo Clinic 16: 388–395

Campbell H A, Link K P 1941 Studies on the haemorrhagic sweet clover disease. IV. The isolation and crystallization of the hemorrhagic agent. J Biol Chem 138: 21–33

Cesbron N, Boyer C, Guillin M C et al 1973 Human coumarin prothrombin: chromatographic, coagulation and immunologic studies. Thromb Diathes Haemorrh 30: 437–450

Church W R, Messier T, Howard P R, Amiral J, Meyer D, Mann K C 1988 A conserved epitope on several vitamin K dependant proteins: location of the antigenic site and influence of metal ions on antibody binding. J Biol Chem 263(13): 6259–6267

Church W R, Bhushan F H, Mann K G et al 1989 Discrimination of normal and abnormal prothrombin and protein C in plasma using a calcium ion-inhibited monoclonal antibody to a common epitope on several vitamin K dependent proteins. Blood 74: 2418–2425

Collentine G E, Quick A J 1942 The interrelationship of vitamin K and dicoumarin. Am J Med Sci 222: 7–12

Coon W W, Willis P W 1974 Hemorrhagic complications of anticoagulant therapy. Arch Int Med 133: 386–392

Dahlback B 1983 Purification of human vitamin K dependent protein S and its limited proteolysis by thrombin. Biochem J 209: 837–846

Dam H 1929 Cholesterinstoffwechsel in Huhneriern and Hunchen. Biochem Zeit 215: 475–492

Dam H 1935 The antihaemorrhagic vitamin of the chick. Biochem J 29: 1273–1285

Dam H 1942 Vitamin K, its chemistry and physiology. Adv Enzymol 2: 285–324

Dam H, Schonheyder F, Tage-Hansen E 1936 Studies on the mode of action of vitamin K. Biochem J 30: 1075

D'Angelo A, Vigano-D'Angelo S, Esmon C et al 1988 Acquired deficiencies of protein S activity during oral anticoagulation, in liver disease, and in disseminated intravascular coagulation. J Clin Invest 81: 1445–1454

Discipio R G, Davie E W 1979 Characterization of protein S, a gamma carboxy glutamic acid containing protein from bovine and human plasma. Biochemistry 18: 899–904

Discipio R G, Hermodson M A, Yates S G 1977 A comparison of human prothrombin, factor IX, factor X and Protein S. Biochemistry 16: 698–706

Dombrose F A, Gittel S N, Zawalich K et al 1979 The association of bovine prothrombin fragment 1 with phospholipid: Quantitative characterization of the calcium ion mediated binding of prothrombin fragment 1 to phospholipid vesicles in a molecular model for its association with phospholipids. J Biol Chem 254: 5027–5040

Eagle H 1937 Recent advances in the blood clotting problem. Medicine 16: 95–138

Esmon C T, Owen W G 1981 Identification of endothelial cell cofactor for thrombin catalyzed activation of protein C. Proc Natl Acad Sci USA 78: 2249–2252

Esmon C T, Sadowski J A, Suttie J W 1975 A new carboxylation reaction: The vitamin K incorporation of $H^{14}CO_3^-$ into prothrombin. J Biol Chem 250: 4744–4748

Fieser L F 1939 Identity of synthetic 2-methyl-3-phytyl-1,4-naphthoquinone and vitamin K1. J Am Chem Soc 61: 2559

Friedman P A, Shia M 1976 Some characteristics of a vitamin K-dependent carboxylating system from rat liver microsomes. Biochem Biophys Res Commun 70: 647

Fujikawa K, Lagaz M E, Davie E W 1972 Bovine factor X-1 and X-2 (Stuart Factor) isolation and characterization. Biochemistry 11: 4882–4891

Fulcher C A, Gardiner J, Griffin J et al 1983 Proteolysis of factor VIII procoagulant protein with thrombin and activated protein C. Thromb Haemostasis 50: 351 (Abstract)

Furie B, Furie B C 1979 Conformation-specific antibodies as probes of the γ-carboxyglutamic acid-rich region of bovine prothrombin: Studies of metal-induced structural changes. J Biol Chem 254: 9766–9771

Furie B C, Mann K B, Furie B 1976 Substitution of lanthanide ions for calcium ions in the activation of bovine prothrombin by activated factor X. J Biol Chem 251: 3235–3241

Furie B C, Blumenstein M, Furie B 1979 Metal binding sites of a γ-carboxyglutamic acid-rich fragment of bovine prothrombin. J Biol Chem 254: 12521–12530

Furie B, Liebman H A, Blanchard R A et al 1984 Comparison of the native prothrombin antigen and the prothrombin time for monitoring oral anticoagulant therapy. Blood 64: 445–451

Furie B, Diuguid C F, Jacobs M et al 1988 Randomized prospective trial comparing the native prothrombin antigen and prothrombin time for monitoring oral anticoagulant therapy. Blood 72(suppl): 366a

Greaves J H, Agres P 1967 Heritable resistance to warfarin in rats. Nature 215: 877–878

Haley P E, Doyle M F, Mann K G 1989 The activation of bovine protein C by factor Xa. J Biol Chem 264: 16303–16310

Hemker H C, Muller A D 1968 Kinetic aspect of the interaction of blood clotting enzymes. V. The reaction mechanism of the extrinsic clotting system as revealed by the kinetics of one-stage estimations of coagulation enzymes. Thromb Diathes Haemorrh 19: 368–382

Hermodson M A, Sutte J W, Link K P 1969 Warfarin metabolism and vitamin K requirement in the warfarin-resistant rat. Am J Physiol 217: 1316–1319

Higgins D L, Mann K G 1983 The interaction of bovine factor V and factor V-derived peptides with phospholipid vesicles. J Biol Chem 258: 6503–6508

Higgins D L, Callahan P J, Prendergast F G et al 1985 Lipid mobility in the assembly and expression of the activity of the prothrombinase complex. J Biol Chem 260: 3604–3612

Hirsh J, Deykin D, Poller L 1986 'Therapeutic range' for oral anticoagulant therapy. Chest 89: 115–155

Howard J B, Nelsestuen G L 1974 Properties of a Ca^{2+} binding peptide from prothrombin. Biochem Biophys Res Commun 59: 757–763

Howard P R, Bovill E G, Mann K G et al 1988 A monoclonal based radioimmunoassay for measurement of protein C in plasma. Clin Chem 34: 324–330

Hull R, Hirsh J, Jay R et al 1982 Different intensities of oral anticoagulant therapy in the treatment of proximal vein thrombosis. N Engl J Med 307: 1676–1681

Isler O and Wiss O 1959 Chemistry and biochemistry of the K vitamins. Vitam Horm 17: 53–90

Jacob F, Monod J 1961 Genetic regulatory mechanisms in the synthesis of protein. J Mol Biol 3: 318–356

Kisiel W, Davie E W 1975 Isolation and characterization of bovine factor VII. Biochemistry 14: 4928–4934

Kisiel W, Davie E W 1981 Protein C. Meth Enzymol 80: 320–332

Landefeld C S, Rosenblatt M W, Goldman L 1989 Bleeding in outpatients treated with warfarin: relation to the prothrombin time and important remediable lesions. Am J Med 87: 153–159

Lehmann J 1942 Svenska Lak-Tidn 39: 1041–1045

Liska D J, Suttie J W 1988 Location of γ-carboxyglutamyl residues in partially carboxylated prothrombin preparations. Biochemistry 27: 8636–8641

Lorusso D J, Suttie J W 1972 Warfarin binding to microsomes isolated from normal and warfarin-resistant rat liver. Mol Pharmacol 8: 197–203

Lowenthal J 1970 Vitamin K analogs and mechanisms of action of vitamin K. In: Deluca H F, Suttie J W (eds) Fat soluble vitamins. University of Wisconsin Press, Madison, p 431

Lowenthal J, Chowdry M N R 1970 Synthesis of vitamin K1 analogs: a new class of vitamin K antagonists. Can J Chem 48: 3957

Lowenthal J, MacFarlane J A 1964 The nature of the antagonism between vitamin K and indirect anticoagulants. J Pharmacol Exp Ther 143: 273–277

Madar D A, Hall T J, Hiskey R G et al 1981 Kinetic and equilibrium metal ion binding behaviour reflected in a metal ion dependent antigenic determinant of bovine prothrombin fragment 1. Biochem J 193: 411–418

Madar D A, Sarasua M M, Marsh H C et al 1982 The relationship between protein–protein and protein–lipid interactions and immunological properties of bovine prothrombin and several of its fragments. J Biol Chem 257: 1836–1844

Magnusson S, Sottrup-Jenson L, Petersen T E 1974 Primary structure of the vitamin K dependent part of prothrombin. FEBS Lett 44: 189–193

Malhotra O P 1981 Dicoumarol induced prothrombins. Ann NY Acad Sci 370: 426–437

Malhotra O P 1989 Dicoumarol-induced prothrombins containing 6, 7 and 8 γ-carboxyglutamic acid residues: Isolation and characterization. Biochem Cell Biol 67: 411–421

Malhotra O P 1990 Dicoumarol-induced γ-carboxyglutamic acid prothrombin: isolation and comparison with 6-, 7-, 8- and 10-γ carboxyglutamic acid isomers. Biochem Cell Biol 68(4): 705–715

Malhotra O P, Nesheim M E, Mann K G 1985 The kinetics of activation of normal and γ-carboxyglutamic acid-deficient prothrombins. J Biol Chem 260: 279–287

Mann K G 1976 Prothrombin. Meth Enzymol 45: 123–155

Mann K G 1984a The biochemistry of coagulation. In: Clinics for Laboratory Medicine, Vol. 4. W B Saunders, Philadelphia

Mann K G 1984b Membrane bound enzyme complexes in coagulation. In: Spaet T J (ed) Progress in Hemostasis and Thrombosis 7: 1–23

Mann K G, Fass D 1983 The molecular biology of blood coagulation. In: Fairbanks V F (ed) Current haematology, vol 2. Wiley, New York, p 347

Mann K G, Nesheim M E, Hibbard L S 1981 The role of factor V in the assembly of the prothrombinase complex. Ann NY Acad Sci 370: 378–388

Matschiner J T, Bell R G, Amelotti J M et al 1970 Isolation and characterization of a new metabolite of phyloquinone in the rat. Biochim Biophys Acta 201: 309–315

Matschiner J T, Zimmerman A, Bell R G 1974 Physiology and biochemistry of prothrombin conversion: the influence of warfarin on vitamin K epoxide reductase. Thromb Diathes Haemorrh (Suppl 57): 45–52

McKee R W, Binkley S B, MacCorquodale D W et al 1939 The isolation of vitamins K_1 and K_2. J Am Chem Soc 61: 1295

McMullen B A, Fujikawa K, Kisiel W et al 1983 Complete amino acid sequence of the light chain of human coagulation factor X: evidence for identification of residue 63 as β hydroxy aspartic acid. Biochemistry 22: 2875–2884

Miletich S P, Broze G J 1987 Human plasma protein Z antigen: range in normal subjects and effect of warfarin therapy. Blood 69: 1580–1586

Nelsestuen G L 1976 Role of γ-carboxyglutamic acid: an unusual protein transition required for the calcium-dependent binding of prothrombin to phospholipid. J Biol Chem 251: 5648–5656

Nelsestuen G L, Suttie J W 1972 The purification and properties of an abnormal prothrombin protein produced by dicoumarol treated cows (a comparison to normal prothrombin). J Biol Chem 247: 8176–8182

Nelsestuen G L, Suttie J W 1973 The mode of action of vitamin K: isolation of a peptide containing the vitamin K dependent portion of prothrombin. Proc Natl Acad Sci USA 70: 3366–3370

Nelsestuen G L, Zytkovicz T H, Howard J B et al 1974 Identification of gamma-carboxyglutamic acid as a component of prothrombin. J Biol Chem 249: 6347–6350

Nelsestuen G L, Broderius M, Martin G 1976 Role of γ-carboxyglutamic acid: Cation specificity of prothrombin and factor X phospholipid binding. J Biol Chem 251: 6886–6893

Nesheim M E, Eid S, Mann K G 1981a Assembly of the prothrombinase complex in the absence of prothrombin. J Biol Chem: 256: 9874–9882

Nesheim M E, Kettner C, Shaw E et al 1981b Cofactor dependence of factor Xa incorporation into the prothrombinase complex. J Biol Chem 256: 6537–6540

Nesheim M E, Canfield W M, Kisiel W M et al 1982 Studies of the capacity of factor Xa to protect factor Va from inactivation by activated protein C. J Biol Chem 257: 1443–1447

Olson R E, Kipfer R K, Li L F 1969 Evidence for a ribosomol site of action for vitamin K. Clin Res 17: 465

O'Reilly R A 1970 The second reported kindred with hereditary resistance to oral anticoagulants. N Engl J Med 282: 1448–1451

Osterud B, Bouma B N, Griffin J H 1978 Human blood coagulation factor IX purification, properties and mechanism of activation by factor XI. J Biol Chem 253: 5946–5951

Overman R S, Stahmann M A, Link K P 1942 Studies on the haemorrhagic sweet clover disease. VIII. The effect of 2-methyl-1,4-naphthoquinone and 1-ascorbic acid upon the action of 3-3'-methylenebis-(4-hydroxycoumarin) on the prothrombin time of rabbits. J Biol Chem 145: 155–162

Poller L, McKernan A, Thomson J M et al 1987 Fixed minidose warfarin: a new approach to prophylaxis against venous thrombosis after major surgery. Br Med J (Clin Res) 295: 1309–1312

Pool J G, O'Reilly A O, Schneiderman L J et al 1968 Warfarin resistance in the rat. Am J Physiol 215: 627–631

Prendergast F G, Mann K G 1977 Differentiation of metal ion induced transitions of prothrombin fragment 1. J Biol Chem 252: 840–850

Prowse C V, Esnouf M P 1977 The isolation of a new warfarin sensitive protein from bovine plasma. Biochem Soc Trans 5: 255–256

Prydz H, Gladhaug A 1971 Factor X: Immunological studies. Thromb Diathes Haemorrh 25: 157–165

Ray G, Chakravarty N N, Roy S C 1962 Studies in prothrombin: the position of vitamin K as a component of prothrombin. Ann Biochem Exp Med 22: 319–328

Roberts H R, Lechter E, Webster W P 1965 Survival of transfused factor X in patients with Stuarts disease. Thromb Diathes Haemorrh 13: 305–313

Robertson P, Hiskey R G, Koehler K A 1978 Calcium and magnesium binding to γ-carboxyglutamic acid-containing peptides via metal ion nuclear magnetic resonance. J Biol Chem 253: 5880–5883

Roderick L M 1931 A problem in the coagulation of the blood: sweet clover disease of cattle. Am J Physiol 96: 413–425

Sadowski J A, Suttie J W 1974 Mechanism of action of coumarins: significance of vitamin K epoxide. Biochemistry 13: 3696–3699

Sadowski J A, Schnoes H K, Suttie J W 1977 Vitamin K epoxidase: properties and relationship to prothrombin synthesis. Biochemistry 16: 3856–3863

Sadowski J A, Bacon D S, Hood S et al 1988 The application of methods used for the evaluation of vitamin K nutritional status in human and animal studies. In: Suttie J W (ed) Current advances in vitamin K research. Elsevier, New York, p 453

Sadowski J A, Hood S J, Dallal G E et al 1989 Phylloquinone in plasma from elderly and young adults: Factors influencing its concentration. Am J Clin Nutr 50: 100–108

Schonheyder F 1935 Anti-haemorrhagic vitamin of the chick: measurement and biological action. Nature 135: 653–654

Shaprio S 1953 The purification of human prothrombin. Angiology 4: 380–390

Solvonuk P E, Jaques L B, Leddy J E et al 1952 Experiments with ^{14}C-menadione (vitamin K3). Proc Soc Exp Biol Med 79: 597–604

Stenflo J 1974 Structural comparison of normal and dicumarol-induced prothrombin. J Biol Chem 249: 5527–5535

Stenflo J, Ganrot P O 1972 Vitamin K and the biosynthesis of prothrombin. I. Identification and purification of a dicoumarol-induced abnormal prothrombin from bovine plasma. J Biol Chem 247: 8160–8166

Stenflo J, Fernlund P, Egan W et al 1974 Vitamin K dependent modifications of glutamic acid residues in prothrombin. Proc Natl Acad Sci USA 71: 2730–2733

Suttie J W 1985 Vitamin K. In: Diplock A T (ed) The fat-soluble vitamins. Technomic Publishing Lancaster, PA, p 239

Suzuki K, Stenflo J, Dahlback B et al 1983 Inactivation of human coagulation factor V by activated protein C. J Biol Chem 258: 1914–1920

Thierry M J, Hermodson M A, Suttie J W 1970 Vitamin K and warfarin distribution and metabolism in the warfarin resistant rat. Am J Physiol 219: 854–859

Thompson A R 1986 Structure, function and molecular defects of factor IX. Blood 67: 565–572

Veltkamp J J 1971 Detection and clinical significance of PIVKA. Mayo Clin Proc 49: 923–924

Walker F J, Esmon C T 1979 The effects of phospholipid and factor Va on the inhibition of factor Xa by antithrombin III. Biochem Biophys Res Comm 90: 641–647

Walls J D, Berg D T, Yan B et al 1989 Amplification of multicistronic plasmids in the human 293 cell line and secretion of correctly processed recombinant human protein C. Gene 81: 139–149

Whitlon D S, Sadowski J A, Suttie J W 1978 Mechanisms of coumarin action: significance of vitamin K epoxide reductase inhibition. Biochemistry 17: 1371–1377

Willingham A K, Matschiner J T 1974 Changes in phylloquinone epoxidase activity related to prothrombin synthesis and microsomal clotting activity in the rat. Biochem J 140: 435–441

Zimmerman A, Matschiner J T 1974 Biochemical basis of hereditary resistance to warfarin in the rat. Biochem Pharmacol 23: 1033–1040

7

Clinical and laboratory aspects of thrombophilia

M. Greaves   F.E. Preston

Although clinical risk factors for thrombosis have long been recognized, prior to the past decade laboratory investigation only rarely identified abnormalities of coagulation of pathogenic and prognostic importance. It is now recognized that deficiency of a natural anticoagulant or the presence in serum of antibody to negatively charged phospholipid may be detected in a proportion of subjects with thrombotic events, and screening for these abnormalities is becoming an important aspect of the work of the coagulation laboratory. This chapter is devoted to the clinical and laboratory aspects of these disorders.

The term thrombophilia (a disturbance of the coagulation mechanisms leading to a prethrombotic state) has now become generally accepted. Whilst in some subjects the thrombotic tendency is symptomatic of another chronic disorder, such as myeloproliferative disease or carcinoma, these are not the principal topics of our discussion, which centres around thrombosis which may occur in those of otherwise apparent good health, and due to inherited or acquired disturbances of coagulation mechanisms which require specialized coagulation laboratory tests for accurate identification.

FAMILIAL THROMBOPHILIA

Inherited deficiencies of antithrombin and of the vitamin K-dependent anticoagulants protein C and S are undoubtedly linked to a high risk of venous thrombosis. The evidence relating to some other deficiency states and defects such as heparin cofactor II deficiency, dys- and hypoplasminogenaemia and dysfibrinogenaemia, and to fibrinolytic defects, is less strong, however.

Antithrombin deficiency

In 1965 Egeberg reported on the association between familial deficiency of antithrombin III (now known as antithrombin) and thromboembolism. His work clearly demonstrated an important physiological role for coagulation inhibitors at a time when most work was directed toward procoagulant factors.

119

Antithrombin is a glycoprotein with a molecular weight of 50 000, synthesized primarily by the liver, and with a plasma concentration of approximately 150 μg/ml. It is the major serine protease inhibitor not only of thrombin but also of factors IXa, Xa, XIa and XIIa. Inhibition of these enzyme activities is achieved through the formation of a 1 : 1 stoichiometric complex involving serine at the active site of the enzyme and arginine of antithrombin. In the absence of heparin the rate of complex formation occurs relatively slowly but in its presence is dramatically potentiated. This observation is of considerable physiological importance since heparan sulphate proteoglycans, located at endothelial cell surfaces, exert a similar accelerating effect through an identical mechanism (Marcum et al 1984). Rosenberg (1989) has suggested that a small fraction of plasma antithrombin is normally bound to heparan sulphate proteoglycans synthesized by vascular endothelial cells. The protease inhibitor would thus be ideally located at a major generation site of intrinsic factor enzymes.

Familial antithrombin deficiency – molecular genetics and classification

Familial antithrombin deficiency is inherited in an autosomal dominant manner (Thaler & Lechner 1981). There have been widely varying estimates of its prevalence ranging from 1/2000 to 1/30 000–40 000 (Abildgaard 1981, Rosenberg 1975, Gladson et al 1988, Vykidal et al 1985). It is probably responsible for 2–5% of episodes of venous thromboembolism occurring in adults below the age of 45 years (Thaler & Lechner 1981).

Initially the classification of familial antithrombin deficiency was based on results obtained by functional and immunological antithrombin assays. Two types were recognized: Type I ('classical') defects are characterized by parallel reductions of both antigenic and functional antithrombin assays and account for 80–90% of inherited antithrombin deficiencies (Prochownik 1989). Most heterozygotes with type I deficiency have levels of 50–70%. In individuals with a type II ('variant') defect a reduced functional concentration is associated with a normal level of immunoreactive antithrombin.

Our understanding of the molecular basis of familial antithrombin deficiencies has been greatly enhanced by the cloning and characterization of the antithrombin gene and its cDNA (Bock et al 1982, Prochownik et al 1983, Chandra et al 1983). The antithrombin molecule has two important functional domains, viz. a heparin binding domain centred on Arg_{47}, and a thrombin binding domain centred on Arg_{393}–Ser_{394} (Prochownik 1989). Type I defects probably arise as a consequence of genetic mutations producing silent antithrombin alleles whilst type II defects result from point mutations in the antithrombin molecule which alter its heparin or thrombin binding characteristics.

It is possible to distinguish between reactive site and heparin binding site defects using crossed immunoelectrophoresis in the presence of heparin

(Lane & Caso 1989). Heparin cofactor assays do not permit this distinction since the assay depends upon both functional domains of the protein.

The distinction between the two main subgroups of the type II variants is of some clinical importance since significant differences exist in respect of their associated thrombotic complications. Where the functional defect is confined to the heparin binding site of the protein as in antithrombin (AT)IIIs Toyama, Tours, Rouen I and II, the incidence of thrombotic episodes in heterozygotes is low (6%). This compares with an incidence of thrombosis of approximately 50% in individuals with type I defect and a similar, and possibly higher incidence in those individuals with an abnormality affecting the thrombin binding site of the molecule (Lane & Caso 1989). This group includes ATIIIs Glasgow, Sheffield, Northwick Park and Hamilton (Lane & Caso 1989, Prochownik 1989).

Clinical features

Antithrombin deficiency most commonly presents as venous thrombosis of the lower limb. The next most common event is pulmonary embolus. Recurrent thrombosis and thrombosis in an unusual site, such as the inferior vena cava or cerebral, mesenteric, portal or renal veins, are also common. A family history of venous thromboembolism is often present but this is not an invariable feature since the defect may reflect a spontaneous mutation. Also, there may be large individual variations in the incidence of thrombotic events amongst affected family members. Thrombophlebitis is less commonly observed than in individuals with protein C or protein S deficiency. Commonest precipitating factors are pregnancy and the puerperium, surgery and prolonged immobilization. In our experience infection can also precipitate a thrombotic event. However, thrombosis may occur spontaneously. Thaler & Lechner (1981), for example, reported that there was no obvious precipitating factor in 36% of thrombotic episodes in 67 patients.

In heterozygotes with antithrombin deficiency there is a strong association between the risk of thrombosis and age. Thaler & Lechner (1981) reported that by the age of 55 years thrombosis had occurred in 85% of heterozygotes. This compares with 10% of affected children below the age of 15 years. More recently Hirsh and his colleagues (1989) have analysed the frequency distribution of thrombosis in ATIII carriers from cross-sectional studies of different families reported in the literature. They confirmed that thrombosis is uncommon in children below the age of 10 years and they suggested that this might relate to the protective effect of high levels of α_2-macroglobulin during this period. Hirsh et al (1989) also calculated that during the first decade of life the risk of thrombosis is 0.5%, i.e. by the age of 10, 5% of all carriers of ATIII deficiency are likely to develop thrombosis. These figures compare with a 65% chance of developing thrombosis during the next 15 years in a previously asymptomatic carrier at the age of 15. This information is not simply of academic interest since it facilitates a more rational approach to the prophylactic use of oral anticoagulant therapy.

Protein C deficiency

Protein C is a vitamin K-dependent glycoprotein, molecular weight 62 000, synthesized by the liver. Following activation it functions as an anticoagulant by degrading the activated forms of factors V and VIII. Activated protein C also destroys platelet prothrombinase activity by degrading platelet-bound factor Va at the receptor for factor Xa. Normally activation of protein C occurs at the vascular endothelial cell surface by a thrombin–thrombomodulin complex.

Prevalence and classification

Familial protein C deficiency and its association with venous thromboembolism was first reported by Griffin et al (1981).

Familial protein C deficiency can be classified into two types on the basis of functional and immunological assays. In the more common type I disorder there is parallel reduction in both types of assay. Type II variants are characterized by normal or near-normal immunoassay levels but reduced functional protein C.

Most heterozygotes with protein C deficiency have levels approximately 50% of normal. The prevalence of hereditary protein C deficiency in the general population remains the subject of considerable debate; Broekmans et al (1983) suggested a figure of 1 in 16 000 and Gladson et al (1988) 1 in 36 000. These figures are at marked variance with those reported by Miletich et al (1987). This group found that 1 in 200–300 of 5000 healthy blood donors (with no history of thrombosis) had levels consistent with type I deficiency. This appeared to indicate that protein C antigen levels are not predictive of a thrombotic risk. There are a number of possible explanations for the marked prevalence differences reported by these different groups. Figures quoted by Broekmans et al (1983) and Gladson et al (1988) were calculated from the incidence of protein C deficiency in patients with venous thrombosis and the prevalence of venous thrombosis in the general population. Results obtained by Miletich and his coworkers (1987) were from healthy young blood donors with symptomatic individuals excluded.

In a study of 319 patients presenting with venous thromboembolism from western Holland Broekmans et al (1983) found that protein C deficiency was present in 2% of all patients but the prevalence was higher (4.8%) in patients less than 41 years of age and higher still in younger patients in whom thrombotic events were recurrent. Similar observations were made by Gladson et al (1988) in a study of West German patients. Here the prevalence of protein C deficiency in those presenting with venous thromboembolism was 4% in adults less than 45 years of age and rising to 12% in young adults with recurrent thrombosis.

Clinical features

Homozygous protein C deficiency. For the diagnosis of homozygous protein C deficiency, protein C should be undetectable and both parents should be heterozygous for the condition (Marlar et al 1989).

Homozygous protein C deficiency is an autosomal recessive disorder that usually presents as purpura fulminans in the neonatal period. To date 17 confirmed cases of severe homozygous protein C deficiency have been described in Europe and the United States. All but one of these infants had purpura fulminans (Marlar et al 1989). In the majority of infants symptoms occur 2–12 hours after birth. These comprise ecchymoses associated with purpuric and necrotic lesions, CNS thrombosis and blindness, due to vitreous or retinal haemorrhage secondary to thrombosis.

As with heterozygous protein C deficiency there is now convincing evidence for a highly variable phenotypic expression of homozygous protein C deficiency (Tripodi et al 1990). The clinical features described above occurred in infants with extremely low levels of protein C. Tuddenham and coworkers (1989), for example, reported two cases of homozygous protein C deficiency who developed thrombotic complications in the second half of their first year of life. More remarkable were the two patients with homozygous protein C deficiency described by Tripodi et al (1990). One had a very low, but detectable, level of protein C and developed venous thrombosis at the age of 28 years, whilst the other, with a similar level of protein C, remains asymptomatic at the age of 38 years. It would therefore appear that protein C levels that are detectable but lower than 10% are compatible with a negative clinical history of thrombosis (Tripodi et al 1990).

Heterozygous protein C deficiency. It has been suggested that on the basis of clinical manifestations protein C deficiency can be inherited in two ways: autosomal dominant and autosomal recessive (Marlar et al 1989). In the autosomal dominant disorder, heterozygotes have recurrent venous thrombosis whereas heterozygotes for the autosomal recessive condition remain asymptomatic.

The thrombotic manifestations of heterozygotes for the autosomal dominant phenotype are similar to those described for antithrombin-deficient individuals in that they are predominantly venous, often recurrent, occur at a young age and may be at an unusual site. In kindreds with an established history of thrombosis the incidence of thrombosis in family members is high. Broekmans (1985) reported that 50% of such individuals had suffered at least one event by the age of 30 years and that 80% had become symptomatic by the age of 40 years. Superficial thrombophlebitis is a common manifestation of protein C deficiency and has been reported in 10–57% of heterozygotes and is the sole manifestation in up to 10% (Dolan et al 1989).

Protein C has a short half-life such that following the administration of oral anticoagulants the level falls in parallel with that of factor VII and in advance of the other vitamin K-dependent clotting factors. In protein C deficiency a further rapid reduction of protein C by warfarin may produce the rare complication of warfarin-induced skin necrosis. This occurs within a few days of starting warfarin therapy and is caused by widespread capillary and superficial venous thrombosis.

Protein S deficiency

Protein S is a vitamin K-dependent protein which functions as a cofactor for activated protein C in the degradation of activated clotting factors Va and VIIIa. It is synthesized not only by the liver but also by vascular endothelial cells. Protein S is also located within alpha granules of platelets.

In plasma, protein S exists in two forms: free protein S and a complex of protein S and C4b-binding protein (C4bBP); 60–65% of protein S is found within the complex and 35–40% is in the free form. Protein S which is complexed with C4bBP is unable to function as a cofactor for activated protein C: free protein S is thus the active moiety.

Laboratory diagnosis of protein S deficiency

In diagnosis both free and bound protein S must be measured. The concentration of C4bBP in the plasma influences the amount of protein S that complexes with it. Thus, if C4bBP is elevated the free protein S level may be reduced even in the presence of a normal total protein S level (Comp et al 1986). For routine laboratories the diagnosis is based on results of immunoassays since, currently, functional assays are not readily available.

Two types of hereditary protein S deficiency have been proposed by Comp et al (1986). In the more common type I deficiency almost all of the available protein S is complexed with C4bBP, resulting in very low levels of free protein S. These individuals may have normal or slightly reduced total protein S antigen levels. Type II deficiency, characterized by low levels of both free and bound protein S, appears to be rare.

Prevalence and clinical features

First described in 1984 by Comp and his coworkers, there have been numerous reports of this disorder which is inherited in an autosomal dominant manner. Prevalence in young adults presenting with venous thromboembolism is within the range of 5–8%. Engesser et al (1987) reported that 55% of affected family members with familial protein S deficiency had suffered at least one thrombotic event and that in 77% of these thrombosis was recurrent. They also showed that the probability of an affected individual being thrombosis free at the age of 35 years was only 32%. Interestingly, the thrombotic risk in these individuals correlated better with the total rather than free protein S antigen levels.

Venous thromboembolism predominates. Superficial thrombophlebitis and deep vein thrombosis are equally common, accounting for approximately 50–70% of thrombotic events, while pulmonary embolism accounted for 23–38% of the thrombotic events (Engesser et al 1987). As is the case with protein C deficiency, venous thrombosis in an unusual location is a feature.

Management of familial thrombophilia

Acute thrombotic episodes are treated by anticoagulation in the conventional way. In order to avoid coumarin-induced skin necrosis in patients with protein C deficiency, warfarin should be introduced without a loading dose and after full heparinization has been achieved. In patients with antithrombin deficiency some difficulty may be encountered in achieving adequate heparinization and relatively large doses may be required. Antithrombin concentrates are now available and their use should be considered in affected patients with an acute event.

There is no general agreement on the long-term management of patients with thrombosis. Following deep vein thrombosis it would seem reasonable to continue with oral anticoagulants for 3–6 months whereas a longer period of treatment would be usual following a pulmonary embolus. The final decision relating to this will be influenced by other factors. For example, lifelong anticoagulant therapy is recommended for a spontaneous pulmonary embolus whilst a shorter period of treatment is usual if there is an obvious precipitating factor. Also, in women of childbearing age, the teratogenic risk of warfarin must be considered.

It is not possible to provide precise guidelines for the prophylactic administration of anticoagulants in individuals with familial thrombotic disorders since there is considerable variability of clinical expression both within and between affected kindreds. This applies particularly to familial protein C and S deficiency states. However, in the event of elective surgery or during periods of prolonged immobilization the prophylactic administration of subcutaneous heparin is strongly recommended for all affected individuals.

The findings of a deficiency of a natural anticoagulant is not in itself an indication for anticoagulant therapy. Healthy affected family members and their medical attendants should be advised about the avoidance of other risk factors and the need for prophylaxis at times of increased risk such as perioperatively and during prolonged periods of immobilization.

The question of prophylactic anticoagulant therapy during pregnancy and the puerperium is an extremely difficult one. The risk of thrombosis is substantially greater in women with antithrombin deficiency than in those with protein C or protein S deficiency and antithrombin deficient women may benefit from the early administration of anticoagulants (Conard et al 1990). A possible regimen is subcutaneous heparin during the first trimester and from week 36–37 of the pregnancy, with warfarin being introduced for the second trimester. Anticoagulant therapy should be continued for approximately 12 weeks after delivery since the risk of thrombosis during this period remains high. Antithrombin concentrate may be used to cover the delivery. In protein C/S deficiency it is difficult to predict the risk of thrombosis and decisions relating to prophylactic anticoagulant therapy will be greatly influenced by the previous obstetric and thrombotic history. It is probably not necessary to institute anticoagulant therapy during the first trimester but again anticoagulant should be continued for 12 weeks after delivery.

Other possible familial thrombotic disorders

Hereditary heparin cofactor II (HCII) deficiency

HCII is a 65 000 molecular weight glycoprotein synthesized by the liver. It is an inhibitor of coagulation with narrow specificity, inhibiting only thrombin efficiently. The rate of inhibition is greatly accelerated by heparin, dermatan sulphate and heparan sulphate. Although there are occasional reports of kindreds with familial HCII deficiency and venous and arterial thrombosis (Tran et al 1985, Sie et al 1985) there is no clear evidence of an association between the inherited defect and thromboembolism. Recently, Bertina et al (1987) concluded that hereditary HCII deficiency is equally prevalent amongst healthy volunteers and patients with thrombotic disease.

Familial plasminogen deficiency

Plasminogen is an inactive proenzyme which is converted into the active serine protease plasmin by the plasminogen activators. There have been a number of reports of thrombosis in both familial plasminogen deficiency and familial dysplasminogenaemia. The former is characterized by a parallel decrease of functional and immunoreactive plasminogen, the latter by a disproportionately lower functional plasminogen level. Although it has been suggested that inherited defects of plasminogen account for 2–3% of unexplained thrombosis in adults younger than 45 years of age (Gladson et al 1988) the relationship between familial plasminogen deficiency and thrombosis is far from clear since in almost all of the reported kindreds the occurrence of thromboembolism has been confined to the propositus.

Dysfibrinogenaemia

In dysfibrinogenaemia a low plasma level of functional fibrinogen is accompanied by a normal protein level. More than 100 kindreds with dysfibrinogenaemia have been described and it has been suggested that this disorder accounts for 1% of unexplained venous thrombosis in young adults (Gladson et al 1988). However, the relationship between thrombosis and dysfibrinogenaemia is not clearly established since only a minority of affected individuals give a history of thromboembolism. One interesting feature of familial dysfibrinogenaemia is that within the same kindred arterial thrombosis may coexist with venous thromboembolism (Mannucci & Tripodi 1988).

Disorders of plasminogen activation

Although there are reports of families in which a thrombotic tendency appeared to relate to defective release of t-PA following venous occlusion or stimulation with deamino-D-arginine vasopressin (DDAVP) (Mannucci & Tripodi 1988) there is as yet no clear evidence to support a relationship between genetically determined abnormalities of tissue-type plasminogen activator (t-PA) and plasminogen activator inhibitor-I (PAI-I) synthesis and release.

Acquired deficiencies of antithrombin, protein C and protein S

In clinical practice a reduction of antithrombin, protein C or protein S is commonly secondary to disease or therapy and this must clearly be recognized if misdiagnosis of congenital deficiency is to be avoided. Some important situations in which a reduction has been seen are listed in Table 7.1. It is apparent that inherited antithrombin deficiency should be diagnosed with caution during an acute thrombotic event, in patients on heparin therapy,

Table 7.1 Acquired deficiency of antithrombin, protein C and protein S

Antithrombin	Protein C	Protein S
Liver disease	Liver disease and	Liver disease
Protein-losing	transplantation	Disseminated
enteropathy	Disseminated	intravascular
Nephrotic syndrome	intravascular	coagulation
Disseminated	coagulation	Warfarin therapy
intravascular	Warfarin therapy	Pregnancy
coagulation	Cardiopulmonary bypass	Systemic lupus
Major surgery	surgery	erythematosus
Acute thrombosis	Haemodialysis	Chemotherapy for
Heparin therapy	Asparaginase therapy	breast cancer
Oestrogen therapy	Chemotherapy for	In association with
Asparaginase therapy	breast cancer	antiphospholipid antibody

in the early postoperative phase and in liver disease. Similarly, during warfarin treatment the diagnosis of inherited deficiency of protein C or S is more difficult. Family studies and the establishment by each laboratory of the ratio of protein C to prothrombin or factor VII in non-deficient subjects stabilized on warfarin help overcome these problems.

ANTIPHOSPHOLIPID ANTIBODIES AND THROMBOSIS

An acquired prethrombotic state has been associated with the presence in serum of antibodies reactive with negatively charged phospholipids. In our screening programme for the identification of prethrombotic states the detection of such antibodies, by use of coagulation-based tests for the lupus anticoagulant or solid-phase assays for anticardiolipin, constitutes a high proportion of our positive test results. In contrast to the inherited thrombophilic states, where arterial occlusive disease is an unusual feature, the thrombotic episodes which have been associated with antiphospholipid antibodies encompass the full range of arterial, venous and microvascular events.

History

Antiphospholipid antibodies have been identified, in their various manifestations, for many decades. Consideration of the history of these antibodies helps clarify the interrelationships between the tests and the associations with various disease states.

In 1906 Wassermann introduced the serological test for syphilis which bears his name, and which uses a lipid extract of sheep or human tissue – the first description of an antiphospholipid antibody (APA). Subsequently developed tests detect reaginic antibodies which react with complex lipid antigens resulting from interaction between the treponeme and the host. In the VDRL purified beef cardiolipin is used as a substrate, cardiolipin being a major phospholipid component of human mitochondria.

In 1952 antibodies to cardiolipin (ACL) were detected in autoimmune disease, particularly systemic lupus erythematosus (SLE): so-called biological false positive tests for syphilis (Haserick & Long 1952). Antiphospholipid antibodies may then be present in autoimmune disease as well as infections. In the same year acquired coagulation inhibitors without an associated haemorrhagic diathesis were found in SLE (Conley & Hartmann 1952) and the misleading term 'lupus anticoagulant' (LA) was coined. Thrombosis is a feature of SLE and it soon became apparent that the antibodies against coagulation-related phospholipids responsible for the LA effect were clinically associated with an increased tendency to thrombotic disease. Despite this association with vascular occlusion rather than haemorrhage and our appreciation that most subjects with 'lupus anticoagulant' have no clinical features of SLE, no alternative and less misleading terminology has been adopted.

From the above it is apparent that the false positive test for syphilis, anticardiolipin antibody and lupus anticoagulant all represent antiphospholipid antibodies, the differences lying in specificity and in the physical presentation of epitopes.

Laboratory testing for antiphospholipid antibodies

Thrombotic events have been described in subjects with prolonged clotting times in phospholipid-dependent tests of coagulation and also in those with antiphospholipid detected as antibody to cardiolipin in solid-phase assays (Hughes 1983, 1988). Clinical observation suggests that the coagulation assays may be more predictive of thrombosis but we have identified many subjects with high-titre anticardiolipin and thrombosis but with normal coagulation tests; the significance of a weak positive anticardiolipin test is, however, in some doubt. It is, then, apparent that in the identification of subjects at risk a comprehensive laboratory approach to diagnosis is essential.

Tests for the lupus anticoagulant

LA inhibits the formation of the phospholipid-dependent complexes in the coagulation cascade. It is thus a common cause of prolongation of the activated partial thromboplastin time (APTT). Several tests have been advocated as being sensitive and specific (Table 7.2) but until recently there has been no consensus on the most appropriate laboratory methodology. Methods have been recommended by a working party of the International Society for Thrombosis and Haemostasis (Green et al 1983) but recent experience would suggest their use would result in a high rate of false negative tests. However, a recent survey in the UK has identified important methodological details in detection of the LA and lead to recommendations for reliable laboratory testing (Machin et al 1990).

Preanalytical variables. Details of sample collection and handling strongly influence results in the LA tests. LA activity can be quenched by platelet phospholipids, and inadequate removal of platelets affects test results. Freezing of samples leads to the formation of platelet fragments. Efficient platelet separation by filtration or double centrifugation is essential prior to

Table 7.2 Commonly used tests for the detection of lupus anticoagulant

APTT	
APTT	with aluminium hydroxide absorption and heat stability (Austen & Rhymes 1975)
KCT	
DTT	(Exner et al 1978)
DRVVT	

testing/storage of plasma if weak inhibitors are to be regularly detected. We avoid delay in transport of samples to the laboratory wherever possible.

Recommended tests and important methodological variables. Whilst the APTT is a useful screening test for LA a weak inhibitor may be missed and it is strongly recommended that further tests should be used in addition (Machin et al 1990). Also, in the APTT sensitivity is reagent dependent and those with a low phospholipid content are undoubtedly most sensitive and should be used preferentially. Furthermore, the classical mixing experiment with 50% plasma for detection of an inhibitor is unreliable as a weak LA may correct under such conditions.

Of the additional tests (Table 7.2) the kaolin clotting time (KCT) and dilute Russell's viper venom time (DRVVT) are particularly sensitive to LA and are recommended. If the KCT is employed specificity may be increased by use of mixtures of test and normal plasma; a 1 : 4 mix of test to normal is recommended and use of the full range of dilutions originally described is probably unnecessary. Specificity in the DRVVT is enhanced by the use of a platelet neutralization procedure in which quenching of the anticoagulant effect by a suspension of freeze-thawed, washed platelets is demonstrated. The Austen and Rhymes modification of the APTT using aluminium hydroxide absorption and heating (Austen & Rhymes 1975) is unreliable and should not be used. The dilute thromboplastin time (DTT) is markedly influenced by coagulation factor deficiencies and specificity is in doubt. Also, use of low thromboplastin dilutions may result in false negatives.

Detailed recommended methods for the APTT, KCT and DRVVT will be published in the near future (Taberner et al 1990). In our laboratory we employ the APTT and DRVVT, with a platelet neutralization procedure, for screening. In difficult cases we also perform relevant coagulation factor assays to exclude inhibitory activity against a single factor. Non-parallelism in the assays for several factors is a frequent feature in the presence of LA.

Practical problems in testing for LA. In many instances anticoagulant therapy has already been instituted at the time of testing. It is advisable to test after discontinuation of anticoagulants wherever possible, although interruption to therapy may not be clinically acceptable. In the presence of a warfarin effect addition of 50% normal plasma may abolish the coumarin defect without correction of that due to a strong LA, and a ratio of >1.1 to control in the DRVVT on a 50% normal plasma mix or of >1.2 in the KCT on a 80% normal : 20% test plasma mix is suggestive of LA. However, confident diagnosis of the presence of LA is not possible in the presence of anticoagulation.

Tests for anticardiolipin

Sensitive immunoassays for antiphospholipid antibodies have been developed and some attempts at standardization made (Harris et al 1987). The binding of an antibody to its target phospholipid is governed by affinity and its type, and also by the physical state of the lipid. Standardization of test conditions is thus at least as important as in coagulation-based assays. Problems with non-specific binding have been highlighted (Peter 1990) and interpretation of low positive results is difficult and concordance between laboratories poor (Harris et al 1987). IgM ACL levels are unreliable in the presence of rheumatoid factor. However, the methodology offers the possibility to examine for cross-reactivity with phospholipids other than cardiolipin and such investigations may provide important information on the pathogenicity of antiphospholipid antibodies. In our laboratory we use an enzyme-linked immunoassay method on microtitre plates to test for IgG and IgM antibodies. Values in excess of three standard deviations in excess of mean normal are considered positive (the distribution is skewed) and interpreted in the light of their reproducibility over several months, coagulation test results and a consideration of the clinical picture.

Conditions associated with the presence of antiphospholipid antibodies

Antiphospholipid antibodies, most commonly ACL but also LA, have been found in association with a variety of disease states and conditions as well as in response to drug exposure (Table 7.3). In many conditions the association is beyond doubt, e.g. in collagen vascular disease and some infections; in others, e.g. recurrent abortion and thrombovascular disease, patient groups have often been highly selected; however, a true relationship seems likely. The observation that antiphospholipid antibodies may arise transiently, in infections and after tissue injury such as that occurring in myocardial infarction, indicates that the significance of a single positive test, particularly a weak positive, is open to considerable doubt. This applies especially to solid-phase methodology such as the standard test for anticardiolipin antibody. Furthermore, we have not uncommonly detected positive tests for lupus anticoagulant preoperatively in patients who appear to be healthy apart from a minor surgical condition unlikely to be relevant to the presence of autoantibody.

Antiphospholipid antibodies and thrombosis

In SLE the presence of APL is associated with an increased tendency to thrombotic events, probably of the order of threefold for LA positivity and a little less in the presence of ACL only, in comparison with SLE sufferers who are negative in the tests (Petri et al 1990). It is now recognized that subjects without features of systematic lupus, or other disease, may suffer thromboembolic events apparently in association with the presence of positive tests for LA, ACL or both. One such case is illustrated in Fig. 7.1.

In one large series (Gastineau et al 1985) the frequency of thrombotic events was approximately 25% in antiphospholipid positive subjects both

Table 7.3   Situations in which antiphospholipid antibodies have been reported

Infections	Acute self-limiting infections
	Syphilis
	Malaria
	HIV infection
Rheumatic and collagen vascular diseases	Systemic lupus erythematosus
	Systemic sclerosis
	Rheumatoid arthritis
	Temporal arteritis
	Psoriatic arthropathy
	Sjogren's syndrome
Disorders of the nervous system and eye	Thrombotic stroke
	Multi-infarct dementia
	Transient cerebral ischaemia and amaurosis fugax
	Sagittal sinus thrombosis
	Chorea
	Guillain–Barré syndrome
	Ischaemic optic neuropathy
	Retinal venous occlusion
	Transverse myelitis
Thrombotic disease	Myocardial infarction and ischaemic heart disease
	After coronary artery bypass graft surgery
	Valvular heart disease
	Peripheral arterial occulsion
	Venous thromboembolic disease
	Microvascular thrombosis
	Renal vascular disease
	Pulmonary hypertension
Obstetric disorders	Recurrent abortion
	Fetal growth retardation
	Early, severe pre-eclampsia
With medication	Chlorpromazine
	Procainamide
	Hydralazine
	Phenytoin
	Quinidine
Miscellaneous conditions	Autoimmune thrombocytopenia
	Autoimmune haemolytic anaemia
	Sickle cell disease
	Behcet's syndrome
	Intravenous drug abuse
	Livedo reticularis
	Skin ulceration

Key references: Alarcon-Segovia et al (1989), Elias & Eldor (1984), Gastineau et al (1985), Hamsten et al (1986), Harris et al (1985), Lockshin et al (1985), Malia et al (1988), Morton et al (1986).

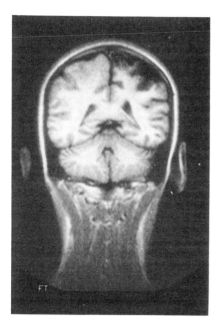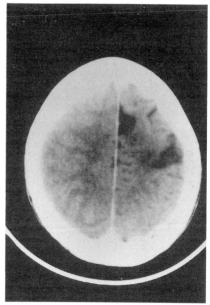

Fig. 7.1   Magnetic resonance imaging scan (left) and computerized axial tomographic scan (right) of the head of a 22-year-old female with hemiparesis. There were no risk factors other than oral contraceptive usage. The KCCT was prolonged. The DRVVT has been repeatedly prolonged, with correction by washed, frozen-thawed platelets. All other tests, including those for anticardiolipin and antinuclear factor, have been negative. Areas of infarction are easily seen.

with and without SLE. The range of vascular occlusive manifestations included deep venous thrombosis, small vein thrombosis, peripheral arterial occlusion as well as cerebrovascular events. We and others have observed thrombotic events in relatively unusual sites in subjects positive for antiphospholipid, such as axillary vein thrombosis, sagittal sinus thrombosis, Budd–Chiari syndrome and retinal vein occlusion; frequently the presence of LA or ACL has been the only abnormal laboratory finding. In rheumatic disorders, especially SLE, thrombocytopenia is strongly associated with elevated ACL titres.

The clinical significance of a positive test

The appearance of ACL transiently during an acute infectious episode suggests that a single positive test is unreliable as a marker for thrombosis. Even in subjects with collagen vascular disease major changes in strength of antibody may be detected over a period of months, and spontaneous resolution has been observed. Furthermore, raised ACL titres observed in some circumstances do not appear to be associated with thrombotic or other events, for example in immune thrombocytopenic purpura and HIV infection. Also, there is disagreement on the thrombotic risk associated with drug-induced APL: in Gastineau's series no thrombotic events were seen in this group (Gastineau et al 1985), whereas others have observed major occlusive events (Triplett et al 1988).

Our impression is that LA is a better predictor of thrombotic risk than is ACL and we are particularly loath to attach significance to low-titre ACL in the absence of LA. Again, the clinical picture and rigorous exclusion of other risk factors are important in interpretation. The relative predictive value of IgG and IgM ACL remains to be determined.

In some situations APL may be generated apparently as a result of tissue injury. This may be the cause of elevated titres of ACL in some young survivors of myocardial infarction (Hamsten et al 1986) and in subjects undergoing coronary artery bypass graft surgery (Morton et al 1986). However, in both situations subsequent thrombotic episodes are more common in the ACL-positive groups.

Obstetric associations

Fetal loss in the first or second trimester, stillbirth and early severe pre-eclampsia have been described in association with APL in SLE but also in women of otherwise good health and with no clinical or serological markers of SLE (Branch et al 1985, Lockshin et al 1985). Placental infarction has been seen in many cases (Fig. 7.2) but is not uniformly present and mechanisms other than thrombosis in the placental vasculature may be operative.

In our laboratory we have found an incidence of 15–20% of LA (positive DRVVT) and a similar incidence of IgG ACL (>3 SD of mean normal) in women with a history of three or more fetal losses in the first or second trimester. LA and ACL occurred independently. The incidence of positive tests was much lower in women with one or two episodes of fetal loss and in over 400 women with normal pregnancy the frequency of LA, IgG and IgM ACL was only approximately 1% for each (Creagh et al 1990).

It is generally considered that the reproducible finding of APL in a woman with recurrent fetal loss is of pathogenic significance and that therapeutic intervention may be helpful, but clinical trials are awaited.

The 'antiphospholipid syndrome'

The observation that subjects without SLE but with APL may develop thrombotic, obstetric and perhaps other clinical problems has led to the concept of a 'primary antiphospholipid syndrome'. This can perhaps be defined as the finding of APL (LA or ACL) on at least two occasions 8 weeks apart in a subject with two or more of: history of recurrent fetal loss (three or more), venous thrombosis, arterial thrombosis, thrombocytopenia, and without clinical or serological evidence of SLE or related disorder

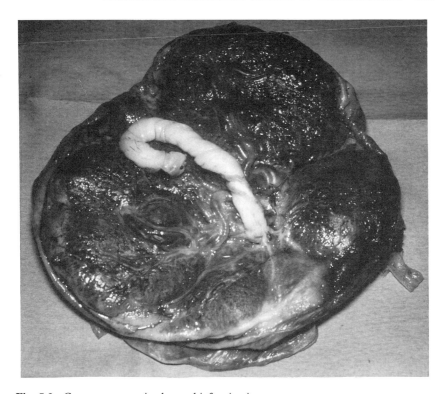

Fig. 7.2 Gross, macroscopic placental infarction is apparent.

(Alarcon-Segovia & Sanchez-Guerrero 1989). In these cases it is considered that the APL is significant in the development of disease, although cause and effect has not been demonstrated. The requirement for two clinical manifestations will exclude many related cases in which only obstetric complications or thrombosis have occurred but these cannot be confidently included in the diagnostic category, although the finding of LA or high-titre (>20 units) ACL may still be of prognostic and therapeutic importance. Arguably, other common associations, especially livedo reticularis, could be included.

Pathogenic mechanisms for thrombosis

The mechanisms whereby antiphospholipid antibody could produce thrombotic vascular occlusion have not yet been determined, but there are many possibilities. Direct damage to the endothelial cell membrane could occur, and we have found cross-reactivity between antibody to cardiolipin and to endothelial cell surface. Platelet activation through membrane interaction is a possibility, and the association between APL and thrombocytopenia is of interest here. Controversy exists as to the ability of

APL sera to inhibit endothelial cell prostacyclin production in vitro; we have found this to be the case. Inhibition of fibrinolysis has been reported and we have recently described marked interference in the protein C/S anticoagulant system by IgG preparations from APL subjects (Malia et al 1990). The requirement for phospholipid in protein C activation provides a basis for this interaction, although the association of arterial as well as venous thrombosis with APL is difficult to explain by such a mechanism.

It is likely that multiple interactions exist, although it must be acknowledged that it remains possible that APL constitutes an epiphenomenon in thrombotic disease and is merely a marker for some as yet undetected defect. Of great interest is the recent report, by two independent groups, that antiphospholipid activity is not directed primarily against negatively charged phospholipid but against a 50-kDa plasma glycoprotein which itself binds to negatively charged phospholipids (Galli et al 1990, McNeil et al 1990). If confirmed these findings could dramatically alter the direction of research into APL and thrombosis.

Clinical management

There are no controlled clinical trials on the management of thrombosis in association with APL. Subjects with major venous or arterial thrombosis require anticoagulant therapy. Recurrent thrombosis on discontinuation of anticoagulants has been described and the finding on APL may suggest that long-term anticoagulation is advisable. However, this must depend on the nature and severity of the presenting episode and the perceived risk : benefit ratio in the individual patient. Other risk factors, such as oral contraceptive usage and smoking, should be avoided. Whether aspirin is effective in prophylaxis remains to be determined but its use could certainly be justified for transient cerebral ischaemic episodes and probably after thrombotic stroke and myocardial infarction. Although the finding of APL may represent an immune mechanism in thrombotic disease immunosuppressive therapy is not indicated unless required for other autoimmune manifestations, as in SLE.

When APL is found incidentally no treatment is indicated. Where abnormal coagulation tests are found preoperatively, the demonstration of LA should allow surgery to proceed safely without haemorrhagic risk provided there is no associated thrombocytopenia. The clinician should, though, be aware of the rare association between APL and coagulation factor inhibitors, particularly against prothrombin, but also factor VIII.

Again, no controlled trials exist for prophylaxis against fetal loss in women with APL. Good results have been claimed for the use of corticosteroids, aspirin, heparin and intravenous immunoglobulin. It is pertinent that a live infant may result from a subsequent pregnancy, without intervention, even in a woman with a very poor obstetric history (Petri et al 1989). The consensus view is that the considerable morbidity associated with corticosteroid usage is best avoided. Our approach, in women with three or more miscarriages and detectable APL on at least two occasions, is to offer prophylaxis with subcutaneous heparin and/or low-dose aspirin for subsequent pregnancies, combined with close liaison with obstetric colleagues and regular assessment of progress using ultrasound scans. More aggressive therapy with higher anticoagulant dosage, steroids or intravenous immunoglobulin could be considered should there be evidence of fetal growth retardation, whilst acknowledging that none of these approaches is yet of proven value.

CONCLUDING REMARKS

A protocol for the investigation of thrombophilia is now available which allows a rational approach to treatment. The indications for testing which we have adopted are listed in Table 7.4 and the tests performed in our laboratory in Table 7.5. However, this still only allows the identification of an underlying mechanism in a minority of affected individuals. We can look forward in the next few years to further major advances in this clinically important area.

ACKNOWLEDGEMENTS

We are indebted for the expertise of Mrs L. Wattam in the preparation of the manuscript. Our thanks to Miss S. L. B. Duncan, Reader in Obstetrics, Sheffield, for supplying Fig. 7.2.

Table 7.4   Indications for screening for thrombophilia

Tests for ATIII, protein C and protein S	Tests for lupus anticoagulant and anticardiolipin
1. Venous thromboembolism presenting at <45 years of age	1. Venous thromboembolism presenting at <45 years of age
2. Recurrent venous thrombosis	2. Arterial thrombosis presenting at <45 years of age in the absence of risk factors
3. Venous thrombosis in an unusual anatomical site	3. In the investigation of some disorders listed in Table 3, e.g. ischaemic optic neuropathy, chorea, livedo reticularis
4. Positive family history of thrombophilia	4. Recurrent (>3) abortion of unknown cause
	5. Early, severe pre-eclampsia
	6. For assessment of thrombotic risk in some cases of SLE

Table 7.5 The laboratory investigation of thrombophilia

A. Relevant screening tests
    Full blood count
    PT
    APTT
    TT
    Reptilase time
    Fibrinogen concentration
    Liver enzymes

B. Tests of specific diagnostic and prognostic value
    Antithrombin assay: Functional
                           Immunological

    Protein C assay: Functional
                           Immunological

    Protein S assay: Total
                           Free

    C4b binding protein assay

    Tests for antiphospholipid antibody

C. Tests of unproven value
    Heparin cofactor II assay
    Euglobulin clot lysis time ($\pm$ venous occlusion)
    Assays for tissue plasminogen activator and inhibitor

The table outlines the investigations employed in our laboratory.
Those in section A are important for the accurate interpretation of the tests in section B.
We perform the investigations listed under C for research purposes.

REFERENCES

Abildgaard U 1981 Antithrombin and related inhibitors of coagulation. In: Poller L (ed) Recent advances in blood coagulation. Churchill Livingstone, Edinburgh 3: 151–173
Alarcon-Segovia D, Sanchez-Guerrero J 1989 Primary antiphospholipid syndrome. J Rheumatol 16: 482–487
Alarcon-Segovia D, Deleze M, Oria C V, Sanchez-Guerrero J et al 1989 Antiphospholipid antibodies and the antiphospholipid syndrome in systemic lupus erythematosus: a prospective analysis of 500 consecutive patients. Medicine 68: 353–365
Austen D E G, Rhymes I L 1975 In: Laboratory manual of blood coagulation. Blackwell Scientific Publications, Oxford
Bertina R M, Van Der Linden I K, Muller H P, Brommer E J P 1987 Hereditary heparin cofactor deficiency and the risk of development of thrombosis. Thromb Haemostasis 57: 196–200
Bock S C, Wion K L, Vehar G A, Lawn R M 1982 Cloning and expression of the cDNA for human antithrombin III. Nucleic Acids Res 10: 8113–8125
Branch D W, Scott J R, Kochenour N K, Hershgold E 1985 Obstetric complications associated with the lupus anticoagulant. N Engl J Med 313: 1322–1326
Broekmans A W 1985 Hereditary protein C deficiency. Haemostasis 15: 233–240
Broekmans A W, Eltkamp J J, Bertina R M 1983 Congenital protein C deficiency and venous thromboembolism: the study of three Dutch families. N Engl J Med 309: 340–343
Chandra T, Stackhouse R, Kidd V J, Woo S L C 1983 Isolation and sequence characterisation of a DNA clone of human antithrombin III. Proc Natl Acad Sci USA 58: 1094

Comp P C, Nixon R R, Cooper M R, Esmon C T 1984 Familial protein S deficiency as associated with recurrent thrombosis. J Clin Invest 74: 2082–2099

Comp P C, Dorey D, Patton D, Esmon C T 1986 An abnormal plasma distribution of protein S occurs in functional protein S deficiency. Blood 67: 504–508

Conard J, Horellou M H, Van Dreden P, Lecompte T, Samama M 1990 Thrombosis and pregnancy in congenital deficiencies in ATIII, protein C or protein S: study of 78 women. Thromb Haemostasis 63: 319–320

Conley C L, Hartmann R C 1952 A haemorrhagic disorder caused by circulating anticoagulant in patients with disseminated lupus erythematosus. J Clin Invest 31: 621–623

Creagh M D, Duncan S L B, McDonnell J, Greaves M 1990 The incidence of the lupus anticoagulant (LA) and anticardiolipin antibodies (ACL) in normal pregnancy. Clin Exp Rheumatol 8: 219

Dolan G, Ball J, Preston F E 1989 Protein C and Protein S. In: Tuddenham E D G (ed) Baillière's Clinical Haematology. International Practice and Research. The Molecular Biology of Coagulation. Baillière Tindall, London, p 4

Egeberg O 1965 Inherited antithrombin III deficiency causing thrombophilia. Thromb Diathesis Haemorrhagica 13: 516–530

Elias M, Eldor A 1984 Thromboembolism in patients with the 'lupus'-type circulating anticoagulant. Arch Intern Med 144: 510–515

Engesser L, Broekmans A W, Briet E, Brommer E J P, Bertina R N 1987 Hereditary protein S deficiency: clinical manifestations. Ann Intern Med 106: 667–682

Exner T, Rickard A, Kronberg H 1978 A sensitive test demonstrating lupus anticoagulant and its behavioural pattern. Br J Haematol 40: 143–151

Galli M, Maussen C, Comfurius P, Hemker H C et al 1990 Isolation and characterisation of a plasmatic factor interacting with anticardiolipin antibodies. Clin Exp Rheumatol 8: 206

Gastineau D A, Kazmier F J, Nichols W L, Bowie E J W 1985 Lupus anticoagulant: an analysis of the clinical and laboratory features of 219 cases. Am J Haematol 19: 265–275

Gladson C L, Sharrer I, Hach V, Beck K H, Griffin J H 1988 The frequency of type I heterozygous protein C deficiency in 141 unrelated young patients with venous thrombosis. Thromb Haemostasis 59: 18–22

Green D, Hougie C, Kazmier F J, Lechner K et al 1983 Report of the working party on acquired inhibitors of coagulation: studies of the 'lupus' anticoagulant. Thromb Haemostasis 49: 143–146

Griffin J H, Evatt B, Zimmerman T S, Kleiss A J, Widenman C 1981 Deficiency of protein C in congenital thrombotic disease. J Clin Invest 68: 1370–1373

Hamsten A, Norberg R, Bjorkholm M, de Faire U, Holm G 1986 Antibodies to cardiolipin in young survivors of myocardial infarction: an association with recurrent cardiovascular events. Lancet 1: 113–116

Harris E N, Gharavi A E, Hegde U, Derue G et al 1985 Anticardiolipin antibodies in autoimmune thrombocytopenic purpura. Br J Haematol 59: 231–234

Harris E N, Gharavi A E, Patel S P, Hughes G R V 1987 Evaluation of the anticardiolipin tests: report of an international workshop held on 4 April 1986. Clin Exp Immunol 68: 215–222

Haserick J R, Long R 1952 Systemic lupus erythematosus preceded by false positive tests for syphilis. Ann Int Med 37: 559–565

Hirsh J, Piovella S, Pini M 1989 Congenital antithrombin III deficiency. Am J Med 87 (suppl 3B): 34–38

Hughes G R V 1983 Thrombosis, abortion, cerebral disease and the lupus anticoagulant. Br Med J 287: 1088–1089

Hughes G R V 1988 An immune mechanism in thrombosis. Q J Med 258: 753–754

Lane D A, Caso R 1989 Antithrombin: structure, genomic organisation, function and inherited deficiency. In: Tuddenham E G (ed) Molecular biology of coagulation. Baillière Tindall, London

Lockshin M D, Druzin M L, Goei S, Qamar T et al 1985 Antibody to cardiolipin as a predictor of fetal distress or death in pregnant patients with systemic lupus erythematosus. N Engl J Med 313: 152–156

Machin S J, Giddings J, Greaves M, Hutton R et al 1990 Detection of the lupus like anticoagulant: current laboratory practice in the United Kingdom. J Clin Pathol 43: 73–79

McNeil H P, Chesterman C N, Krilis S A 1990 Antiphospholipid antibodies are directed against a complex antigen which includes a lipid-binding plasma glycoprotein. Clin Exp Rheumatol 8: 209

Malia R G, Greaves M, Rowlands L M, Lawrence A C K et al 1988 Anticardiolipin antibodies in systemic sclerosis: immunological and clinical associations. Clin Exp Immunol 73: 456–460

Malia R G, Kitchen S, Greaves M, Preston F E 1990 The inhibitory effect of antiphospholipid antibodies on the natural anticoagulant protein C/protein S pathway. Br J Haematol (in press)

Mannucci P M, Tripodi A 1987 Laboratory screening of inherited thrombotic syndromes. Thromb Haemostasis 57: 247–251

Mannucci P M, Tripodi A 1988 Inherited factors in thrombosis. Blood Rev 2: 27–35

Marcum J A, McKenney J B, Rosenberg R D 1984 Acceleration of thrombin–antithrombin complex formation in rat hind quarters via naturally occurring heparin-like molecules bound to the endothelium. J Clin Invest 74: 341–350

Marlar R A, Montgomery R R, Broekmans A W 1989 Diagnosis and treatment of homozygous protein C deficiency. Report of the working party on homozygous protein C deficiency of the sub-committee on protein C and protein S. International Committee on Thrombosis and Haemostasis. J Pediatr 114: 528–534

Miletich J, Sherman L, Broze G 1987 Absence of thrombosis and subjects with heterozygous protein C deficiency. N Engl J Med 317: 991–996

Morton K E, Gavaghan T P, Krilis S A, Daggard G E et al 1986 Coronary artery bypass graft failure: an autoimmune phenomenon? Lancet 2: 1353–1357

Peter J B 1990 Cardiolipin antibody assays. Lancet 335: 1405

Petri M, Rheinschmidt M, Whiting-O'Keefe Q, Hellmann D et al 1989 Russell viper venom test for the lupus anticoagulant is a more specific associate of thrombosis than anticardiolipin antibody. Clin Exp Rheumatol 6: 210

Prochownik E V 1989 Molecular genetics of inherited antithrombin III deficiencies. Am J Med 87(suppl 3B): 15–18

Prochownik E V, Markham A F, Orkin S H 1983 Isolation of a cDNA clone for human antithrombin III. J Biol Chem 128: 8389–8394

Rosenberg R D 1975 Actions and interactions of antithrombin and heparin. N Engl J Med 292: 146–151

Rosenberg R D 1989 Biochemistry of heparin antithrombin interactions, and the physiologic role of the natural anticoagulant mechanism. Am J Med 97(suppl 3B): 2–9

Sie P, Pichou J, Dupouy D, Boneu B 1985 Constitutional heparin co-factor II deficiency associated with recurrent thrombosis. Lancet 2: 414–416

Taberner D A, Giddings J, Greaves M, Hutton R et al 1990 The lupus anticoagulant working party of the BCSH Haemostasis and Thrombosis Task Force of the British Society for Haematology. Guidelines on testing for the lupus anticoagulant (in preparation)

Thaler E, Lechner K 1981 Antithrombin III deficiency and thromboembolism. Clin Haematol 10: 369–390

Tran T H, Narbet G A, Duckert F 1985 Association of heparin co-factor II deficiency with thrombosis. Lancet 2: 413–414

Triplett D A, Brandt J T, Musgrave K A, Orr C A 1988 The relationship between lupus anticoagulants and antibodies to phospholipid. JAMA 259: 550–554

Tripodi A, Franchi F, Krachmalnicoff A, Mannucci P M 1990 Asymptomatic homozygous protein C deficiency. Acta Haematol 83: 152–155

Tuddenham E G D, Takse T, Thomas A E et al 1989 Homozygous protein C deficiency with delayed onset of symptoms at 7–10 months. Thromb Res 53: 475–484

Vykidal R, Korninger C, Kyrir P A et al 1985 The prevalence of antithrombin III deficiency in patients with a history of venous thromboembolism. Thromb Haemostasis 54: 744–745

8

Haemophilia: diagnosis and management

A.L. Bloom   I.R. Peake

During the five years that have elapsed since the fourth edition of this book similar aspects of haemophilia remain important but there have been some notable advances in genetic diagnosis and in therapy which will be described in this chapter.

HAEMOPHILIA DIAGNOSIS

Phenotypic diagnosis

The diagnosis of haemophilia in the child and adult is based on measurement of plasma factor VIII or IX levels. A range of assays is available including clotting, chromogenic and immunological assays, the latter being only applicable in cases where the disease results from both qualitative and quantitative deficiency of the appropriate factor. Prenatal diagnosis by measurement of factor VIII or IX in fetal blood obtained in the 2nd trimester (18–20 weeks) by either fetoscopy or ultrasound scan-guided cordocentesis has been the mainstay of prenatal diagnosis in the haemophilias (Mibashan et al 1989). Experience of over 300 cases at King's College London has underlined the accuracy of the techniques, their only drawback being the lateness of any ensuing elective termination.

Genotypic diagnosis

The advent of molecular biology and genetics has resulted in important advances in the diagnosis of the carrier state in the haemophilias and has also resulted in prenatal diagnostic procedures which may be performed at 8–10 weeks gestation on chorionic villus sample (CVS) material. Diagnosis based on DNA (gene) analysis is of two sorts.

1. Gene tracking using intragenic or extragenic (linked) DNA polymorphisms, generally detected as restriction fragment length polymorphisms (RFLPs).
2. Detection of the precise genetic defect responsible for the disease in an affected member and subsequently in possible carriers or a male fetus at risk.

In the following few pages the present situation with regard to genotypic diagnosis in haemophilia A and B are reviewed. For more detailed descriptions the reader is referred to Tuddenham (1989), Chapter 5 of this book and Giannelli (1989). The most dramatic advance in the techniques of DNA analysis has been the introduction of polymerase chain reaction (PCR)-based procedures whereby selected short regions of DNA can be amplified to such an extent that they can be readily visualized and analysed without the need for radiolabelled DNA probes. PCR is taking over from Southern blotting procedures in many cases and the reader is strongly recommended to read several reviews on the theory and application of the technique (Peake 1989, Macintyre 1989, Eisenstein 1990).

Haemophilia A

RFLP analysis. Five intragenic and two linked RFLPs have been described for the factor VIII gene which are useful in tracking haemophilia A within affected families (Table 8.1). The intragenic RFLPs are all diallelic, and overall, taking into account linkage disequilibrium, some 70–75% of females are heterozygous for at least one of them. The fragments given in Table 8.1 are those seen with the appropriate probe and an example of a family study with the BclI RFLP is given in Figure 8.1. PCR techniques for the detection of the BclI RFLP, where a DNA fragment of 142 base pairs (b.p.) containing the polymorphic BclI site is amplified, have also been described (Kogan et al 1987). The presence (or absence) of the polymorphic site is revealed by digestion of the amplified fragment with BclI giving bands of 99 and 43 b.p. if the site is present (Fig. 8.2). A similar procedure has also been described for the XbaI RFLP (Kogan et al 1987).

The heterozygosity rates for the factor VIII RFLPs has been shown to vary between different ethnic populations. For example, the BglI RFLP has not been detected in Chinese populations, while it is more frequent in American blacks (38%) compared with American whites (24%). The two

Table 8.1 Factor VIII gene RFLP

Enzyme	Probe	Fragments (k.b.)	Heterozygosity (%)	Reference
BclI	p114.12	1.1/0.8	42	Gitschier et al (1985)
BglI	c-DNA	20/5	24	Antonarakis et al (1985)
XbaI	p486.2	6.2/4.8(1.4)	49	Wion et al (1986)
MspI	p624.3	7.5/4.3	43	Youssoufian et al (1987)
HindIII	p114.12	2.7/2.6	42	Ahrens et al (1987)
BglII	DX13(L)	5.8/2.8	50	Harper et al (1984)
TaqI MspI	ST14(L)	Various	70	Oberle et al (1985)

(L), linked probe.
Heterozygosity (%) for white European/North American populations.
Data compiled from published and unpublished reports by IRP for ISTH SSC factor VIII/IX Subcommittee.

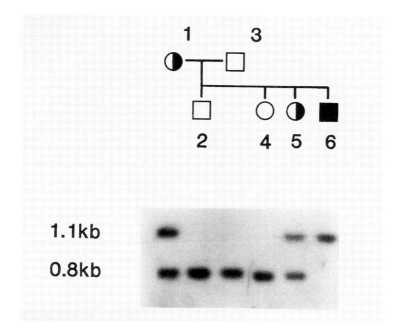

Fig. 8.1 Haemophilia A family study using the intragenic BclI RFLP detected by probe p114.12 and Southern blotting (Gitschier et al 1985). Patient 5 is diagnosed as a carrier and patient 4 as a non-carrier.

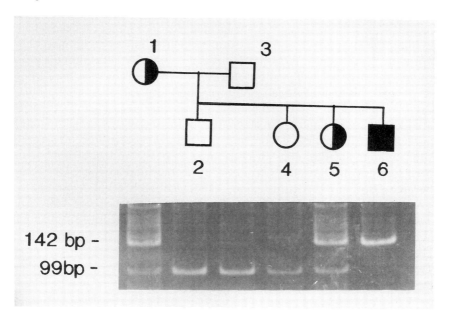

Fig. 8.2 Haemophilia A family study (as in Fig. 8.1). The intragenic BclI RFLP has been detected by digestion of PCR amplified DNA (Kogan et al 1987).

linked RFLPs used in haemophilia A studies (DX13/BglII and ST14/TaqI/ MspI) are both highly informative, particularly ST14, which is multiallelic. However, studies have shown a cross-over rate of up to 5% between the DX13 and ST14 loci (DXS15 and DXS52) and the factor VIII gene locus, so necessitating probability assessment in carrier studies and prenatal diagnosis.

Detection of specific defects. The size (181 k.b.) and complexity (26 exons) of the factor VIII gene have meant that the detection of the specific defect within a particular haemophilia A patient has, in most cases, proved to be a difficult task. Factor VIII gene deletions (either partial or total) have been reported and occur in some 5% of severely affected patients, some of whom have developed inhibitors to factor VIII as a result of replacement therapy. However, there appears to be little correlation between the size and location of the deletion and the occurrence of an inhibitor. Restriction enzyme analysis has revealed a series of point mutations almost entirely detected by the enzyme TaqI (cutting site TCGA). This appears to be due to the propensity for C to T transitions within CpG dinucleotides (probably as a result of deamination of methylated cystosine). Thus within the TaqI site a change from TCGA to TTGA occurs and, if the CGA is in frame, this results in an arginine to Stop codon mutation (e.g. at Arg 1941, Arg 2116, Arg 2147, Arg 2209 and Arg 2307 in the factor VIII molecule). The frequency of this change is underlined by the fact that the same mutation has been reported within several unrelated severely affected individuals. Clearly the introduction of a Stop codon within the normally transcribed region of the gene will result in a truncated peptide being produced which is either inactive, poorly secreted from the cells or has a very limited half-life in the circulation. C to T transitions at the same site but within the non-coding DNA strand will result in Arg (CGA) to Gln (CAA) in the coding strand and this change has also been reported (e.g. Gitschier et al 1986).

PCR amplification and direct analysis of specific areas of the factor VIII gene known to contain sequences coding for important functional domains in the factor VIII molecule have met with limited success. Recently Arg to Cys mutations at thrombin cleavage sites (Arg 372 and Arg 1689) have been reported, both resulting from a C to T transition so that CGC (Arg) becomes TGC (Cys) (Pattinson et al 1989, O'Brien & Tuddenham 1989). These patients have circulating levels of non-functional factor VIII (Arg 372 mutation < 1.0 u/dl VIIIC) or factor VIII with reduced functional activity (Arg 1689 4 u/dl VIIIC) i.e. CRM + haemophilia. An Arg 372 to His mutation has also been reported in a mild haemophiliac (Arai et al 1989). It is likely that further PCR studies will identify defects in other important areas of the factor VIII protein.

Haemophilia B

RFLP analysis. Seven intragenic and one linked RFLPs have proved of use in the tracking of the affected factor IX gene in haemophilia B families (Table 8.2). An overall heterozygosity rate of better than 90% has been reported for the intragenic RFLPs within white European and North American populations. However, considerable ethnic variation in heterozygosity for several of the RFLPs has been reported. Indeed the TaqI, XmnI and DdeI RFLPs are not detected in Japanese populations, and at only low levels in Chinese and Malays. The TaqI, XmnI, MspI and BamHI RFLPs are a result of point mutations and are generally detected by Southern blotting with appropriate probes, although PCR-based methods are being developed. DdeI detects a polymorphism resulting from the presence or absence of a 50-b.p. intron insert sequence. The HhaI RFLP can only be detected by digestion of PCR-amplified DNA, since in the original genomic DNA a cytosine in the HhaI recognition site (GCGC) is methylated, so preventing HhaI cleavage. PCR amplified sequences are not methylated. HhaI is a particularly useful RFLP since it has a high heterozygosity rate (48%) and is in complete linkage equilibrium with the TaqI, XmnI and DdeI RFLPs (Winship et al 1989). The MnlI RFLP arises as a result of an alanine/threonine dimorphism at amino acid 148 in the factor IX activation peptide. Because of this the polymorphism may also be detected in an immunological assay using specific monoclonal antibodies (Thompson et al 1988). The linked SstI RFLP, detected by a probe at the DXS99 locus, has a high frequency both in white European and North Americans (49%) and in the Japanese (50%), where it is the only informative genetic marker for the factor IX gene described so far. Its recombination rate with the factor IX gene is probably less than 5%.

Detection of specific defects. The human factor IX gene is considerably smaller than that for factor VIII, with eight exons and a length of 33.5 kb. Use of a range of cDNA and genomic probes and, more recently, PCR amplification of each exon followed by DNA sequencing or chemical cleavage

Table 8.2 Factor IX gene RFLP

Enzyme	Probe	Fragments (k.b.)	Heterozygosity (%)	Reference
TaqI	VIII	1.8/1.3	43	Giannelli et al (1984)
XmnI	VIII	11.5/6.5	37	Winship et al (1984)
DdeI	XIII	1.75/1.7	36	Winship et al (1984)
MspI	c-DNA	5.8/2.4	36	Freedenberg et al (1987)
BamHI	VIII	25/23	4	Hay et al (1986)
SstI	DXS99(L)	8.8/5.9	49	Mulligan et al (1987)
MnlI	(PCR)	–	43	Graham et al (1989)
HhaI	(PCR)	–	48	Winship et al (1989)

(L), linked probe.
(PCR), detected by PCR reaction.
MnlI also detected by monoclonal antibodies (Ala/Thr dimorphism).
Heterozygosity (%) for white European/North American population.
Data compiled from published and unpublished reports by IRP for ISTH SSC factor VIII/IX Subcommittee.

analysis has resulted in a considerable list of defects. Some 21 patients with total or partial factor IX gene deletions have been reported (Giannelli 1989), and of these 18 developed inhibitors to factor IX. Of the remaining individuals, one had circulating levels of factor IX protein (exon d is deleted but this allowed for a normal splice of exon c to exon e, resulting in a molecule with the first growth factor domain missing). In a second case where exons e and f were deleted, factor IX antigen was detectable in the patient's urine. The number of point mutations and small deletions detected within the factor IX genes of patients with haemophilia B has increased dramatically with the advent of PCR as mentioned above and a full description of the defects described is outside the scope of this chapter. For example, a number of mutations which cause premature termination of factor IX synthesis have been observed as a result of either a base substitution resulting in a Stop codon (e.g. haemophilia B Malmo 3 Arg 248 to Stop), or a small deletion resulting in a frame shift. A comprehensive list of point mutations throughout the factor IX gene has recently been published by Giannelli (1989), and it is now clear that expert laboratories are now able to detect the genetic defect in the majority of patients referred to them. Significantly some 30% of point mutations appear to involve C to T transitions. Once detected the defect can be used as an absolute marker in family studies and in prenatal diagnosis.

HAEMOPHILIA TREATMENT

Five important aspects of therapy will be reviewed: the present status of viral infection in the haemophiliac, especially the hepatidides and human immunodeficiency virus infection; the development of new factor concentrates including recombinant clotting factors; the treatment of von Willebrand's disease; the management of patients with factor inhibitors; and the outlook for gene transfer therapy.

Viral infections in haemophilia

Hepatitis

The background knowledge concerning hepatitis was reviewed in the last edition of this series. With regard to hepatitis B (HBV) the effectiveness of immunization with both plasma-derived and recombinant vaccine has been confirmed. It should be noted that antibody response tends to fall off with age and where possible effectiveness should be checked by means of quantitative antibody assay. It is important that susceptibility to hepatitis B is checked in all patients by serological testing, and vaccination or re-vaccination offered as appropriate. Vaccination should also be offered to susceptible house contacts and haemophilia centre staff.

As the problem of hepatitis B became a little more contained, concern about non-A non-B (NANB) hepatitis strengthened with the realization of high incidence of chronic liver disease in spite of earlier optimistic reports. Epidemiological studies of hepatitis in haemophiliacs had suggested that NANB hepatitis is caused by two viruses. Further evidence may follow the identification of the hepatitis C virus (HCV). Using techniques of molecular biology and gene cloning with nucleic acid derived from infectious plasma, Choo et al (1989) developed a construct which coded for a protein reacting with hepatitic serum. Further extension of the original construct and expression in yeast allowed the development of an antigen suitable for use in a hepatitis C antibody test (see Zuckerman 1989 for review). Although confirmatory tests are needed preliminary results suggest that anti-HCV is present in 0.5% of the normal blood donor population (Kuhnl et al 1989, Janot et al 1989), a finding consistent with previous epidemiological data relating to NANB post-transfusion hepatitis. Thus haemophiliacs treated with unheated pooled blood products should all be infected, a supposition in keeping with clinical data. Preliminary serological data (Table 8.3) indicate that about 60–80% of treated haemophiliacs are positive for HCV antibodies (Roggendorf et al 1989, Noel et al 1989, Ludlam et al 1989). It is not clear why all patients treated with older large pool concentrates are not seropositive; initial test systems may not be sufficiently sensitive, some patients may not respond by antibody production and of course there may be other NANB hepatitis viruses. The term hepatitis D (HDV) is reserved for the Delta virus infection but no doubt others will be described in due course. As one might expect, raised incidence of HCV antibodies was detected in intravenous drug abusers (Mortimer et al 1989) and in patients with chronic liver disease (Esteban et al 1989). Worrying from the point of view of haemophiliacs are reports of high incidence of HCV antibodies in patients with hepatocellular carcinoma (Bruix et al 1989, Colombo et al 1989) independently of infection with HBV or excess alcohol intake.

Treatment for HCV (NANB) hepatitis

The above considerations make it important that a treatment for hepatitis is developed as soon as possible. Recombinant interferon alpha and human lymphoblastoid interferon have been shown to be effective in chronic

Table 8.3 Hepatitis C antibody tests: initial reports

| Author (1989) | Patients tested | Percentage positive overall | | | |
		Haem A	Haem B	vWD	Overall
Esteban et al	97	68	71	58	70
Roggendorf et al	211	–	–	–	78
Noel et al	400	63	75	–	61
Ludlam et al	61	85	90	80	85

Estimates in donor populations = ˜ 0.13 – 1.2%, mean about 0.5%.

hepatitis B (Thomas & Scully 1985). Jacyna et al (1989) report a favourable effect of interferon in seven patients with NANB hepatitis in a randomized controlled trial. Aspartate transaminase levels were reduced and the authors concluded that treatment may prevent progression to cirrhosis. These findings are encouraging but the need for ongoing treatment is not known. This is an important consideration not least because of the unpleasant side effects of interferon therapy.

HIV infection

Epidemiological features. Since the introduction of sensitive and specific tests for antibodies to the human immunodeficiency virus (HIV) the pattern of infection in haemophiliacs has become apparent. A majority of patients treated with large pool factor VIII concentrates imported from the United States during the years 1979–1984 were infected but domestic concentrates and those produced in other countries also became contaminated.

At one time it was thought that the accession rate of HIV-positive haemophiliacs to symptoms of immunodeficiency lagged behind that of other risk groups. More recent epidemiological data (Ragni et al 1987) do not support this conclusion but further data indicate that the rate of progression to AIDS is strongly dependent upon age (Darby et al 1989, Goedert et al 1989). According to Goedert et al older adults seemed to be disproportionately affected during the earlier phases of HIV disease and cytomegalovirus infection appears to be associated with a more rapid progression to HIV disease (Webster et al 1989). The ultimate proportion of HIV antibody-positive haemophiliacs who become symptomatic remains to become apparent but to date overall about 40% have done so within 5–6 years of seroconversion (Table 8.4). Similar conclusions were reached by Ward and colleagues (1989) in patients infected with HIV from ordinary blood transfusion. In 1985 AIDS overtook intracranial bleeding as the commonest cause of death in haemophilia in the UK.

Most haemophiliacs and their partners are counselled regarding sexual transmission of HIV. In UK some 29 out of 493 (6%) of partners at risk have seroconverted. This proportion is similar to that found in a recent study of partners of non-haemophiliacs without other risk factors (De Vincenzi 1989). In another more optimistic study in haemophiliacs (Van

Table 8.4 Aids incubation period in haemophilia

Author	Time since seroconv.	Symptoms (%)	AIDS (%)
Ragni et al (1987)	>5y	34	12
Giesecke et al (1988)	6y	40	7
Stain et al (1989)	>5y	48	18

der Ende et al 1988) the number of partners (13) was too small to draw valid conclusions.

Further information of epidemiological importance may develop by the application of the polymerase chain reaction (PCR) for amplification of HIV-specific DNA. Using this technique HIV-specific DNA has been detected in newborns from HIV-infected mothers (Laure et al 1988) and, more worrying with regard to haemophiliacs and their partners, in seronegative individuals from very high-risk groups (Loche & Mach 1988). The significance of the latter observations is not yet fully apparent but it is well established that HIV antibody does not develop in a proportion of recipients of known infected batches (lots) of factor VIII. Perhaps a proportion of such patients have been infected with HIV but have not mounted an antibody response. It should be noted that PCR is an ultrasensitive technique and false positives from laboratory cross-contamination is a hazard. Furthermore the detection of viral DNA does not necessarily indicate the presence of replicative virus; RNA amplification may be more relevant in this respect.

Similar considerations apply to the widespread use of the test for screening blood for transfusion and preparation of factor VIII concentrates, or for the testing of the final products.

Clinical and therapeutic aspects. The clinical course of HIV infection in haemophilia is similar to that seen in other risk groups. Concomitant sexually transmitted diseases are of course no more prevalent in haemophilia than in the general population. Kaposi's sarcoma (KS) is unusual but has been reported. It was thought that the presence of HLA DR5 phenotype and repeated CMV infection could have been important codeterminants of KS in this case (de Biasi et al 1989).

To date the only effective specific treatment for HIV infection is azidothymidine (Zidovudine). There is little doubt that this is of some benefit in patients with AIDS but marrow toxicity on full dosage may limit treatment in these patients. It is not yet clear if Zidovudine in reduced dosage will prolong life in asymptomatic HIV-infected patients or in those with falling T4 cell counts. These aspects are presently under study, for instance in a joint UK–French (MRC–INSERM) trial. Preliminary unpublished results of studies in the USA suggest a role for this form of treatment and many physicians would now regard a steady fall of T4 cells as an indication for Zidovudine therapy in asymptomatic HIV-infected patients. One important indication for Zidovudine therapy in haemophiliacs is thrombocytopenia when this is thought to be of autoimmune nature (ITP) and not a part of more general HIV-induced marrow disease (Flegg et al 1989, Hymes et al 1988). Marrow examination, covered by factor VIII therapy, is an important aspect of assessment, and if the findings are consistent with ITP the platelet count may be corrected by Zidovudine therapy.

Parvovirus B19 infection

Although not usually considered to be a serious infection parvovirus B19 is receiving increasing attention as a complication of haemophilia therapy. B19 infection commonly occurs in normal people, especially in children, and causes a self-limiting mild disorder – erythema infectiosum. The virus has a curious predilection for marrow red cell precursors and causes aplastic crises in haemolytic anaemas as well as persistent anaemia in immuno-compromised persons. In pregnant women it can lead to fetal infection with hydrops fetalis and fetal death. Persons infected with B19 may have inter-mittent viraemia and this becomes a potential problem in blood donors and hence in blood products such as factor VIII and IX concentrates, especially as the virus is thermoresistant. Serological evidence of parvovirus infection was detected in haemophiliacs treated with unheated (Mortimer et al 1983) and heat-treated factor VIII concentrate (Corsi et al 1988) whilst sympto-matic B19 infection has been observed after therapy with factor IX concen-trate heated at 80°C for 72 hours (Lyon et al 1989). Parvovirus B19 can be acquired as a nosocomial infection and this could represent a potential risk to health care workers, especially to those who are pregnant. The subject is reviewed by Anderson & Torok (1989).

Blood products for haemophilia therapy

The realization that blood and blood products transmit infectious diseases led to the development of screening of donated blood and viricidal procedures for 'sterilizing' factor concentrates. These were originally developed for hepatitis viruses but serendipitously were found to be more effective against HIV. Screening procedures include self-selection of donors and serological tests such as those for hepatitis B antigen and HIV antibody. Until recently no serological tests were available that would detect carriers of NANB hepatitis. In some countries surrogate tests, e.g. of alanine amino transferase levels, were used with arguable effectiveness. Hopefully the new tests for hepatitis C antibodies (see above) will help further to eliminate dangerous donations.

Processes designed to sterilize factor concentrates are of three main types:

1. Heat.
2. Chemical.
3. Immunoaffinity separation of viruses from factor.

Heat treatment

The effect of heat treatment depends on:

a. Temperature and duration.
b. Presence of moisture.

c. Protein stabilizers (which may also stabilize viruses).
d. Presence of organic solvents which may dissolve viral lipid envelopes.

The presence of moisture is very important. Dry heat is less effective, other things being equal, than heating in aqueous solution or in water vapour under pressure.

Thus concentrate pasteurized at 60°C for 10 hours in aqueous solution seems to be as sterile (Schimpf et al 1987) as that heated in the dry state at 80°C for 72 hours (report of Study Group 1988) but the yield is very much lower. On the other hand concentrates heated in the dry state at lower temperatures such as 60°C and 68°C have been found to transmit hepatitis viruses and in some cases HIV (see below). A method involving heating concentrate in an organic solvent heptane slurry reduces but does not abolish the risk of transmission of NANB hepatitis (Kernoff et al 1987). One advantage of an effective stringent dry heat process is that it is applied to the product in the final vial, thus safeguarding against in-process cross-contamination.

Chemical processes

β-Propiolactone with ultraviolet light has been successfully used to sterilize factor IX–prothrombin complex concentrates but this process inactivates factor VIII. More recently the use of organic solvent and detergent combinations have been described, particularly tri(n-butyl) phosphate (TNBP) and either sodium cholate or Tween 80 to inactivate lipid-enveloped viruses. This seems to be effective against hepatitis viruses and HIV (Horowitz et al 1988).

Immunoaffinity purification

The purification of factor VIII using solid-phase antibodies was originally undertaken as a preliminary to gene cloning but has since been developed on a commercial scale for therapeutic concentrates. Plasma or preliminary concentrate is passed over solid-phase immunoadsorbent to which has been bound monoclonal antibodies to factor VIII or von Willebrand's factor (vWF). The factor VIII–vWF complex or factor VIII alone binds to solid phase, and other plasma constituents including viruses pass through and are thereby separated. The immobilized factor VIII is washed, eluted from the solid phase and further purified by chromatographic methods. At an appropriate stage a sterilization process is introduced, e.g. solvent/detergent in the case of Hemofil M (Baxter) or pasteurization in the case of Monoclate P (Armour). The process is capable of producing very pure factor VIII with specific activity of about 3000 u/mg, which is close to the theoretical maximum but for stability and other pharmaceutical reasons it is formulated for therapeutic use in pasteurized human albumin to a final specific activity of about 15 u/mg. As far as is known there seems to be little carry-over of mouse proteins from the monoclonal antibodies and the materials seem to be secure from hepatitis viruses and HIV.

Assessment of viral safety

The availability of serological tests for hepatitis B and HIV infection simplifies the assessment of safety of an individual concentrate from these viruses provided that the patients have not previously been exposed to other materials within a reasonable incubation period. Thus with regard to HIV a concentrate subjected to dry heat at 60°C for only 30 hours has been associated with several seroconversions and a handful of cases have been associated with other concentrates (Mariani et al 1987, MMWR 1988).

The assessment of safety from NANB viruses may be assisted by the HCV antibody test discussed above, but this will not entirely solve the problem because of the probable existence of other hepatitis viruses. Assessment in patients previously unexposed (PUPs) to blood or blood products will therefore continue to be needed. The recommended method has been updated by Mannucci & Colombo (1989) but it should be noted that even with a series of 30 patients according to the statistical rule of three the risk of transmission is still 0–10%.

The risk of transmission of any given virus in concentrates prepared from large pools of plasma is obviously also related to the prevalence of infection in the donor population and the effectiveness of screening. For HIV in USA the antibody prevalence is 1 in 7500 and the suggested virus prevalence after screening is 1 in 130 000 (Cumming et al 1989). Thus for plasma pools of 20 000 per lot, 15% of lots would be infected. In the UK the corresponding figures are much lower. Antibody prevalence is 1 in 50 000, viral prevalence is about 1 in 800 000 and plasma pools are about 8000. Thus only about 1% of batches of factor VIII concentrate would be infected. These types of considerations must be taken into account in assessing safety from a particular virus.

It is unlikely that any plasma-derived concentrate can be guaranteed free from all live viruses and of course occasional failure of quality-control processes may occur. For this reason all susceptible patients, house contacts and health care workers should be counselled accordingly and offered vaccination against hepatitis B.

Factor VIII concentrates and immune modulation

Apart from the immunocompromising effect of HIV infection it has been claimed that protein or other non-viral contaminants of factor concentrates may down-regulate immune function. In vitro effects on peripheral blood mononuclear cells include down-regulations of Fc receptors (Mannhalter et al 1988), inhibition of IL2 production (Thorpe et al 1989) and impaired mixed lymphocyte reactions and phytohaemagglutinin transformation (Schreiber et al 1987). In vivo effects include reduction of T4 cells, reduced production of γ-interferon by peripheral blood cells and reduced cutaneous hypersensitivity (Madhok et al 1986, Ruffault et al 1988).

It has been claimed that this down-regulation of immune function may be important clinically or may further aggravate the effects of HIV infection (Brettler et al 1989). This possibility has been put forward to justify the use of expensive highly purified concentrates such as those prepared by monoclonal antibody immunoaffinity. However, clinical immune impairment was not a feature of haemophilia in the heyday of therapy with crude concentrates such as cryoprecipitate, the evidence for immune benefit of highly purified products in clinical practice is not convincing and the long-term effect of their content of human albumin remains to be assessed. At the present time therefore this problem is not resolved.

Recombinant factor VIII (rFVIII)

As described in the previous edition of this series, the cloning and expression of factor VIII was reported by two groups in 1984. This was a remarkable achievement because of the low concentration of factor VIII, its high molecular weight, and low concentration and availability of mRNA. Expression in a mammalian cell system was necessary to achieve glycosylation and for effective production in Chinese hamster ovary cells co-expression or presence of vWF was needed. vWF stabilizes factor VIII, promotes the association of heavy and light chains and protects factor VIII from proteolysis (see Kaufman 1989 for review). The assessment of rFVIII included its coagulation and amidolytic activity, neutralization by human anti-FVIII and reaction with monoclonal anti-FVIII, binding to vWF, inactivation patterns by thrombin and protein C, electrophoretic pattern, absence of neoantigenic sites on animal inoculation, and sequence data. The expressed material is purified using a monoclonal antibody immunoaffinity technique and the final product must be free of murine and hamster proteins. It is deficient of vWF and like plasma-derived pure factor VIII must be formulated in pasteurized human albumin. Regretfully, therefore, it is not devoid of human blood derivatives.

To date two companies, Baxter Healthcare and Cutter Biologicals, have entered rVIII into experimental and clinical trials. Early studies in haemophilic dogs showed that it has virtually identical properties to plasma-derived FVIII (pdFVIII) (Giles et al 1988b) and this has now been confirmed in clinical trials (White et al 1989, Harrison & Bloom 1990). Efficacy trials, home treatment and assessment of its use in major surgery are now under way. No doubt rFVIII will be licensed for therapy, but its economic role in haemophilia therapy remains to be assessed. For haemophilia B recombinant factor IX has been a less attractive commercial proposition because plasma levels needed by concentration are about 50 times higher than those of factor VIII, whilst patients are fewer in number. Furthermore the post-translational modifications such as γ-carboxylation have been difficult. Nevertheless, therapeutic rFIX will no doubt be produced and like monoclonal plasma derived factor IX concentrate could have distinct advantages over current IX-PCC with regard to the incidence of thrombotic complications.

Treatment of factor VIII inhibitors

This subject has been reviewed recently by Bloom (1987) and Kasper (1989). It is intended to comment here only on selected recent advances.
Treatment of inhibitors can be divided into two main types:

1. Treatment designed to suppress the development of antibody to factor VIII or to induce immune tolerance
2. Treatment of acute bleeding episodes.

Induction of immune tolerance

Nilsson and colleagues (1988) have described an apparently successful regime. This is based on a number of developments.

a. Extracorporeal immunodepletion of factor VIII or IX inhibitors using solid-phase staphylococcal protein A.
b. The exhibition of an immunosuppressive agent, cyclophosphamide, whilst at the same time administering high dose of factor VIII (or IX).
c. The administration of high-dose intravenous IgG, given originally to replace that removed by the protein A column but serendipitously found to potentiate the immunotolerating process.

For details the original description should be consulted (Nilsson et al 1988), but the regime was successful in 9/11 patients with haemophilia A and 3/4 patients with haemophilia B. It was found that a new species of non-neutralizing antibodies developed in the successfully treated patients.
The results of using this regime need to be confirmed. Many patients with inhibitors are infected with HIV and this may be considered by some to be a drawback for the use of cytotoxic drugs and complicated extracorporeal circuits. In addition there is a suggestion that HIV infection itself may be associated with a decline of inhibitor potency (Ragni et al 1989).

Treatment of acute bleeding episodes

The use of conventional factor VIII bypassing materials and activated and non-activated PCC has been reviewed by Bloom (1987). A consensus of clinical trials indicated that non-activated PCC was effective in about 50% of episodes, activated PCC in about 65% compared to a placebo effect of albumin in about 25% of episodes, but the degree of effect was not as great as that seen in non-inhibitor patients treated with factor VIII, and the influence of heat-treatment processes on the effectiveness of these materials has not been assessed. These constraints and the reports of thrombotic episodes in patients treated with PCC has prompted the search for alternative forms of factor VIII bypassing agents.

a. The observations reviewed by Bloom (1987) and Kasper (1989) that phospholipid protects factor VIII from interaction with inhibitor has prompted the development of phospholipid and factor VIII preparation for use in patients but clinical studies have not yet been reported.

b. Giles and colleagues (1988a) noted that phospholipid and factor Xa could be a determinant of thrombogenicity of PCC and have developed a carefully formulated mixture which is currently undergoing pre-clinical trials for efficacy in inhibitor patients.

c. According to conventional coagulation theory factor VIIa acts independently of the intrinsic system. It is dependent on tissue factor and may induce local haemostasis at the site of injury in haemophilia without systemic effect. Hedner & Kisiel (1983) used pdVIIa for successful management of two inhibitor patients. The method has been placed on a more realistic basis by the development at NOVO Industri by Thim et al (1988) of recombinant human VIIa in transfected baby hamster kidney cells. It is almost fully carboxylated and with similar glycosylation to human pdVIIa. Successful use of rVIIa has been reported in massive doses for synovectomy (Hedner et al 1988) and in more modest dose for treatment of sublingual haematoma with no adverse effects (Macik et al 1988). About 30–40 patients have been treated to date in a multicentre international trial with encouraging results. Personal experience indicates that to be effective levels of factor VIIC greater than 6 u/ml must be achieved and unexpectedly there is considerable shortening of the APTT. To date, however, there have been no untoward effects and no evidence of intravascular coagulation.

d. With a similar theoretical background to the use of rVIIa, recombinant tissue factor could also be a possible therapeutic means of bypassing factor VIII inhibitor (see O'Brien 1989 for review).

Use of these materials should be restricted at the moment to expert centres. Disaster could follow uncritical sequential ad hoc trials in dangerously ill patients – for instance, materials which contain a trace of tissue factor could trigger intravascular coagulation if given before or after rVIIa.

It should be noted that rVIIa does not contain stabilizing human blood derivatives and if proved to be effective it could represent an acceptable form of treatment for Jehovah's Witnesses.

Treatment of von Willebrand's disease (vWD)

Until recently deamino-D-arginine vasopression (DDAVP) was the initial treatment of choice for most patients with type I and some with type IIa vWD suffering from moderate bleeding episodes. More severe bleeding or treatment of other types of vWD usually necessitates the use of alternative materials, of which cryoprecipitate was the most effective.

Recent developments have caused some reservations regarding these recommendations. Single-donor cryoprecipitate is not subjected to sterilization procedures. Although the risk of HIV transmission in most countries is now small due to donor screening the risk has not been eliminated entirely. More important is the risk of transmission of hepatitis. DDAVP is also not without problems since there have been recent reports of coronary occlusion after its use (Van Dantzig et al 1989). Since patients with heterozygous vWD do not seem to be protected from coronary artery disease it seems unwise to use DDAVP in patients over 40 years of age or with other risk factors (Mannucci & Lusher 1989).

Difficulties now arise for the specific management of vWD. Most factor VIII concentrates do not correct the bleeding time. Some may contain apparently adequate amounts of vWF antigen and ristocetin cofactor but the high-molecular-weight forms are depleted (Fricke & Yu 1989). The highly purified concentrates prepared by monoclonal antibody and recombinant technology contain little if any vWF. The choice of adequate replacement therapy is therefore limited. Adequate factor VIII levels may be sufficient for controlling secondary haemostasis after surgery but for primary haemostasis only one commercial factor VIII/vWF preparation sterilized by pasteurization in aqueous solution (Hemate P, Behring) has been shown to be effective (Schimpf et al 1987). Hopefully this apparent therapeutic shortfall will be met by product development.

The future of haemophilia therapy

It is not the intention here to guess the contents of the next edition of this series. Haemophilia has been cured by liver transplant (Bontempo et al 1987) but this is hardly a practical proposition for most patients. In the short and medium term haemophilia therapy will no doubt move in the direction of highly purified and recombinant products, but more fundamental treatment by genetic manipulation is in the offing. Human factor IX has been expressed in the milk of sheep rendered transgenic by targetted gene transfer to the mammary gland (Clark et al 1989). Although this is unlikely to represent a therapeutic breakthrough it points the way to potentially more useful gene transfer and eventually to site-directed recombination for effective cure (Weatherall 1989).

REFERENCES

Ahrens P, Kruse T A, Schwartz M et al 1987 A new HindIII restriction fragment length polymorphism in the hemophilia A locus. Hum Genet 76: 127–128

Anderson L J, Torok T J 1989 Human parvovirus B19. N Engl J Med 316: 918–922

Antonarakis S E, Waber P G, Kittur S D et al 1985 Hemophilia A: detection of molecular defects and of carriers by DNA analysis. N Engl J Med 313: 842–848

Arai M, Inaba H, Higuchi M et al 1989 Direct characterisation of factor VIII in plasma: detection of a mutation altering a thrombin cleavage site (arginine 372-histidine). Proc Natl Acad Sci USA 86: 4277–4281

Bloom A L 1987 The treatment of factor VIII inhibitors. In: Verstraete M, Vermylen J, Lijnen H R, Arnout J (eds) Thrombosis and haemostasis. International Society on Thrombosis and Haemostasis and Leuven University Press, Leuven, pp 447–471

Bontempo F A, Lewis J H, Gorenc T J et al 1987 Liver transplant in hemophilia A. Blood 69: 1721–1724

Brettler D B, Forsberg A D, Levine P H, Petillo J, Lamon K, Sullivan J L 1989 Factor VIII: C concentrate purified from plasma using monoclonal antibodies: human studies. Blood 73: 1859–1863

Bruix J, Barrera J M, Calvet X et al 1989 Prevalence of antibodies to hepatitis C virus in Spanish patients with hepatocellular carcinoma and hepatic cirrhosis. Lancet 2: 1004–1006

Choo Q-L, Kuo G, Weiner A J, Overby L R, Bradley D W, Houghton M 1989 Isolation of a c-DNA clone derived from a blood borne non-A, non-B viral hepatitis genome. Science 244: 359–362

Clark A J, Bessos H, Bishop J O, Brown P et al 1989 Expression of human anti-hemophilic factor IX in the milk of transgenic sheep. Biotechnology 7: 487–492

Colombo M, Kuo G, Choo Q-L et al 1989 Prevalence of antibodies to hepatitis C virus in Italian patients with hepatocellular carcinoma. Lancet 2: 1006–1008

Corsi O B, Azzi A, Morfini M, Fanci R, Rossi Ferrini P 1988 Human parvovirus infection in haemophiliacs first infused with treated clotting factor concentrates. J Med Virol 25: 165–170

Cumming P D, Wallace E L, Schorr J B, Dodd R Y 1989 Exposure of patients to human immunodeficiency virus through the transfusion of blood components that test antibody-negative. N Engl J Med 321: 941–946

Darby S C, Rizza C R, Doll R, Spooner R J D, Stratton I M, Thakarar B 1989 Incidence of AIDS and excess mortality associated with HIV in haemophiliacs in the United Kingdom: report on behalf of the directors of haemophilia centres in the United Kingdom. Br Med J 298: 1064–1068

de Biasi R, Miralglia E, Mastrullo L, Rocino A, Pisani M, Ruocco V 1989 Kaposi's sarcoma as clinical manifestation of the acquired immunodeficiency syndrome in a hemophilic patient. Haematologia 74: 305–308

De Vincenzi and European Study Group 1989 Risk factors for male to female transmission of HIV. Br Med J 298: 411–415

Eisenstein B I 1990 The polymerase chain reaction: a new method of using molecular genetics for medical diagnosis: N Engl J Med 322: 178–183

Esteban J I, Esteban R, Vicadomiu L et al 1989 Hepatitis C virus antibodies among risk groups in Spain. Lancet 2: 294–297

Flegg P J, Jones M E, MacCallum L R, Williams K G, Cook M K, Brettle R P 1989 Effect of Zidovudine on platelet count. Br Med J 298: 1074–1075

Freedenberg D L, Chen S-H, Kurachi K et al 1987 MspI polymorphic site within the factor IX gene. Hum Genet 76: 262–264

Fricke W A, Yu M W 1989 Characterization of von Willebrand factor in factor VIII concentrates. Am J Hematol 31: 41–45

Giannelli F 1989 Factor IX. In: Tuddenham E G D (ed) The molecular biology of coagulation. Baillière's Clinical Haematology 2: 821–848

Giannelli F, Anson D S, Choo K H et al 1984 Characterisation and use of an intragenic polymorphic marker for detection of carriers of haemophilia B (factor IX deficiency). Lancet 1: 239–241

Giesecke J, Schllia-Tomba G, Berglund O, Berntorp E, Schulman S, Stigendal L 1988 Incidence of symptoms and AIDS in 146 Swedish haemophiliacs and blood transfusion recipients infected with human immunodeficiency virus. Br Med J 297: 99–102

Giles A R, Mann K G, Nesheim M E 1988a A combination of factor Xa and phosphatidylcholine-phosphatidylserine vesicles by passes factor VIII in vivo. Br J Haematol 69: 491–497

Giles A R, Tinlin S, Hoogendoorn H, Fournez M A, Ng P, Pencham N 1988b In vivo characterization of recombinant factor VIII in a canine model of haemophilia A (factor VIII deficiency). Blood 72: 335–339

Gitschier J, Drayna D, Tuddenham E G D et al 1985 Genetic mapping and diagnosis of haemophilia A achieved through a BclI polymorphism in the factor VIII gene. Nature 314: 738–740

Gitschier J, Wood W I, Shuman M A et al 1986 Identification of a missense mutation in the factor VIII gene of a mild haemophiliac. Science 232: 1415–1416

Goedert J J, Kessler C M, Aledort L M et al 1989 A prospective study of human immunodeficiency virus type I infection and the development of AIDS in subjects with hemophilia. N Engl J Med 321: 1141–1148

Graham J B, Kunkel G R, Tennyson G S et al 1989 The Malmo polymorphism of factor IX: establishing the genotypes by rapid analysis of DNA. Blood 73: 2104–2107

Harper K, Winter R M, Pembrey M E et al 1984 A clinically useful DNA probe closely linked to haemophilia A. Lancet 2: 6–8

Harrison J F M, Bloom A L 1990 The pharmacokinetics of recombinant factor VIII. Semin in Haematol (in press)

Hay C W, Robertson K A, Yong S-L et al 1986 Use of a BamHI polymorphism in the factor IX gene for the determination of hemophilia B carrier status. Blood 67: 1508–1511.

Hedner U, Kisiel W 1983 Use of human factor VIIa in the treatment of two hemophilia A patients with high titer inhibitors. J Clin Invest 71: 1836–1841

Hedner U, Glazier S, Pingel K et al 1988 Successful use of recombinant factor VIIa in patient with severe haemophilia A during synovectomy. Lancet 2: 1193

Horowitz M S, Rooks C, Horowitz B, Hilgartner M W 1988 Virus safety of solvent/detergent-treated anti-haemophilic factor concentrate. Lancet 2: 186–189

Hymes K B, Greene J B, Karpatkin S 1988 The effect of azidothymidine on HIV-related thrombocytopenia. N Engl J Med 318: 516–517

Jacyna M R, Brooks M G, Loke R H T, Main J, Murray-Lyon I M, Thomas H C 1989 Randomised controlled trial of interferon alfa (lymphoblastoid interferon) in chronic non-A non-B hepatitis. Br Med J 198: 80–82

Janot C, Courouce A M, Maniez M 1989 Antibodies to hepatitis C virus in French blood donors. Lancet 2: 796–797

Kasper C K 1989 Treatment of factor VIII inhibitors. Prog Haemostasis Thromb 9: 57–86

Kaufman R J 1989 Genetic engineering of factor VIII. Nature 342: 207–208

Kernoff P B A, Miller E J, Savidge G F, Machin S J, Dewar M S, Preston F E 1987 Reduced risk of non-A, non-B hepatitis after a first exposure to 'wet heated' factor VIII concentrate. Br J Haematol 67: 207–211

Kogan S C, Doherty M, Gitschier J 1987 An improved method for prenatal diagnosis of genetic diseases by analysis of amplified DNA sequences: application to hemophilia A. N Engl J Med 317: 985–990

Kuhnl P, Seidl S, Stangel W, Beyer J, Sibrowski W, Flik J 1989 Antibody to hepatitis C virus in German blood donors. Lancet 2: 324 (c)

Laure F, Courgnaud V, Rouzioux C et al 1988 Detection of HIV DNA in infants and children by means of the polymerase chain reaction. Lancet 2: 538–541

Loche M, Mach B 1988 Identification of HIV-infected seronegative individuals by a direct diagnostic test based on hybridisation to amplified viral DNA. Lancet 2: 418–421

Ludlam C A, Chapman D, Cohen B, Litton P A 1989 Antibodies to hepatitis C virus in haemophilia. Lancet 2: 560–561

Lyon D J, Chapman C S, Martin C et al 1989 Symptomatic parvovirus B19 infection and heat-treated factor IX concentrate. Lancet 1: 1085

Macik B G, Hohneker J, Roberts H R, Griffin A M 1989 Use of recombinant activated factor VII for treatment of a retropharyngeal hemorrhage in a hemophilic patient with a high titer inhibitor. Am J Hematol 32: 232–234

Macintyre 1989 The use of the polymerase chain reaction in haematology. Blood Rev 3: 201–210

Madhok R, Gracie A, Lowe G D O et al 1986 Impaired cell mediated immunity in haemophilia in the absence of infection with human immunodeficiency virus. Br Med J 293: 978–980

Mannhalter J W, Ahmad R, Liebl H, Gottlichter J, Wolf H M, Eibl M M 1988 Comparable modulation of human monocyte functions by commercial factor VIII concentrates of varying purity. Blood 71: 1662–1668

Mannucci P M, Colombo M 1989 Revision of the protocol recommended for studies of safety from hepatitis of clotting factor concentrates. Thromb Haemostasis 61: 532–534

Mannucci P M, Lusher J 1989 Desmopressin and thrombosis. Lancet 2: 675–676

Mariani G, Ghirardini A, Mandelli F et al 1987 Heated clotting factors and seroconversion for human immunodeficiency virus in three hemophilic patients. Ann Int Med 107: 113

Mibashan R S, Peake I R, Nicolaides K H 1989 Prenatal diagnosis of hemostatic disorders. In: Alter B P (ed) Perinatal hematology. Methods in Hematol 21: 64–107

MMWR 1988 Safety of therapeutic products used for hemophilic patients. Morbidity Mortality Weekly Rep 37: 441–450

Mortimer P P, Luan N L C, Kelleher J F, Cohen B J 1983 Transmission of serum parvovirus-like virus by clotting factor concentrates. Lancet 2: 482–484

Mortimer P P, Cohen B J, Litton P A et al 1989 Hepatitis C virus antibody. Lancet 2: 798

Mulligan L, Holden J J A, White B N 1987 A DNA marker closely linked to the factor IX (haemophilia B) gene. Hum Genet 75: 381–383

Nilsson I M, Berntorp E, Zettervall O 1988 Induction of immune tolerance in patients with haemophilia and antibodies to factor VIII by combined treatment with intravenous IgG, cyclophosphamide and factor VIII. N Engl J Med 318: 947–950

Noel L, Guerois C, Maisonneuve P, Verroust F, Laurian Y 1989 Antibodies to hepatitis C virus in haemophilia. Lancet 2: 560

Oberle I, Camerino G, Heilig R et al 1985 Genetic screening for haemophilia A (classic haemophilia) with a polymorphic probe. N Engl J Med 312: 682–686

O'Brien D P 1989 The molecular biology and biochemistry of tissue factor. In: Tuddenham E G D (ed) Clinical haematology: the molecular biology of coagulation. Baillière Tindall, London, pp 801–820

O'Brien D P, Tuddenham E G D 1989 Purification and characterisation of factor VIII 1689 Cys: a nonfunctional cofactor occurring in a patient with severe hemophilia A. Blood 73: 2117–2122

Pattinson J K, McVey J H, Boon M et al 1990 CRM + haemophilia A due to a missense mutation (372-Cys) at the internal heavy chain thrombin cleavage site. Br J Haematol 75: 73–77

Peake I R 1989 The polymerase chain reaction. J Clin Pathol 42: 673–676

Ragni M V, Winkelstein A, Kingsley L, Spero J A, Lewis J H 1987 Update of HIV seroprevalence, seroconversion, AIDS incidence and immunologic correlates of HIV infection in patients with hemophilia A and B. Blood 70: 786–790

Ragni M V, Bontempo F A, Lewis J H 1989 Disappearance of inhibitor to factor VIII in HIV-infected hemophiliacs with progression to AIDS or severe ARC. Transfusion 29: 447–449

Roggendorf M, Deinhardt F, Rasshofer R et al 1989 Antibodies to hepatitis C virus. Lancet 2: 324–325

Ruffault A, Genetet N, Berthier A M et al 1988 Interferon production in severe haemophiliacs with and without HIV antibodies. J Interferon Res 8: 89–94

Schimpf K, Mannucci P M, Kreutz W et al 1987 Absence of hepatitis after treatment with a pasteurized factor VIII concentrate in patients with hemophilia and no previous transfusions. N Engl J Med 316: 918–922

Schreiber A B, Gillette R, Hrinda M E 1987 In vitro immune parameters of Monoclate R, a monoclonal antibody purified human plasma factor VIII: C therapeutic preparation. Thromb Haemostasis 58: 346 (absract)

Stain C, Pabinger-Fasching I, Guggenberger K et al 1989 High risk of acquired immune deficiency syndrome (AIDS) and of AIDS related complex (ARC) in hemophiliacs seropositive for more than 5 years. Thromb Haemostasis 61: 354–356

Study Group of UK Haemophilia Centre Directors 1988 Effect of dry-heating of coagulation factor concentrates at 80°C for 72 hours on transmission of non-A, non-B hepatitis. Lancet 2: 814–816

Thim L, Bjoern S, Christensen M et al 1988 Amino acid sequence and posttranslational modifications of human factor VIIa from plasma and transfected baby hamster kidney cells. Biochemistry 27: 7785–7793

Thomas H C, Scully L J 1985 Anti-viral therapy in chronic hepatitis B infection. Br Med Bull 41: 374–386

Thompson A R, Chen S-H, Smith K J 1988 Diagnostic role of an immunoassay-detected polymorphism of factor IX for potential carriers of hemophilia B. Blood 72: 1633–1638

Thorpe R, Dilger P, Dawson N J, Barrowcliffe T W 1989 Inhibition of interleukin-2 secretion by factor VIII concentrates: a possible cause of immunosuppression in hemophiliacs. Br J Haematol 71: 387–391

Toole J J, Knopf J L, Wozey J M et al 1984 Molecular cloning of a c-DNA encoding human antihemophilic factor. Nature 312: 342–347

Tuddenham E G D 1989 Factor VIII and haemophilia A. In: Tuddenham E G D (ed) The molecular biology of coagulation. Baillière's Clin Haematol 2: 849–877

Van Dantzig J M, Duren D R, Ten Cate J W 1989 Desmopressin and myocardial infarction. Lancet 1: 664

Van der Ende M E, Rothbarth P, Stibbe J 1988 Heterosexual transmission of HIV by haemophiliacs. Br Med J 297: 1102–1103

Ward J W, Bush T J, Perkins H A et al 1989 The natural history of transfusion-associated infection with human immunodeficiency virus: factors influencing the rate of progression to disease. N Engl J Med 321: 947–951

Weatherall D J 1989 Gene therapy: getting there slowly. Br Med J 198: 691–692

Webster A, Lee C A, Cook D G et al 1989 Cytomegalovirus infection and progression towards AIDS in haemophiliacs with human immunodeficiency virus infection. Lancet 2: 63–66

White G C II, McMillan C W, Kingdon H S, Shoemaker C B 1989 Use of recombinant antihemophilic factor in the treatment of two patients with classic hemophilia. N Engl J Med 320: 166–170

Winship P R, Anson D S, Rizza C R et al 1984 Carrier detection in haemophilia B using two further intragenic restriction fragment length polymorphisms. Nucleic Acids Res 12: 8861–8872

Winship P R, Rees D J G, Alkan M 1989 Detecting polymorphisms at CpG dinucleotides using the polymerase chain reaction procedure: application to the diagnosis of haemophilia B carriers. Lancet 1: 631–634

Wion K L, Tuddenham E G D, Lawn R M 1986 A new polymorphism in the factor VIII gene for prenatal diagnosis of haemophilia A. Nucleic Acids Res 14: 4535–4542

Youssoufian H, Phillips D G, Kazazian H H et al 1987 MspI polymorphisms in the 3' flanking region of the human factor VIII gene. Nucleic Acids Res 15: 6212

Zuckerman A J 1989. The elusive hepatitis C virus: a cause of parenteral non-A, non-B hepatitis. Br Med J 299: 871–873

9

Prophylaxis of deep vein thrombosis

A.G.G. Turpie

Deep vein thrombosis and pulmonary embolism are among the most common and serious complications occurring in hospitalized patients. Using objective diagnostic techniques, it has been established that venous thromboembolism occurs much more frequently than was previously suspected. If routine prophylaxis is not used, many hospitalized patients develop deep vein thrombosis as a complication of other illness or following surgery. A large proportion of them will develop long-term sequelae including the post-phlebitic syndrome with resultant recurring pain and swelling or chronic ulceration of the legs. These long-term sequelae are particularly common in patients undergoing orthopaedic surgical procedures such as elective hip replacement in whom there is a significant incidence of proximal vein thrombi (Wessler 1975). Pulmonary embolism is also a serious threat in such patients. In the United States, it has been estimated that, each year, pulmonary embolism occurs in more than 500 000 patients of whom approximately 200 000 will die (Bell & Simon 1982). Almost half of those patients who die will be terminally ill or have incurable diseases but the remainder of the deaths occur in patients who would otherwise have recovered completely. The majority of patients who die from pulmonary embolism do so early after presentation and, therefore, usually before the diagnosis can be made and the treatment commenced. More than half of such patients have no clinical evidence of preceding thromboembolic events, although there is often evidence of prior minor embolic episodes at autopsy in those who die. Similarly, many major deep vein thrombi are silent. Since the clinical diagnosis of deep vein thrombosis is notoriously unreliable and since the majority of pulmonary emboli arise from thrombi in the deep veins of the legs, prevention of venous thrombosis would be the most effective way of preventing death from pulmonary embolism. It has been estimated that routine effective prophylaxis in patients undergoing elective general surgery, for example, could prevent 4000–8000 postoperative deaths annually in the United States (Salzman & Hirsh 1987). In addition, effective primary prophylaxis will significantly reduce the frequency of chronic venous insufficiency.

RISK FACTORS AND INCIDENCE OF VENOUS THROMBOSIS

A number of clinical circumstances increase the risk of venous thromboembolism is hospitalized patients, including trauma, increasing age, obesity, malignant disease, heart disease, prolonged immobility or lower limb paralysis, use of oral contraceptives, and a history of prior venous thromboembolism. Several of these risk factors may co-exist in individual patients and multiply the risk. The magnitude of the problem of venous thrombosis in various diagnostic categories of hospitalized patients is shown in Table 9.1. Using objective diagnostic tests in the absence of prophylaxis, venous thrombosis has been shown to occur in approximately 20–50% of patients undergoing elective general surgical procedures, 40–60% of patients undergoing elective hip replacement and even higher in patients undergoing surgery for fractured hip. In addition, patients hospitalized with myocardial infarction or stroke have a high frequency of deep vein thrombosis, ranging from 20% to 60%. Without prophylaxis, fatal pulmonary embolism occurs in less than 1% of general surgical patients. The incidence of fatal pulmonary embolism is much higher in orthopaedic patients, ranging from 1–2% in patients undergoing elective hip replacement to 4–5% in patients having surgery for fracture of the hip. In the orthopaedic patients, fatal pulmonary embolism remains the major cause of postoperative death (Sheppeard et al 1981).

PREVENTION OF VENOUS THROMBOEMBOLISM

Two approaches can be used to prevent venous thromboembolism in high-

Table 9.1 Frequency of venous thrombosis diagnosed by objective tests

Category	Incidence
Elective surgery	
Major abdominal	20–35
Thoracic	26–65
Gynaecological	7–45
Retropubic prostatectomy	24–51
Transurethral prostatectomy	7–10
Hip replacement	40–65
Knee replacement	40–65
Emergency surgery	
Hip fracture	48–74
Neurosurgical patients	
Brain tumour, head trauma, subarachnoid haemorrhage	19–28
Medical	
Myocardial infarction	23–38
Stroke	20–60

risk patients. These are: early detection of subclinical venous thrombosis by screening high-risk patients; and the use of primary prophylactic methods.

Early detection of subclinical thrombosis

The rationale for the use of sensitive objective methods of the early diagnosis of venous thromboembolism as a method of prophylaxis depends upon their ability to detect asymptomatic subclinical disease and permit early effective treatment. Screening high-risk patients with non-invasive tests for venous thrombosis has been shown in an early analysis to be effective in the prevention of fatal pulmonary embolism but it is not cost-effective because the strategy includes the cost of the tests plus the cost of treating patients who develop the disease (Salzman & Davies 1980). Furthermore, it is not known whether all patients with subclinical venous thrombosis following general surgery should receive full-dose intravenous heparin therapy followed by long-term secondary prophylaxis. Screening has major limitations as an approach to the prevention of venous thromboembolism following orthopaedic surgery since it has been recently determined that the combination of leg scanning and impedance plethysmography lacks enough sensitivity for the detection of venous thrombosis after hip surgery to be useful (Cruickshank et al 1989). In this study, the use of either screening test or a combination had a sensitivity of 49.6% and a specificity of 93.9% for all venographically demonstrated venous thrombosis. In addition, in contrast to symptomatic patients, the sensitivity of impedance plethysmography for proximal vein thrombosis was less than 30%, probably because the thrombi were small and non-occlusive at the time of venography.

Primary prophylaxis

The ideal method of prophylaxis should be safe, effective and acceptable to patients, nurses and medical staff and should be easily administered, inexpensive and simple to monitor. The methods of primary prevention of venous thromboembolism which have been evaluated in prospective clinical trials are shown in Table 9.2. These include low-dose heparin, low-molecular-weight heparin, oral anticoagulants, platelet function-suppressing drugs, dextran and physical methods.

Low-dose heparin

Low-dose heparin is the most commonly used method of venous thrombosis prophylaxis. In the late 1960s it was first reported that small doses of heparin, while insufficient to prolong the whole blood clotting time, were effective in reducing the frequency of clinically detectable venous thrombosis. Numerous clinical trials using objective methods to diagnose venous thromboembolism have now confirmed the effectiveness of low-dose

Table 9.2   Primary prophylaxis for venous thromboembolism

Anticoagulants
Heparin
Heparin–dihydroergotamine
Low-molecular-weight heparin
Vitamin K antagonists

Platelet inhibitors
Aspirin
Hydroxychloroquine

Dextran

Physical methods
Intermittent pneumatic compression
Graduated compression stockings
Electrical calf muscle stimulation

---

subcutaneous heparin in preventing venous thrombosis among high-risk patients. There have been over 20 randomized, prospective trials comparing heparin in doses of 5000 units 8-hourly or 12-hourly subcutaneously with placebo or no treatment for the prevention of venous thrombosis in patients undergoing general abdominothoracic or gynaecological surgery. The results of these studies have been consistent and in more than 3000 patients the incidence of deep vein thrombosis was reduced from approximately 30% in control patients to less than 7% in those treated with low-dose heparin. In a recent meta-analysis of all reported placebo-controlled and open-label prospective trials of low-dose heparin prophylaxis in general surgical patients reported by Collins et al (1988), low-dose heparin was shown to produce a risk reduction of venous thrombosis of 67% ± 4% (Fig. 9.1). This difference is both clinically and statistically highly significant ($P<0.0001$). However, not all patients undergoing general surgery were protected to the same extent; for example, in patients with malignant disease, the incidence of venous thrombosis is about two times as high as in patients with non-malignant disorders, and the protective effect of low-dose heparin, while statistically significant, is less than that in patients with non-malignant disorders. There was no evidence in the meta-analysis that the three times daily regimen was more efficacious than the twice daily regimen in this group of patients. The odds reduction for the 8-hour was 72% ± 5% compared with 63% ± 5% for the 12-hour regimen (Collins et al 1988).

Orthopaedic patients undergoing elective hip or knee joint replacement are at particularly high risk of developing venous thromboembolism. There have been a number of studies evaluating low-dose heparin prophylaxis in these patients. The evidence from the individual studies is less persuasive that low-dose heparin is as effective as in general surgical patients. However, the recent meta-analysis by Collins et al (1988) showed a risk reduction with low-dose heparin in a dose of either 5000 units 8-hourly or 12-hourly of 68% ± 7% for all thrombi, and in the studies in which separate information

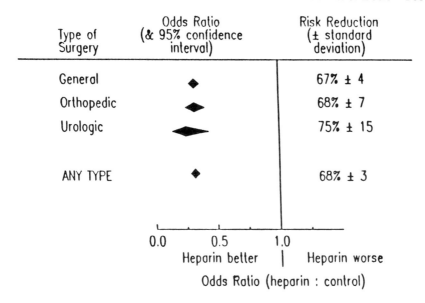

Fig. 9.1 Apparent effects of perioperative subcutaneous heparin on reported rates of deep vein thrombosis in randomized trials in general, orthopaedic and urological surgery. Reprinted, by permission of the New England Journal of Medicine (318: 1166, 1988).

for proximal deep vein thrombosis was available the reduction was 56% ± 12% (Fig. 9.1). As was the case in general surgery, there was no difference in efficacy between the two heparin regimens. The odds reduction for the 8-hour regimen was 68% ± 10% compared with 68% ± 11% for the 12-hour regimen. In orthopaedic patients, however, fixed low-dose heparin prophylaxis is not ideal since 20–25% of patients who receive this regimen will develop deep vein thrombosis. The best results with subcutaneous heparin were reported by Leyvraz et al (1983) using an adjusted dosage regimen in which patients undergoing elective hip replacement were randomly allocated to receive either a fixed dose of subcutaneous heparin, 3500 units 8-hourly or a dose adjusted to maintain the activated partial thromboplastin time, performed 6 hours after the morning dose, of 32–36 seconds. Using this regimen, the frequency of deep vein thrombosis was reduced from 39% in the fixed-dose group to 13% in the adjusted dose group. Taberner et al (1989) confirmed the improved efficacy of an adjusted heparin regimen over fixed low-dose heparin 5000 units 8-hourly in patients having surgery for fracture of the hip or elective hip replacement. The individual studies of low-dose heparin prophylaxis in patients undergoing urological surgery were likewise less convincing for a benefit compared with general surgery patients but the meta-analysis by Collins et al (1988) confirmed a significant risk reduction of 75% ± 15% in such patients (Fig. 9.1). Thus, in urological and orthopaedic surgery, as well as in general surgery, the reported studies provide significant evidence for an important decrease in the frequency of deep vein thrombosis by low-dose heparin.

In medical patients with acute myocardial infarction, congestive heart failure and in patients with thrombotic stroke, there is convincing evidence that low-dose heparin prophylaxis is effective in significantly reducing the incidence of venous thromboembolic disease (Wray et al 1973, McCarthy et al 1977). In one large study reported by Halkin et al (1982), low-dose heparin decreased hospital mortality in medical patients.

The efficacy of low-dose heparin in the prevention of both fatal and non-fatal pulmonary embolism is post-operative and medical patients is of major importance. The effect of low-dose heparin prophylaxis on the incidence of pulmonary embolism has been evaluated in six studies, and in five of these postoperative pulmonary embolism was significantly reduced in the treated patients (International Multicenter Trial 1975, Scurr et al 1979, Sagar et al 1975, Kiil et al 1978, Gruber et al 1977, 1980). The most important of the studies was the large multicentre trial coordinated by Kakkar (International Multicentre Trial 1975) involving more than 4000 patients where there was convincing evidence that the incidence of both fatal and non-fatal pulmonary embolism was strikingly reduced by low-dose heparin. The meta-analysis by Collins et al (1988) confirmed the efficacy of low-dose heparin in the prevention of fatal and non-fatal pulmonary embolus (Fig. 9.2). In the evenly randomized trials, the reduction in fatal pulmonary embolism was 64% ± 15%.

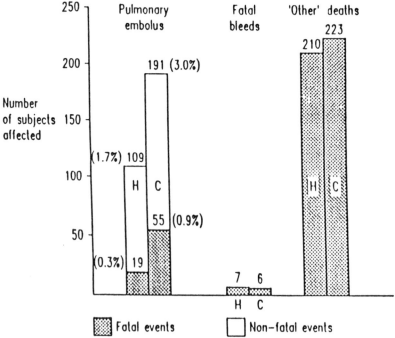

Fig. 9.2 All available data on pulmonary embolus and mortality from evenly randomized trials of perioperative subcutaneous heparin in general, orthopaedic and urological surgery. Reprinted, by permission of the New England Journal of Medicine (318: 1168, 1988).

Low-dose heparin has been used in combination with dihydroergotamine, a vasoconstrictor, which has been reported to reduce stasis by inducing vasoconstriction of the copacitant vessels of the leg. A number of randomized studies have been reported on the combination treatment and there is evidence that it is more effective than heparin alone in the prevention of deep vein thrombosis in general surgical and orthopaedic patients (Gent & Roberts 1986). Because of its pharmacological action, patients with overt vasospastic disorders, ischaemic heart disease or peripheral vascular disease should not be given dihydroergotamine because of the possibility of arterial vasospasm complicating treatment.

A potential complication of low-dose heparin prophylaxis is bleeding. The reported frequency of clinically significant bleeding in the randomized trials has varied. In most reports, bleeding was not found to be significant, but in a minority of studies a clear increase in the percentage of patients who develop postoperative haematomas or other postoperative bleeding occurred, but this bleeding was considered to be of minor clinical significance. Collins et al (1988) reported clear and consistent evidence of an increased risk of bleeding with subcutaneous heparin but that major bleeding due to low-dose heparin prophylaxis was uncommon, and that there was no excess in deaths from bleeding compared with controls (Fig. 9.2).

Low-molecular-weight heparin

There is experimental evidence that low-molecular-weight heparin fractions are as effective as standard heparin in preventing venous thrombosis and that they produce less bleeding (Levine & Hirsh 1988). Low-molecular-weight heparin fractions produce less inhibition of platelet function than standard heparin, a property that could account for the reduced haemorrhagic effects. There have been several reports in humans on the benefits of low-molecular-weight heparin fractions or heparinoids in the prevention of thromboembolic disease (Levine & Hirsh 1988). A number of reports of randomized double-blind trials of low-molecular-weight heparin or heparinoid prophylaxis have been recently reported demonstrating their effectiveness in patients undergoing elective general surgery (Kakkar & Murray 1985, Caen 1988), elective hip surgery (Turpie et al 1986, Planes et al 1988) and in patients with thrombotic stroke (Turpie et al 1987). In recent studies, low-molecular-weight heparins have been shown to be more effective when compared with unfractionated heparin in some high-risk groups (Planes et al 1988, European Fraxiparin Study Group 1988). Low-molecular-weight heparin prophylaxis is discussed in detail separately in Chapter 10.

Oral anticoagulants

More than 20 studies have been carried out to evaluate the effectiveness of oral anticoagulants in preventing venous thrombosis in high-risk patients, including general surgical and orthopaedic patients. However, less than half of the studies included concurrent control patients or objective endpoints to diagnose venous thromboembolism (Hull & Hirsh 1981). In each of the controlled studies, oral anticoagulants significantly reduced the frequency of venous thromboembolism, including fatal pulmonary embolism (Salzman & Hirsh 1987). Although side effects varied, several studies reported an increase in the incidence of major bleeding. Therefore, although oral anti-coagulants are effective in preventing venous thromboembolism, particu-larly in orthopaedic patients, their routine use has not gained general acceptance due to the perceived increased likelihood of bleeding complica-tions. One approach to reduce the risk of bleeding that has been evaluated is the use of very low perioperative and early postoperative doses of oral anticoagulants, increasing to more conventional doses when the risk of haemorrhage is reduced (Francis et al 1983). This method has been shown to reduce the frequency of bleeding without reducing prophylactic efficacy in patients having elective orthopaedic surgery but is not cost-effective for widespread clinical use. An alternative approach is to commence oral anti-coagulant therapy postoperatively but this may result in a reduction in the efficacy (Powers et al 1989). Mini-dose warfarin using 1 mg has been shown by Poller et al (1987) to significantly reduce the frequency of venous thrombosis in gynaecological patients with minimal bleeding risk. This approach has great potential and requires further evaluation.

Dextran

Dextran is a glucose polymer that was originally introduced as a volume expander with antithrombotic properties (Lambie et al 1970, Data & Nies 1974). Results of studies evaluating dextran for the prevention of deep vein thrombosis in surgical patients are conflicting, with some reports, especially in patients undergoing hip surgery, indicating significant benefit and others showing no benefit (Salzman & Hirsh 1987). The major side effect of dextran is volume overload, which can result in cardiac failure; also, allergic reactions have been described but are relatively uncommon. Excessive bleeding has been reported in some patients. Since dextran is relatively expensive and must be given by intravenous infusion, it is not an ideal prophylactic agent.

Physical methods

Because stasis is a major factor in the development of deep vein thrombosis, a number of simple techniques designed to increase blood flow from the legs have been evaluated for the prevention of venous thrombosis in postoperative and other immobilized patients. These measures include early ambulation, leg elevation, physiotherapy, elastic stockings, and graduated compression stockings. More advanced methods for pro‧ blood flow include electrical calf muscle stimulation and inter‧ pneumatic compression.

Simple physical methods. Several studies have reported the results of simple physical methods to prevent venous thrombosis in general surgical patients, which include leg elevation, elastic stockings, a combination of elastic stockings and intensive physiotherapy, and graduated compression stockings (Hull & Hirsh 1981). The results indicated that neither elastic stockings alone nor leg elevation alone reduced the frequency of post-operative venous thrombosis by more than a third. However, several trials have shown a significant reduction in postoperative venous thrombosis through the use of graduated compression stockings (Colditz et al 1986). Thus, a combination of simple measures provides some benefit, and the use of graduated pressure stockings, particularly in low-risk patients, is effective.

Electrical calf muscle stimulation. Electrical calf muscle stimulation which prevents venous stasis by contracting the calf muscles has been evaluated for venous thrombosis prophylaxis in several randomized studies and has been shown to reduce the frequency of leg-scan detected venous thrombosis. Electrical calf muscle stimulation is, however, impractical because it may be used only when patients are anaesthetized and is unlikely to help patients who remain immobilized for long periods (Hull & Hirsh 1981).

Intermittent pneumatic compression. Intermittent pneumatic compression of the legs has been tested extensively for the prevention of postoperative venous thrombosis. A number of devices have been developed, which include a variety of cuffs, boots and stockings utilizing different inflation cycle times and pressures. Intermittent compression has been shown to empty the deep calf veins of blood and to increase pulsatile blood flow in the femoral veins. Pneumatic compression has also been shown to increase systemic fibrinolytic enzyme activity, which may contribute to venous thrombosis prevention.

Several studies using a fast compression cycle have shown a significant reduction in leg-scan-detected venous thrombosis among postoperative patients, including patients undergoing general, abdominothoracic, hip or knee surgery. In studies in which a slow cycle compression was used, the reduction in venous thrombosis was less impressive particularly in patients with malignancy (Coe et al 1978, Salzman et al 1980, Nicolaides et al 1980). Pneumatic compression may have special application for patient groups in whom anticoagulant drugs have been found to be ineffective, for example patients undergoing prostatectomy, or who are contraindicated, for example neurosurgical patients (Turpie et al 1989). Intermittent calf compression is, therefore, a promising method of preventing venous leg thrombosis. It is as effective as low-dose heparin and may offer a safe alternative in selected patient groups who are at increased risk of bleeding (Colditz et al 1986).

Platelet-suppressant drugs

Venous thrombosis occurs as a result of fibrin formation and deposition, but the presence of platelet aggregates at sites of some early venous thrombi suggests that platelets play a role in initiating the process. It is possible, therefore, that drugs that suppress platelet function may help prevent venous thrombosis in some high-risk patients. Of the antiplatelet drugs that have been tested in prospective clinical trials for the prevention of deep vein thrombosis, aspirin is the only one that has been used extensively in practice. However, the conclusions from the aspirin studies have been inconsistent. Early reports on the use of aspirin to prevent postoperative venous thrombosis after general abdominothoracic surgery indicated no benefit. Several reports in patients undergoing surgery for fractured hip, elective hip replacement and total knee replacement found aspirin to be beneficial in reducing the frequency of postoperative venous thrombosis (Turpie 1981). There is evidence from one of the elective hip studies that the benefit of aspirin for the prevention of venous thrombosis may be confined to male patients (Harris et al 1974). However, with increasing clinical experience of the use of aspirin as an antithrombotic drug, it is likely that the difference between males and females reported may not be confirmed. Of greater interest is the controversy between the use of low- or high-dose aspirin, an issue which has not yet been resolved.

PRACTICAL APPROACH TO PREVENTION OF VENOUS THROMBOEMBOLISM

Because of the incidence and significance of venous thromboembolism, in the United States the National Heart, Lung and Blood Institute and the National Institutes of Health Office of Medical Applications of Research convened a Consensus Development Conference on the prevention of venous thrombosis and pulmonary embolism to help resolve questions that related to various prophylactic measures in high-risk groups of patients. The Consensus Development panel reviewed data on the risk of venous thrombosis and pulmonary embolism in various patient groups, and evidence for the efficacy and safety of different forms of prophylaxis, and made recommendations for prophylaxis in the various patient groups (National Institutes of Health Consensus Development Conference Statement 1986).

In patients undergoing general surgery, the Consensus Development Conference recommended low-dose heparin 5000 units subcutaneously every 8 or 12 hours until the patient is ambulatory as the treatment of choice. Dextran, external pneumatic compression and graduated compression stockings were all suggested as alternatives for this group of patients. In patients undergoing orthopaedic procedures the Consensus Development Conference recommended low-dose warfarin, dextran or adjusted-dose heparin. In addition, graduated compression stockings or external pneumatic compression were also recommended, particularly in combination with other modalities. For patients undergoing urological procedures, external pneumatic compression was recommended because of the possibility that low-dose heparin may be ineffective in this group. In gynaecology and obstetrics, low-dose heparin or external pneumatic compression was recommended, with dextran as an alternative. In neurosurgical patients, external pneumatic compression was recommended as the treatment of choice. In medical conditions such as congestive heart failure, acute myocardial infarction or pulmonary infections, low-dose heparin was recommended and in chronic medical conditions low-dose warfarin was the recommended treatment of choice.

An alternative approach to the Consensus Development Recommendation is to classify patients into three risk categories, low risk, medium risk and high risk, and to recommend prophylaxis according to risk. Low-risk patients are those under 40 years of age undergoing surgery less than 30 minutes in duration with no other risk factors; moderate risk patients are defined as those over the age of 40 undergoing surgery for more than 30 minutes and patients with myocardial infarction or heart failure; and the high-risk group are defined as patients over the age of 40 with previous deep vein thrombosis, extensive malignant disease or major orthopaedic surgery or paralytic stroke. The frequency of venous thromboembolism in these risk categories is shown in Table 9.3.

Prophylaxis may be recommended on the basis of these three risk categories. The low-risk patients should have graduated compression stockings or early ambulation. Moderate-risk patients, which comprise the majority of hospitalized patients requiring prophylaxis, should have heparin in a dose of 5000 units 12-hourly subcutaneously or external pneumatic compression. Dextran is an alternative for this group of patients. The high-risk patients are those in whom the need for prophylaxis is essential. Several alternatives are available. Low-dose heparin in a dose of 5000 units 8-hourly or 12-hourly or a combination of low-dose heparin plus dihydroergotamine may be effective. Dextran, external pneumatic compression or a combination of low-dose heparin with external pneumatic compression may be used. Increasingly, the use of warfarin with the aim to increase the

Table 9.3 Frequency of thromboembolic event according to risk

Event	Low risk (%)	Medium risk (%)	High risk (%)
Calf vein thrombosis	1–2	10–40	40–80
Proximal vein thrombosis	0.4	2–8	10–20
Clinical pulmonary embolism	0.2	1–8	5–10
Fatal pulmonary embolism	0.002	0.1–0.4	1–5

international normalized ratio (INR) to 2.0–3.0 by the fifth postoperative day is an attractive alternative for this group of patients.

Prevention of venous thromboembolism during pregnancy

Thrombosis prophylaxis during pregnancy poses a special problem. Although venous thromboembolism is uncommon in pregnancy and in the puerperium, pulmonary embolism is a leading cause of maternal mortality second only to complications of abortion (Evans et al 1968, Kierkegaard 1983). The estimated frequency of venous thromboembolic disease related to pregnancy differs widely among reports largely due to the use of different diagnostic criteria for the detection of deep vein thrombosis and pulmonary embolism and because the incidence varies according to the period within the pregnancy and the method of delivery. Although venous thromboembolism is uncommon in uncomplicated pregnancy, it has been estimated that the increased risk of a thromboembolic event during the pregnant state is five fold compared with non-pregnant women not taking oral contraceptives (Tooke & McNicol 1961). The estimated risk of deep vein thrombosis during pregnancy is between 0.1 and 0.6 per thousand postpartum (Kierkegaard 1983, Treffers et al 1983) and is five times more frequent in the postpartum period and is significantly more common following Caesarian section compared to vaginal delivery (Treffers et al 1983). Pulmonary embolism, although less common than deep vein thrombosis, occurs more frequently in the pregnant population than non-pregnant women. The death rate from pulmonary embolism has been estimated to be 0.1 per 10 000 vaginal deliveries and 0.7–1.6 per 10 000 deliveries by Caesarian section (Bonnar 1981).

Prospective evaluation of methods of venous thrombosis prophylaxis during pregnancy is limited to descriptive or cohort studies. The most thoroughly documented and widely used form of venous thrombosis prophylaxis during pregnancy is anticoagulant therapy with low-dose heparin. Because of potential problems associated with anticoagulant therapy during pregnancy, it is imperative that proper selection of patients for thrombosis prophylaxis is used. In addition, the risks and benefits of prophylaxis during pregnancy must be thoroughly weighed and careful consideration given to the methods of prophylaxis chosen. In uncomplicated pregnancy, although there is a slight increase in the risk of venous thromboembolism compared with the non-pregnant state, there is no indication for thrombosis prophylaxis. Prophylaxis is indicated in high-risk pregnant patients, which include patients with a previous history of venous thromboembolism (Aaro & Juergens 1971), patients with congenital protein C or S deficiency (Broekmans et al 1985) or antithrombin III deficiency (Hirsh et al 1989) and patients with a number of non-specific risk factors such as obesity, heart disease or lower limb paralysis (Editorial 1979).

The use of anticoagulants for prophylaxis during pregnancy is controversial because they have the potential to produce adverse effects in the mother and the fetus (Ginsberg & Hirsh 1989a, 1989b, Ginsberg et al 1989a, 1989b). Heparin does not cross the placenta and therefore will not produce complications in the fetus (Flessa et al 1965), whereas oral anticoagulants cross the placenta, enter the fetal circulation and are teratogenic (Becker et al 1975). Contrary to that previously reported, heparin does not cause adverse fetal or infant outcomes and the adverse effects can be explained on the basis of maternal comorbid conditions (Ginsberg & Hirsh 1989a). On the other hand, oral anticoagulants have been proven to be associated with increased risk of fetal wastage and congenital malformations (Maeck & Ziliacus 1948, Ginsberg & Hirsh 1989a).

A practical clinical approach for thrombosis prophylaxis in high-risk patients during pregnancy is the use of low-dose heparin, 5000 units 12-hourly until the third trimester of pregnancy, when the dose of heparin should be increased to prolong the mid-interval activated partial thromboplastin time to $1^{1}/_{2}$ times the control. Oral anticoagulant prophylaxis should be avoided for venous thromboembolism during pregnancy but may be administered in the postpartum period for two to three weeks. The concentration of warfarin excreted in breast milk is insufficient to cause any significant effect in the fetus (McKenna et al 1983, Lao et al 1985). An alternative approach in medium- to high-risk pregnant patients is to monitor them with serial testing using impedance plethysmography or B-mode ultrasound to detect the presence of deep vein thrombosis.

Heparin prophylaxis is required in patients with inherited antithrombin III, protein C or protein S deficiency, particularly in patients with a history of previous thrombi. Although the dose has not been clearly established, low-dose heparin in the initial stages of pregnancy is a reasonable approach combined with screening with an increase in the dose in the second and third trimester of pregnancy. Low-dose heparin is often ineffective in patients with antithrombin III deficiency, and titrated heparin with supplemental antithrombin III infusion has been shown to be successful (Hellgren et al 1982). Low-molecular-weight heparin has not been formally evaluated for the prevention of venous thrombosis in pregnancy but has been used successfully in the treatment of venous thrombosis in a limited number of patients with contraindications to unfractionated heparin, such as patients with heparin-induced thrombocytopenia (Omri et al 1989, deBoer et al 1989).

REFERENCES

Aaro L A, Juergens J L 1971 Thrombophlebitis associated with pregnancy. Am J Obstet Gynecol 109: 1129
Becker M H, Genieser N B, Finegold M et al 1975 Chondrodysplasia Punctata. Is maternal warfarin a factor? Am J Dis Child 129: 356–359
Bell W R, Simon T L 1982 Current status of pulmonary thromboembolic disease: pathophysiology, diagnosis, prevention and treatment. Am Heart J 103: 239–262

Bonnar J 1981 Venous thromboembolism and pregnancy. Clin Obstet Gynaecol 8: 456
Broekmans A W, Bertina R M, Reinalda-Poot J et al 1985 Hereditary protein-S deficiency and venous thromboembolism. Thromb Haemostasis 53: 273–277
Caen J P 1988 A randomized double-blind study between a low molecular weight heparin Kabi 2165 and standard heparin in the prevention of deep vein thrombosis in general surgery: a French multicenter trial. Thromb Haemostasis 59: 216–220
Coe N P, Collins R E C, Klein L A et al 1978 Prevention of deep vein thrombosis in urological patients: a controlled, randomized trial of low-dose heparin and external compression boots. Surgery 83: 230–234
Colditz G A, Tuden R L, Oster G 1986 Rates of venous thrombosis after general surgery: combined results of randomised clinical trials. Lancet 2: 143–146
Collins R, Scrimgeour A, Yusuf S et al 1988 Reduction in fatal pulmonary embolism and venous thrombosis by perioperative administration of subcutaneous heparin. N Engl J Med 318: 1162–1173
Cruickshank M K, Levine M N, Hirsh J et al 1989 An evaluation of impedance plethysmography and ^{125}I-fibrinogen leg scanning in patients following hip surgery. Thromb Haemostasis 62: 830–834
Data J L, Nies A S 1974 Dextran 40. Inn Intern Med 81: 500–504
deBoer K, Heyboer H, Ten Cate J W et al 1989 Low molecular weight heparin treatment in a pregnant woman with allergy to standard heparins and heparinoid (letter). Thromb Haemostasis 61: 148
Editorial 1979 Thromboembolism in pregnancy. Br Med J 6179: 1661.
European Fraxiparin Study Group 1988 Comparison of a low molecular weight heparin and unfractionated heparin for the prevention of deep vein thrombosis in patients undergoing abdominal surgery. Br J Surg 75: 1058–1063
Evans G L, Dalen J E, Dexter L 1968 Pulmonary embolism during pregnancy. JAMA 206: 320–326
Flessa H C, Kapstrom A B, Glueck M J et al 1965 Placental transport of heparin. Am J Obstet Gynecol 93: 570–573
Francis C W, Marder V J, Evarts C M et al 1983 Two-step warfarin therapy: prevention of postoperative venous thrombosis without excessive bleeding. JAMA 249: 374–378
Gent M, Roberts R S 1986 A meta-analysis of the studies of dihydroergotamine plus heparin in the prophylaxis of deep vein thrombosis. Chest 89(suppl): 396S–400S
Ginsberg J S, Hirsh J 1989a Use of anticoagulants during pregnancy. Chest 95: 156S–160S
Ginsberg J S, Hirch J 1989b Anticoagulants during pregnancy. Am Rev Med 40: 79–86
Ginsberg J S, Kowalshuk J, Hirsh J et al 1989a Heparin therapy during pregnancy. Arch Intern Med 149: 2233–2236
Ginsberg J S, Hirsh J, Turner C et al 1989b Risks to the fetus of anticoagulant therapy during pregnancy. Thromb Haemostasis 61: 197–203
Gruber U F, Duckert F, Fridrich R et al 1977 Prevention of postoperative thromboembolism by dextran 40, low doses of heparin or xantinol nicotinate. Lancet 1: 207–210
Gruber U F, Saldeen T, Brokop T et al 1980 Incidences of fatal postoperative pulmonary embolism after prophylaxis with dextran 70 and low-dose heparin: an international multicentre study. Br Med J 1: 69–72
Halkin H, Goldberg J, Modan M et al 1982 Reduction of mortality in general medical in-patients by low dose heparin prophylaxis. Ann Intern Med 96: 561–565
Harris W H, Salzman E W, Athanasoulis C et al 1974 Comparison of warfarin, low-molecular weight dextran and subcutaneous heparin in prevention of venous thromboembolism following total hip replacement. J Bone Joint Surg 56A: 1552–1562
Hellgren M, Tengborn L, Abildgaard U 1982 Pregnancy in women with congenital antithrombin III deficiency: experience of treatment with heparin and antithrombin. Gynaecol Obstet Invest 14: 127–141
Hirsh J, Piovella F, Pini M 1989 Congenital antithrombin III deficiency: incidence and clinical features. Am J Med 87(suppl 3B): 34S–38S
Hull R, Hirsh J 1981 Advances and controversies in the diagnosis, prevention and treatment of venous thromboembolism. Prog Hematol 12: 73–123
International Multicenter Trial 1975 Prevention of fatal postoperative pulmonary embolism by low doses of heparin. Lancet 2: 45–51

Kakkar V V, Murray W J G 1985 Efficacy and safety of low-molecular weight heparin (CY216) in preventing postoperative venous thromboembolism: a cooperative study. Br J Surg 72: 786–791

Kierkegaard A 1983 Incidence and diagnosis of deep vein thrombosis with pregnancy. Acta Obstet Gynecol Scand 62: 239–243

Kiil J, Kiil J, Axelsen F et al 1978 Prophylaxis against postoperative pulmonary embolism and deep vein thrombosis by low-dose heparin. Lancet 1: 1115–1116

Lambie J M, Barber D C, Dhall D P et al 1970 Dextran 70 in prophylaxis of postoperative venous thrombosis: a controlled trial. Br Med J 2: 144–145

Lao T T, DeSwiet M, Letsky E et al 1985 Prophylaxis of thromboembolism in pregnancy: an alternative. Br J Obstet Gynecol 92: 202–206

Levine M N, Hirsh J 1988 Clinical use of low molecular weight heparins and heparinoids. Semin Thromb Haemostasis 14: 116–125

Leyvraz P F, Richard J, Bachmann F et al 1983 Adjusted versus fixed-dose subcutaneous heparin in the prevention of deep vein thrombosis after total hip replacement. N Engl J Med 309: 954–958

Maeck J V S, Ziliacus H 1948 Heparin in the treatment of toxemia of pregnancy. Am J Obstet Gynecol 55: 326–331

McCarthy S R, Turner J J, Robertson D et al 1977 Low dose heparin as a prophylaxis against deep vein thrombosis after acute stroke. Lancet 2: 800–801

McKenna R, Cale E R, Vasan U 1983 Is warfarin sodium contraindicated in the lactating mother? J Pediatr 103: 325–327

National Institutes of Health Consensus Development Conference Statement 1986 Prevention of venous thrombosis and pulmonary embolism. JAMA 256: 744–749

Nicolaides A N, Fernandes E, Fernandes J, Pollock A V 1980 Intermittent sequential pneumatic compression of the legs in the prevention of venous stasis and postoperative deep venous thrombosis. Surgery 87: 69–76

Omri A, Delaloye J F, Andersen H et al 1989 Low molecular weight heparin Novo (LHN-1) does not cross the placenta during the second trimester of pregnancy. Thromb Haemostasis 61: 55–56

Planes A, Vochelle N, Mazas F et al 1988 Prevention of postoperative venous thrombosis: a randomized trial comparing unfractionated heparin with low molecular weight heparin in patients undergoing total hip replacement. Thromb Haemostasis 60: 407–410

Poller L, McKernan A, Thomson J M et al 1987 Fixed minidose warfarin: a new approach to prophylaxis against venous thrombosis after major surgery. Br Med J 295: 1309–1312

Powers P J, Gent M, Jay R et al 1989 A randomized trial of less-intense warfarin or acetylsalicylic acid in the prevention of venous thromboembolism after surgery for fractured hip. Arch Intern Med 149: 771–774

Sagar S, Massey J, Sanderson J M 1975 Low dose heparin prophylaxis against fatal pulmonary embolism. Br Med J 4: 257–259

Salzman E W, Davies G C 1980 Prophylaxis of venous thromboembolism: analysis of cost-effectiveness. Ann Surg 191: 201

Salzman E W, Hirsh J 1987 Prevention of venous thromboembolism. In: Colman R W, Hirsh J, Marder V J, Salzman E W (eds) Hemostasis and thrombosis 2E, Lippincott, Philadelphia, pp 1252–1265

Salzman E W, Ploetz J, Bettman M et al 1980 Intraoperative external pneumatic compression to afford long-term prophylaxis against deep vein thrombosis in urological patients. Surgery 87: 239–242

Scurr J H, Ibrahim S Z, Faber R G et al 1979 The efficacy of graduated compression stockings in the prevention of deep vein thrombosis. Br J Surg 64: 371–373

Sheppeard H, Henson J, Ward D J et al 1981 A clinic-pathological study of fatal pulmonary embolism in a specialist orthopaedic hospital. Arch Orthop Trauma Surg 99: 65–71

Taberner D A, Poller L, Thomson J M et al 1989 Randomized study of adjusted versus fixed low dose heparin prophylaxis of deep vein thrombosis in hip surgery. Br J Surg 76: 933–935

Tooke J E, McNicol G P 1961 Thromboembolic disorders associated with pregnancy and the pill. Clin Haematol 10: 613

Treffers P E, Huidekoper B L, Weenink G H 1983 Epidemiological observations of thromboembolic disease during pregnancy and in the puerperium, in 56,022 women. Int J Gynaecol Obstet 21: 327–331

Turpie A G G 1981 The effectiveness of drugs that modify platelet function in peripheral venous thrombosis and pulmonary embolism. Clin Pharmacol Ther 224–233

Turpie A G G, Levine M N, Hirsh J et al 1986 A randomized controlled trial of low molecular weight heparin (enoxaparine) to prevent deep vein thrombosis in patients undergoing elective hip surgery. N Engl J Med 315: 925–929

Turpie A G G, Levine M N, Hirsh J et al 1987 A double-blind randomized trial of ORG 10172 low molecular weight heparinoid in the prevention of deep vein thrombosis in thrombotic stroke. Lancet 1: 523–526

Turpie A G G, Hirsh J, Gent M et al 1989 Prevention of deep vein thrombosis in potential neurosurgical patients: a randomized trial comparing graduated compression stockings alone or graduated compression stockings plus intermittent pneumatic compression with control. Arch Int Med 149: 679–681

Wessler S 1975 Venous thromboembolism: scope of the problem. In: Wessler S, Fratantoni J (eds) Prophylactic therapy of deep vein thrombosis and pulmonary embolism. Proceedings of a conference. DHEW publication no. (NIH) 76–866. Bethesda, MD, US Department of Health Service, National Institutes of Health, pp 1–10

Wray R, Maurer B, Shinningford J 1973 Prophylactic anticoagulant therapy in the prevention of calf-vein thrombosis after myocardial infarction. N Engl J Med 288: 815–817

10

Low-molecular-weight heparins and related glycosaminoglycans in the prophylaxis and treatment of venous thromboembolism

M. Samama   P. Desnoyers

Knowledge of the biological function and mechanism of action of the different glycosaminoglycans as they relate to coagulation and the thrombogenicity of the vascular wall, combined with the development of techniques allowing extraction, purification and fractionation, has led to characterization of their chemical structures and demonstration of similarities and differences between heparin and the various glycosaminoglycans. Of this biochemical family, heparin is the best-known and the most studied compound.

All the glycosaminoglycans are copolymers of uronic acid and a sugar amine (hexosamine) (Fig. 10.1). An arbitrary classification into five principal groups has been made according to the uronic acid and sugar amine as follows:

1. Hyaluronic acid
2. Heparin and heparan sulphate
3. Chondroitin-4-sulphate and chondroitin-6-sulphate
4. Keratan sulphate
5. Dermatan sulphate

All the glycosaminoglycans except for hyaluronic acid have a large number of O-sulphate groups conferring strong electronegative charge to the molecule, on which their biological properties largely depend.

Apart from heparin the glycosaminoglycans are all present in connective tissue, where they play an important role in the elasticity of vessels and in the maintenance of their structural integrity.

Heparan sulphate is probably bound to receptors in the cellular membrane where it may interact with matrix macromolecules such as fibronectin or collagen. Along with dermatan sulphate it is the most important glycosaminoglycan in vascular wall tissue.

Chondroitin sulphates have been identified in different tissues, particularly cartilage and the intervertebral discs.

Heparin, heparan sulphate and dermatan sulphate, which are the only molecules possessing iduronate residues, are also the only ones with antico-

A

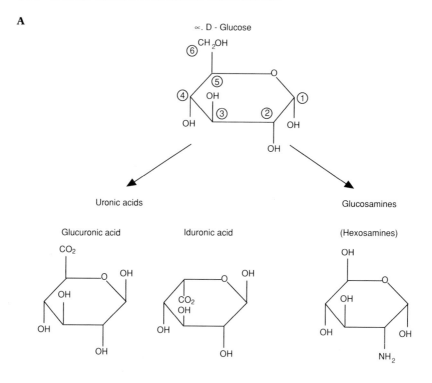

B

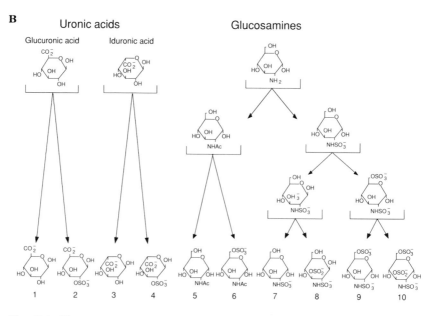

Fig. 10.1 Hexose structure involved in heparin composition. (**B** Reproduced with permission from Choay J, Petiton M 1986 The chemistry of heparin: a way to understand its mode of action. Med J Aus 144: HS 7–10. © Medical Journal of Australia 1986.)

agulant properties in vivo and in vitro. They are generally extracted from porcine intestinal mucosa or bovine pulmonary material.

THE DISCOVERY OF HEPARIN

There are few drugs which, 70 years after their discovery, still stimulate as much interest as heparin, which increasingly occupies a principal role in the modern therapeutic armamentarium. Official credit for its discovery is given to Jay McLean although the route towards its discovery had been paved before by numerous workers in various fields such as histology, physiology and biochemistry.

Jay McLean was an orphan without financial resource and had moved to the Johns Hopkins Institute to train in the laboratories of Professor Howell, the master of American physiology at the time. Using fractionation with organic solvents, he succeeded in 3 months in showing that in the ether extraction of animal brain the cephalin fraction had pro-coagulant properties. He then proposed to Howell that he would carry out the same fractionation on dog liver: these results confirmed the existence of a pro-coagulant fraction similar to the cerebral cephalins but also demonstrated the existence of an additional fraction insoluble in boiling alcohol which possessed anticoagulant properties and which he named antithrombin.

At the end of the summer in 1916 McLean came to the end of his training period and had to finish his research. Thereafter he would follow as a mere spectator the progress of work which he had initiated.

Howell, helped by Holt, continued McLean's work and, unhappy with the term antithrombin, he gave the substance the name Heparin in 1918, the name recalling through its Greek origins the liver from which it had been extracted. After difficult purification, Howell isolated heparin in 1923 in the form of brown-coloured fragments at a titre of 5 units/mg. In 1925 a titre of 40 units was achieved and then in 1928 a product with 100 units/mg was obtained in very small quantities. At this point Howell's contribution ended. To Charles Best, already very well known for his work on insulin, credit is due for transforming in just under 10 years a rare and expensive reagent into an easily obtained drug with valuable therapeutic applications (Baird 1989).

HEPARIN FRACTIONS

Cleavage by the endoglucosidase of the precursor macromolecule of heparin in mast cells, leads to different length chains, explaining the variation in molecular weight found in commercial preparations. An identical situation is found with heparan sulphate. In addition to this heterogeneity in chain length, however, heparin is equally heterogeneous in terms of its affinity for its principal cofactor, antithrombin III (AT III). Indeed, two-thirds of heparin molecules, of standard or unfractionated heparin, have a low affinity for AT III. In order to reduce the variation in molecular weight and to increase the number of molecules with affinity for AT III, attempts have been made to depolymerize the long chains of heparin using various procedures: enzymatic cleavage, peroxidation, depolymerization by nitric acid and gel chromatography. These techniques have allowed isolation of fractions which, still polydispersed but whose molecular weights range between 2000 and 12 000 daltons, the mean molecular weight being around 5000 daltons. These compounds studied since 1976 (Johnson et al) have been named low-molecular-weight heparins (LMWH).

We will consider in turn the pharmacological, pharmacokinetic and clinical properties of LMWH, of dermatan sulphate and of heparan sulphate, then of a heparinoid (ORG 10172) with particular reference to their properties in the prophylaxis and treatment of venous thromboembolic disease.

LOW-MOLECULAR-WEIGHT HEPARINS

It was recognized from the onset that the properties of these new types of fractionated heparins were different from those of their parent preparations. Indeed, whilst standard heparin possesses activity directed against thrombin (activated factor II) equivalent to that against activated Stuart factor (factor Xa), the reduction in molecular weight brings with it a slight loss of activity against Xa but a much more marked loss in activity against factor IIa, so that the ratio of the anti-Xa activity/anti-IIa activity which is close to 1 for non-fractionated heparin is between 2 and 5 for the LMWHs.

The structure of low-molecular-weight heparins

Heterogeneity

Unfractionated heparin is a heterogeneous mixture composed of long-chain saccharides bearing sulphate groups which play a significant role in its anticoagulant activity. In these polysaccharide chains there are both regular and irregular sequences (Fig. 10.2) of saccharide units and the minimum sequence needed for binding to AT III in order to obtain anticoagulant activity has been identified. This is a pentasaccharide unit which has been synthesized (Choay et al 1983). In addition, amongst the molecules containing the pentasaccharide group, those which possess less than 18 saccharide units and a molecular weight under 5000 daltons have no inhibitory activity except against factor Xa, whereas the longer chains can also neutralize the action of thrombin as well as activated factor X.

This difference in behaviour of standard heparin linked to chain length may be explained by the fact that neutralization of thrombin activity requires the formation of a ternary complex and a long polysaccharide chain which is able to bind together both thrombin and AT III. In contrast, however, short chains which produce conformational changes in AT III allow only

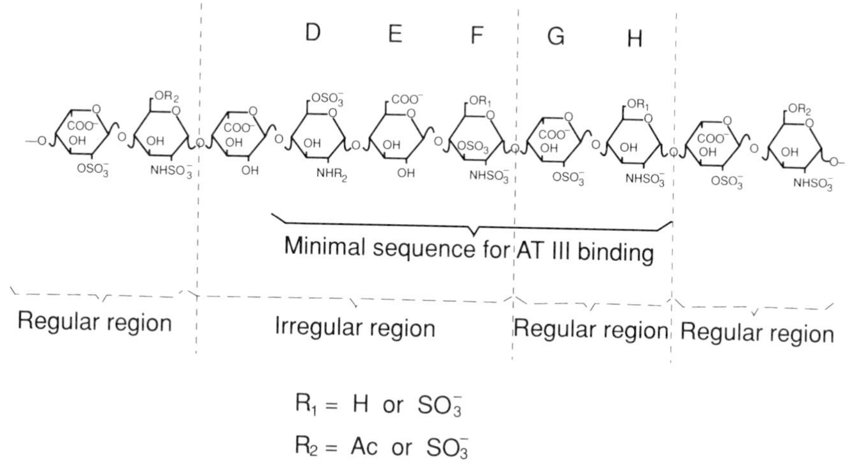

Fig. 10.2   Heparin basic molecular sequences: regular and irregular regions.

neutralization of activated factor X but not of thrombin (Holmer et al 1981). The long chains with a high affinity for AT III may on occasion contain more than one pentasaccharide group. It is possible to identify in total four molecular groups; those with less than 18 saccharide units and those with more, and for each of these two groups those which possess high affinity for AT III and those which only possess low affinity. Within each of these two groups of molecules with affinity for AT III the inhibitory activity tends to increase with molecular weight. Isolation of well-characterized fragments rather than heterogeneous fractions should allow a more precise study of anti-IIa and anti-Xa activities of these molecules.

Problems of quantification of low-molecular-weight heparins

Initially LMWH were titrated against the 4th International Standard of unfractionated heparin, either using amidolytic or coagulation methods. However, because of different kinetics of biological activity (Barrowcliffe et al 1985) comparison between unfractionated heparin and LMWHs is difficult and there is need for an international LMWH standard to reduce these problems (Bara & Samama 1986, Barrowcliffe et al 1988a). This standard is now available and has a titre of 168 IU anti-Xa/mg and 68 IU anti-IIa/mg (ratio anti-Xa/anti-IIa about 2.5) assayed using chromogenic substrate methods. However, the three LMWHs currently marketed in France (Table 10.1), although derived from an almost identical standard heparin, differ in chemical composition. Because of this there has been discussion concerning the validity of the international standard of LMWH (Fareed et al 1988, Hemker 1989). In addition anti-Xa activity does not appear to run in parallel with antithrombotic activity. Although it is acceptable to express the activity of standard heparin in USP units according to the European or American pharmacopoeia this is not recommended for LMWH. At present it is therefore advised that the titre of pharmaceutical preparations of LMWH be expressed in international anti-Xa and anti-IIa units as compared to the first international standard of LMWH and by assays based on chromogenic substrates.

Pharmacological properties of low-molecular-weight heparin

The antithrombotic activity of LMWH has been evaluated in comparison with that of unfractionated heparin on animal models of venous or arterial thrombosis.

Activity against venous thrombosis

In the rabbit the most often used model is jugular venous thrombosis by stasis and injection of procoagulant fractions (human serum according to the classical model of Wessler, factor Xa, thromboplastin, thrombin and activated or non-activated prothrombin concentrates. The LMWHs with a mean molecular weight around 5000 daltons have an antithrombotic action similar to that of standard heparin. Even so, on a weight basis, approximately twice the quantity of LMWH must be used to obtain an antithrombotic activity identical to that of non-fractionated heparin (Bara et al 1986). In contrast to non-fractionated heparin, however, which at antithrombotic

Table 10.1 Comparative activity of various low-molecular-weight heparins

	Code	Molecular weight (daltons)	Activity (according to manufacturer)	Unit package (anti-Xa, International Units)	Anti-Xa activity* (mg raw material) (anti-Xa, International Units)	Anti-IIa activity (mg raw material)
Enoxaparine (Lovenox®)	PK 10169	4500–5000 (3000–8000)	20 mg	2000	100	30
Tedelparine (Fragmine®)	KABI 2165	4000–6000 (2000–9000)	2500 IU anti-Xa amidolytic	2500	122	60
(Fraxiparine®)	CY 216	4500 (2000–8000)	7500U anti-Xa/IC	3100	97	30

* Values obtained in a collaborative study performed by five laboratories using the same methods and reagents, versus the first international standard for low-molecular-weight heparin. Anti-Xa activity was determined in a purified system using human antithrombin III (Kabi-vitrum).

concentrations is associated with prolongation of the APTT (activated partial thromboplastin time) through increasing the anti-IIa and anti-Xa activity, the LMWHs do not cause significant changes in the APTT despite possessing anti-Xa activity similar to that of standard heparin.

The effectiveness of the LMWHs in preventing extension of experimentally produced thrombosis was determined by comparing their ability to inhibit deposition of labelled fibrinogen on non-radioactive autologous thrombus preformed in the jugular vein of the rabbit (Boneu et al 1985). In this animal the LMWHs showed themselves to be effective not only in the prevention of experimental thrombosis but equally in the inhibition of thrombus propagation through fibrinogen deposition.

In the rat antithrombotic activity was measured using the number of laser-induced lesions necessary to obtain total occlusion of mesenteric vessels. Antithrombotic activity was assessed at fixed time intervals following subcutaneous injection of LMWH and lasted for more than 48 hours following injection, whereas the anticoagulant effect measured using both anti-Xa and anti-IIa activity lasted only during the first 6 hours following injection (Bender et al 1988). These results confirmed those of previous studies carried out following intravenous administration of doses of 0.1 and 0.25 mg/kg (Andriuoli et al 1985) and following subcutaneous injection of a dose of 2 mg/kg, where standard heparin was found to be less effective than LMWH in preventing venous thrombosis after ligation of the inferior vena cava (Doutremepuich et al 1987).

In the sheep, in an attempt to find a potential use for LMWH in open cardiac surgery or in haemodialysis, Aiach et al in 1984 used a model of extracorporeal circulation and administered either an LMWH at a dose of 2 mg/kg or unfractionated heparin at different doses. The highest of these doses produced anti-Xa activity identical to that of the LMWH, and the lowest dose the same anti-IIa activity as the LMWH. The LMWH was as effective in preventing thrombosis in the extracorporeal circulation as standard heparin at the higher dose but clots were seen with the lower dose of standard heparin. Although the depolymerization of standard heparin diminishes the anti-APTT activity it does not affect the antithrombotic properties which seem therefore not to be totally related to this activity.

Activity against arterial thrombosis

In the dog the antithrombotic properties of an LMWH enoxaparin were assessed by measuring the inhibition of thrombus formation following transluminal stimulation of the coronary artery with an anodic current. Enoxaparin possessed antithrombotic properties at doses as low as 0.62 mg/kg s.c. which, at a dose of 2.5 mg/kg, were equivalent to a dose of 10 mg/kg s.c. of standard heparin.

On the other hand no relationship could be found between the antithrombotic properties and the activity against factor Xa, and in the doses used the LMWH failed to demonstrate any anticoagulant activity. Fractions of LMWH might therefore be thought of as arterial antithrombotic agents devoid of appreciable anticoagulant activity (Mestre et al 1985).

Haemorrhagic effects

As early as 1982 Carter et al compared the antithrombotic and haemorrhagic effects of different heparin fractions and demonstrated that for an equivalent anti-Xa activity these fractions produced much less marked prolongation of the APTT and of the thrombin time than standard heparin.

In the rabbit they were able to demonstrate using ^{51}Cr blood cell labelling as a sensitive measure of blood loss and an optimal dose threshold that the LMWHs were less likely to cause haemorrhage and possessed greater antithrombotic activity than standard heparin.

These results were confirmed by numerous authors, and in particular by Bergqvist et al (1985), who measured blood loss from mesenteric arterioles and venules in the rabbit following injection of LMWH of different molecular weights.

The mechanism of this reduction in haemorrhagic potential seen in the experimental animal has been the centre of considerable debate and has most often been attributed to a reduction in anti-IIa activity. Other mechanisms may, however, be involved:

1. Salzman et al (1980) suggested that standard heparin which has a weak affinity for AT III might have a greater effect on platelet function than the LMWH with a high affinity for AT III. Fernandez et al (1986a) suggested a relationship between increased bleeding and inhibition of platelet aggregation, in the presence of acid-soluble collagen at low concentration.
2. More recently Barrowcliffe et al (1988b) have suggested that prolongation of the bleeding time is related to a significant release of lipoprotein lipase. The LMWHs have a lesser ability to cause lipoprotein lipase release than standard heparin and hence, possibly, less haemorrhagic potential.
3. A third mechanism proposed is that vascular permeability may be less increased by LMWH, but this hypothesis needs further study.

Binding to the vascular endothelium

The binding of standard heparin, and of LMWHs labelled with ^{125}I or tritium, has been studied on primary cultures of endothelial cells from the umbilical vein. A slow, saturable and reversible binding was found although the reversal was only partial with the LMWH which bound less than standard heparin to the vascular wall. This fact possibly explains their greater bioavailability (Barzu et al 1985).

In a study of genetically diabetic KK mice with C57 black mice as controls, increased production of Type III collagen in relation to Type I and increased biosynthesis of fibronectin was demonstrated using skin flaps in culture. Administration of LMWH to the KK mice normalized these figures for Type III collagen and fibronectin. These results suggest that the LMWHs may be able to control expression of intracellular matrix macromolecules (Asselot et al 1989).

Binding to proteins

In addition to their anticoagulant properties, standard heparin and LMWHs are capable of binding to a large number of proteins of various functions, because of the anionic structure of the molecules conferred by the sulphate and carboxylic groups. In comparative studies looking at heparin, heparan sulphate, dermatan sulphate and other glycosaminoglycans it has been suggested that there may be common binding sites on certain proteins and that the binding strength may be related more to the charge and length of polysaccharide chain than to the specific saccharide sequence of the chains (Lane 1989).

Plasma proteins bound to heparin. Antithrombin is the most abundant plasma protein capable of high-affinity binding to heparin: this interaction appears specific as antithrombin binds solely at the level of the pentasaccharide present in only 30% of commercial preparations. Three binding sites appear to be involved.

A second heparin-dependent thrombin inhibitor was purified from human plasma and called cofactor II (Tollefsen et al 1982). This possessed 25–30% sequence homology with the other members of the 'serpine' family. The region Lys 101–Arg 106 corresponds to the antithrombin sequence containing Arg 47 and Trp 49 which have been implicated in heparin binding.

Heparin binds also to thrombin, this binding being essential for inhibition of the enzyme by antithrombin. This does not, however, appear to be a high-affinity binding site.

Histidine-rich glycoprotein (HRG) binds to heparin in the presence of divalent cations, neutralizing its anticoagulant activity. This reaction is pH dependent (Peterson et al 1987). The kinetics of heparin binding indicate that the mechanism whereby HRG modulates heparin anticoagulant activity involves simultaneous competition both with the inhibitor and the protease.

Finally, heparin binds to the plasma lipoproteins, this binding being dependent on the length of the polysaccharide chain, pH, ionic strength, and the presence of divalent cations. There would appear to be only two binding sites, the first being near to the centre of the protein (residues 142–147) and the second between residues 243 and 272 (Weisgraber et al 1986).

Platelet proteins binding to heparin. Platelets contain a large number of proteins which bind heparin, in particular platelet factor 4 (PF 4) which neutralizes its anticoagulant activity (Loscalzo et al 1985). β-thromboglobulin (β-TG) appears to have a binding ability weaker than that of PF 4. The LMWHs have anti-Xa activity which appears to be poorly neutralized by platelet factor 4 in contrast to standard heparin (Lane et al 1984).

Extracellular matrix proteins binding to heparin. Fibronectins play an important role in cell movement and adhesion, scar formation and in the organization of the cytoskeleton. They bind to heparin by means of a large number of sites, the binding being dependent on divalent cations.

Vitronectin (Preissner et al 1986) appears to possess a heparin binding site found between residues Arg 342 and Arg 375 (Suzuki et al 1984).

Several heparin binding sites have been described for thrombospondin, a protein present both in plasma and platelets. These have been found in particular in the N-terminal region of the molecule (Lawler & Hynes 1987).

The triple helix conformation of collagen appears to be necessary for heparin binding. In addition, the C-terminal fragment obtained following collagenase digestion appears to have greater affinity for heparin than the N-terminal fragment (Keller et al 1986).

Lipolytic activity

Some sulphated polysaccharides, particularly the LMWHs, may have their antithrombotic effect through release of an endogenous anticoagulant in vivo. Certainly, release of lipoprotein lipase and of hepatic triglyceride lipase has been found following injection of LMWH in man (Barrowcliffe 1986). As with standard heparin the LMWHs are capable of inducing lipoprotein lipase and hepatic lipase release. The release of lipoprotein lipase decreases, however, as a function of the molecular weight of the heparin in contrast to the hepatic lipase (Millot et al 1987). Given that hepatic triglyceride lipase may inhibit coagulation caused by factor Xa, Gray et al in 1987 proposed that this enzyme which was released following injection of sulphated polysaccharides may be responsible in part for the anticoagulant effect ex vivo and may contribute to the antithrombotic activity. Another anticoagulant factor may be released, as it has been demonstrated that the extrinsic pathway inhibitor (EPI) or lipoprotein coagulation inhibitor (LACI) is found at increased levels following heparin injection (Sandset et al 1988).

Pharmacokinetic properties of the low-molecular-weight heparins

Unfractionated heparin is cleared from the organism by two mechanisms, the first being saturable and is predominant at low doses (<100 units anti-Xa/kg), and the second which is non-saturable and involved particularly at higher doses, when the first mechanism is saturated. The metabolism of

LMWH has been studied initially in animals, particularly the rabbit, after radiolabelling with [125]I. In this animal, the saturable mechanism only contributes a small part to LMWH clearance, which implicates the non-saturable mechanism to a great extent at all doses studied (Boneu et al 1987). At low doses, for example, standard heparin is cleared much faster than Fraxiparine (CY 216) whereas at very high doses the latter is cleared more rapidly (Briant et al 1989). LMWHs are cleared principally by the renal route through a non-dose-dependent mechanism, hence the problem risk of overdosage in severe renal failure (Caranobe et al 1985, Palm & Mattsson 1987). The LMWHs are cleared therefore through a significantly different mechanism than standard heparin. This possibly explains the apparent prolongation of the anticoagulant effect of the LMWHs at therapeutic doses.

The tissue distribution of one LMWH was studied in the rat using fluoresceine labelling. No fluorescent material was detected in cuts from aorta, lung, spleen or cardiac muscle, whereas significant fluorescence was found in hepatic cuts, with a peak reached between the second and third hour following administration and disappearing at the 12th hour. In the kidneys, intense fluorescence is seen in the cortical region with a peak at 45 minutes. This is much weaker in the medullary zone, where it disappears after approximately 45 minutes (Guizzardi et al 1987).

The pharmacokinetics of LMWH have been studied in man using measurements of biological amidolytic anti-Xa and anti-IIa activities. The half-life of anti-Xa activity is between 3 and 4 hours following intravenous or subcutaneous injection, this differing significantly from that of standard heparin which, dependent on the dose, is between 1 and 1.5 hours (Bratt et al 1986, Matzch et al 1987, Bara & Samama 1988). In contrast to standard heparin there may be a difference with some LMWHs (enoxaparine for example) between the half-lives of anti-Xa and anti-IIa activity, the half-life of anti-IIa activity being shorter than that of anti-Xa (Bara et al 1985, Frydman et al 1988) (Table 10.2).

Although earlier studies (Follea et al 1986) following intravenous administration of heparin to patients with chronic renal failure had demonstrated that the clearance mechanism for LMWH in therapeutic doses was not saturable and that the kidney played only a minor role in this clearance, Boneu et al 1988 observed that in patients with renal failure the biological half-life of LMWH is twice as long as in healthy volunteers.

By subcutaneous injection of 30–40 mg of different heparin fragments it has been demonstrated that the bioavailability of the LMWH and the half-life for anti-Xa clearance are approximately four times greater than those of standard heparin when given at a dose of 29 mg (Bara et al 1984). Total clearance is less rapid than for standard heparin and is not altered by increasing the dose. This difference may be explained by weaker cellular uptake of LMWH.

As compared to the intravenous route, the absolute bioavailability from

Table 10.2   Comparative pharmacokinetics of various low-molecular-weight heparins

LMWH	Authors	Dosage	Subject number	Clearance of anti-Xa activity (min)		Bioavail-ability (%)
				i.v. route	s.c. route	
Enoxaparine (Lovenox®)	Aiach et al (1983)	25 mg 75 mg	10	180 –	– 360	
	Bara et al (1984)	30 mg 60 mg Unfrac-tionated heparin	6	129 ± 7 135 ± 9 51 ± 6	– 330 ± 32 180 ± 91	98
	Bara et al (1985)	40 mg Unfrac-tionated heparin	8	277 35	275 177	91 25
	Frydman et al (1988)	20 mg 40 mg 60 mg 80 mg	8		252 ± 132 261 ± 64 222 ± 48 217 ± 48	
Tedelparine (Fragmine®)	Bratt et al (1985b)	40 IU/kg 60 IU/kg Unfrac-tionated heparin 40 IU/kg	8	126 ± 21 139 ± 28 57 ± 12		
	Bratt et al (1986)	120 IU/kg	6	119 ± 17	228 ± 40	87 ± 6
(Fraxi-parine®)	Rostin et al (1990)	100 U.IC/kg	12	136 ± 45	228 ± 90	88.5 ± 16.9

subcutaneous administration is greater than 90% whereas this figure is only around 30% for non-fractionated heparin. The reason for this is still debated: mechanisms suggested include decreased neutralization of LMWH by platelet factor 4 and by different plasma proteins, reduced binding to endothelial cells, and decreased catabolism. The greatest bioavailability of LMWH as compared to standard heparin was demonstrated for low doses. Recent work in the rabbit has demonstrated that by greatly increasing the dose of unfractionated heparin given bioavailability is increased, explaining why in changing from intravenous to subcutaneous administration of the drug in man it is usually only necessary to increase slightly the dose (Briant et al 1989).

The volume of distribution, as calculated following a single-dose subcu-taneous injection, is only slightly greater than the total blood volume, representing approximately 10% of body mass. The distribution of LMWH is in most cases therefore confined to the intravascular space.

Finally, the activity peak appears between the third and fifth hour following subcutaneous administration, with a highly significant correlation between peak anti-Xa activity (mg or IU/ml) and the dose injected.

In man the relationship between plasma anti-Xa activity and the patient's weight is highly significant for the same dose (Bara et al 1987b, Vitoux et al 1988a).

Mechanism of action of low-molecular-weight heparins

Anticoagulant and antithrombotic activities of the heparins

The anticoagulant activity of standard heparin acts either through two intermediary cofactors, AT III and the second heparin cofactor (HC II), or by a direct antithrombin action unrelated to these two factors, although this latter mechanism is weak. Heparin activity may be found at the surface of the vascular endothelium. This holds also for dermatan sulphate and heparan sulphate in particular, both of which have anticoagulant properties and act through one or other of the two intermediary cofactors mentioned. The therapeutic action of heparin has its physiological equivalent of action therefore at the level of the vascular endothelium (Fig. 10.3).

During the coagulation process in the adult, AT III is involved in the neutralization of approximately 65% of thrombin formed whereas cofactor II binds only to 10%, the remainder being neutralized by α_2-macroglobulin. In contrast, however, in the presence of heparin, the proportion of thrombin neutralized by AT III increases considerably, only a small proportion being bound to cofactor II and to α_2-macroglobulin (Hemker et al 1986). The antithrombotic role of α_2-macroglobulin is more significant in the child than in the adult.

In vitro studies of the effect of the heparins and their derivatives on coagulation have used models of either intrinsic or extrinsic coagulation pathway. These demonstrated the clinical phenomenon that the APTT (intrinsic coagulation) is more sensitive to non-fractionated heparin than the prothrombin time (extrinsic coagulation).

In either case, the study of thrombin generation and of its neutralization has been helped by the use of an inhibitor preventing factor Xa generation (and hence thrombin production), avoiding the resulting difficulties which would otherwise have occurred in measuring the decay of thrombin already formed (Hemker et al 1986).

These studies, along with those of different authors, have brought to light two essential points:

1. The three principal activated factors IIa, IXa and Xa are inhibited by the AT III/heparin complex, but this inhibition requires much higher concentrations of heparin if the activated factors are bound to phospholipids.
2. The inhibition of factor Xa or IIa when added to plasma is not strictly

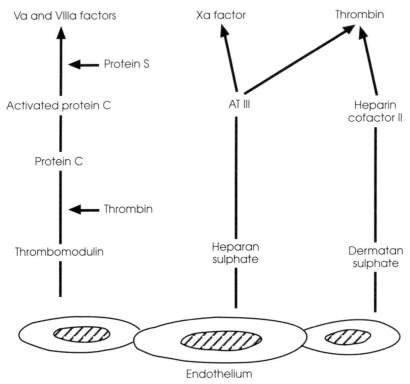

Fig. 10.3 Anticoagulant activity associated with the endothelial cells of the vascular tree. Action of AT III, proteins C and S.

parallel to that seen with the same factors when formed during the coagulation process.

It seems appropriate at this stage to point out that the prophylactic action of heparin at low doses occurs by means of an inhibition of thrombin generation and/or of thrombin itself. Thus heparin, when bound to AT III, may inhibit the first traces of thrombin formed and prevent activation of factors V and VIII, hence reducing prothrombinase generation (Beguin et al 1988, Ofosu et al 1988b). An interesting point is that factor VIIIa when formed 'protects' factor IXa against the action of heparin in the intrinsic coagulation pathway. Factor VIIIa inhibition therefore leaves factor IXa much more vulnerable. Factor IXa, however, is capable of activating factors V and VIII. It has recently been demonstrated that factor Xa possesses enzymatic activity through activation of factor V which is as great as that of thrombin itself (Monkovic & Tracy 1990). The first traces of formed thrombin equally are involved in platelet activation which in turn contributes to the coagulation cascade. The degree of potentiation of the thrombin/AT III reaction by sulphated polysaccharides could serve as an index of antithrombotic activity. In addition, it is useful to note the results obtained with a synthetic pentasaccharide which has the advantage over heparin of possessing only anti-Xa activity. This pentasaccharide, which is capable of inhibiting thrombin generation, has real antithrombotic activity on the rabbit model of venous stasis. The doses of pentasaccharide necessary to obtain biological activity (inhibition of thrombin generation) and experimental activity (antithrombotic) expressed in anti-Xa units, are much higher than those needed for LMWH and standard heparin (Walenga et al 1986).

The ex vivo activity equivalent to experimental antithrombotic activity is an inhibition of thrombin generation to 50% or less. Ofosu et al (1988a) noted that doubling the catalytic activity of heparins on thrombin in plasma ex vivo is equivalent to antithrombotic activity in vivo. One of the fundamental differences of LMWH as compared to standard heparin may be lesser neutralization by platelet factor 4 released in situ following platelet activation.

It is likely therefore that antithrombin activity is essential in order to obtain the antithrombotic and anticoagulant effects of heparin. In contrast, however, the anti-Xa activity, which for some authors has only minimal or a zero role to play in the antithrombotic activity of heparin, may in reality have a much more significant effect in vivo taking into account results obtained with the pentasaccharide and results from therapeutic trials.

Authors who argue that anti-Xa activity does not play a significant role highlight the fact that the quantity of factor Xa generated during coagulation is much larger than that necessary for thrombin generation. This suggests that only with near complete inhibition of factor Xa generation might there be an effect on coagulation, at least in vitro. This is further supported by the fact that substances with anti-Xa activity alone, such as the pentasaccharide, only cause prolongation of the TCA at extremely high concentrations. In favour of the role of anti-Xa activity in the antithrombotic action of heparin one must consider the results obtained in haemodialysis with CY 222 by Lane et al (1986), who demonstrated a significant relationship between anti-Xa activity and inhibition of fibrinopeptide A generation. Furthermore Cadroy (1988) showed that it was possible to inhibit an experimental model of thrombosis using only the pentasaccharide. Finally, in recent work, one of us has demonstrated that the same derivative which has little activity on preformed prothrombinase, was nevertheless able to inhibit prothrombinase generation, as do the heparins (Bendetowicz et al 1990) (Fig. 10.4).

Low-molecular-weight heparins and fibrinolysis

The profibrinolytic activity of the polysaccharides has been known for some 40 years. Vinazzer et al in 1982 demonstrated that standard heparin was able to increase the potential for fibrinolysis as measured by the euglobulin lysis time whereas LMWHs were devoid of such activity. This activation of fibrinolysis appeared to depend on the molecular weight of the heparin and

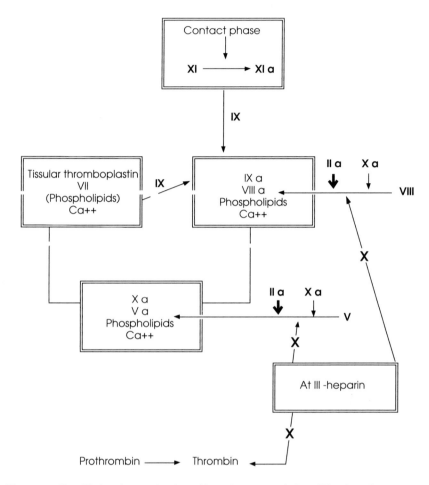

Fig. 10.4 Simplified action mechanism of heparin on coagulation. (Thanks to its antithrombin (anti-IIa) and anti-Xa action, heparin–AT III complex inhibits the first amount of generated thrombin, essential to factors V and VIII activation. Antithrombin action plays a leading part with regard to anti-Xa activity).

also on the degree of sulphation. Nevertheless, certain LMWHs following intravenous or subcutaneous administration are able to increase the level of tissue plasminogen activator (tPA) and of the derivative of fibrin, B beta 15–42, without changing levels of protein C antigen (Fareed et al 1985). These results were confirmed by a recent double-blind randomized crossover study against placebo (Agnelli et al 1988) carried out on volunteers who received a single intravenous dose of either placebo or 5000 IU of standard heparin or LMWH (Kabi 2165) at doses of 5000 or 10 000 IU anti-Xa. Whereas both placebo and LMWH at a dose of 5000 IU anti-Xa were devoid of activity, standard heparin and LMWH at a dose of 10 000 IU anti-Xa caused a significant increase in levels of tPA one hour after injection, lasting for approximately one hour. Curiously, however, the areas of lysis on fibrin plates were unchanged, nor were levels of tPA inhibitor (PAI), plasminogen, fibrinogen, or α_2-antiplasmin. In contrast, other studies failed to demonstrate changes in fibrinolytic activity when circadian variation was taken into account (Grimaudo et al 1988).

The mechanism of this profibrinolytic ability, which is still debated, would appear to be based more on release of tPA than on inhibition of PAI. Finally it was shown that there was a significant reduction in the weight of thrombus formed in subjects as compared to controls using treatment with a LMWH (CY 222). In addition the fibrinolytic activity of treated clots was higher despite being of lower weight; this could be regarded as indirect evidence of tPA binding to the thrombus (Doutremepuich et al 1988). We should note finally the unusual observation by Vairel et al (1983), who demonstrated that the association between LMWH and ε-amino caproic acid resulted in LMWH losing antithrombotic activity in an experimental model.

Clinical studies with low-molecular-weight heparins

A large number of clinical trials using LMWHs have been the subject of recent reviews (Levine & Hirsh 1988, Samama et al 1989).

Prophylaxis of deep vein thrombosis

General surgery. The first indication for the use of LMWH was in the prophylaxis of thromboembolic events in general surgery. Results are now available from dozens of randomized studies both open or double-blind and involving over 7000 patients. Inclusion criteria are generally subjects aged greater than 40 years undergoing general surgery (abdominal, thoracic, gynaecological, urological, etc.) requiring general anaesthesia for more than 30 minutes. The therapeutic protocols have differed from one study to the other but most frequently LMWHs have been compared to control groups receiving subcutaneous standard heparin at a dose of 5000 IU two or three times per day or, in rare cases, placebo. The first injection is carried out 2 hours before surgery except in the case of one study where it was administered 12 hours before (Bergqvist et al 1988). The principal studies are summarized in Table 10.3.

Diagnosis of postoperative deep venous thrombosis was made using fibrinogen labelled with ^{125}I after blocking thyroid uptake. In positive cases ascending venography was carried out as often as possible, but follow-up of possible thromboembolic events was not always carried out after the end of the studies which had a mean duration of approximately 7 days. The number of patients in each study was generally too small to detect an effect on overall mortality or on mortality related to pulmonary embolism (Collins

Table 10.3   Leading trials of low-molecular-weight heparins in general surgery

Authors	LMWH	n	Control	n	Thrombotic events (%)		Bleeding	Hb decrease
					LMWH	Control		
Kakkar (1984)	Fraxiparine® 1850 APTT	501	–	–	3.4		n.s.	n.s.
Kakkar & Murray (1985)	Fraxiparine® 7500 U/IC	199	UF 5000 IU × 2	196	2.5	7.5*	n.s.	n.s.
Encke & Breddin (1988)	Fraxiparine® 7500 U/IC	957	UF 5000 IU × 3	941	2.8	4.5	n.s.	n.s.
Samama et al (1988)	Enoxaparine (Lovenox®)							
	20 mg	167	UF	167	3.8	7.6	n.s.	n.s.
	40 mg	124	5000 IU	123	2.8	2.8	n.s.	n.s.
	60 mg	157	× 3	147	2.9	3.7	n.s.	$p = 0.03$
	Tedelparine (Fragmine®)							
Bergqvist et al (1986)	5000 IU	217	UF 5000 IU × 2	215	6	4.2	$p < 0.01$	n.s.
Koller et al (1986)	2500 IU	73	5000 IU × 2	73	2.8	2.9	n.s.	n.s.
Caen (1988)	2500 IU	195	5000 IU × 2	190	3.1	3.7	n.s.	n.s.
Bergqvist et al (1988)	5000 IU	505	5000 IU × 3	497	5.5	8.7*	oozing	n.s.
Ockelford et al (1989)	2500 IU	120	Placebo	128	4.1	16.9*	n.s.	n.s.
Adolf et al (1989)	LMWH–novo (Logiparine) 1500 APTT	202	5000 IU × 3	202	10.8	11.4	n.s.	n.s.

UF, unfractionated heparin.
* Statistically significant difference.

et al 1988). However, one large multicentre Italian study (STEP) randomized and double-blind (Pezzuoli et al 1989) compared a daily subcutaneous injection of 7500 U/IC of CY 216 to placebo in general surgical patients.

The study reported on a group of 4498 patients aged above 40 years. Twenty-three of the 26 patients who died underwent autopsy. Pulmonary embolus was the direct cause of death in two patients from the treatment group (0.009%) and in four patients from the control group (0.18%, n.s.). It should be noted that during this study the frequency of pulmonary embolus was much lower than that seen in the International Multicentre Trial coordinated by Kakkar (Anonymous 1975). It is possible that the risk of thromboembolism was much lower in the Italian study, this perhaps being confirmed by the fact that total mortality in the STEP study was much less than in the Kakkar study. Both peri- and postoperative haemorrhage were significantly more frequent in the treatment group but did not lead to changes in further management of patients.

All of these studies concluded that LMWH was at least equal if not superior in effect to standard heparin when administered subcutaneously for the prophylaxis of deep venous thrombosis in general surgery (Potron et al 1989). Because of their pharmacokinetic properties LMWHs can be administered in single daily doses and by subcutaneous injection. They are therefore straightforward to use whilst allowing greater comfort for both patient and staff.

In addition there is no greater associated risk of haemorrhage than with standard heparin assuming that the optimal treatment dose is established for each LMWH. Perioperative bleeding has been observed with almost all the LMWHs when the dose used has been too high. As early as 1986 one trial had to be stopped prematurely following the high incidence of haemorrhagic events where too high a dose was used (Koller et al 1986).

The encouraging results from general surgery led clinicians to consider the possibility of prevention of thrombosis in orthopaedic surgery.

Orthopaedic surgery. The risk of deep venous thrombosis is particularly high in fractures of the neck of the femur and in hip and knee replacements, the incidence of thrombosis varying between 30% and 70%. An overview of comparative studies using LMWH and non-fractionated heparin or dextran demonstrated LMWH to be more effective but at doses almost twice that used in general surgery (Table 10.4).

The risk of haemorrhage remains low with the dose used, a most important factor in this type of surgery (Dechavanne et al 1989). In France, the recommended prophylactic treatment used in orthopaedic surgery followed the results of the American consensus and consists of the administration of standard heparin subcutaneously at a dose adapted according to the APTT in order to obtain a mild reduction in coagulability. The use of LMWH either at a standard dose or varied according to the weight of the patient may probably obviate the need for daily biological monitoring with non-fractionated heparin. If the results available at present were to be confirmed in subsequent studies on a larger number of patients this would bring about new interest regarding the possible superiority of LMWH over standard heparin. It appears, however, that at least for enoxaparine there is a

Table 10.4 Leading trials of low-molecular-weight heparins in orthopaedic surgery

Authors	LMWH	n	Control	n	Thrombotic events (%)		Bleeding	Hb decrease
					LMWH	Control		
Turpie et al (1986)	Enoxaparine (Lovenox®) 30 mg × 2	50	Placebo	50	12*	24	n.s.	n.s.
Planes et al (1988)	40 mg	113	UF 5000 IU × 3	124	7.5*	25	n.s.	n.s.
Barre et al (1987)	Tedelparine (Fragmine®) 2500 IU × 2	40	UF adjusted dosage (APTT)	40	17.5	10	n.s.	n.s.
Eriksson et al (1988)	2500 IU × 2	49	Dextran 70	49	20*	45	n.s.	n.s.
Decha-vanne et al (1989)	2500 IU × 2 2500 IU × 2 5000 IU after	41 41	UF adjusted dosage (APTT)	40	4.3* 7.3	10	n.s. n.s.	n.s. n.s.
Matzsch et al (1988)	LMWH–novo (Logiparine) 35 IU/kg	50	Dextran 70	50	28	39	n.s.	n.s.
Chiapuzzo et al (1988)	OP 2123 (Fluxum)	70	UF 5000 IU × 3	70	7.1	10	n.s.	n.s.

UF, unfractionated heparin. *Statistically significant difference.

relationship between the plasma level of anti-Xa and clinical results: indeed the incidence of haematoma is only 5.3% when the level of anti-Xa assayed 12 hours following subcutaneous injection is less than or equal to 0.2 IU/ml plasma, whereas when the level is above 0.2 IU/ml this figure reaches 24.5%. Similarly, the incidence of postoperative deep venous thrombosis is low (6.3%) if the minimum level of factor anti-Xa (still measured 12 hours following injection) is greater than 0.1 IU/ml. If the level is less than or equal to 0.05 IU/ml the percentage incidence of deep venous thrombosis rises to 18.8%. These results suggest that when enoxaparine is administered by a single subcutaneous daily injection the level of factor anti-Xa at 12 hours should not exceed 0.2 IU/ml if haemorrhagic problems are to be avoided but must be greater than 0.05 IU to have good effect (Levine et al 1989).

Medical patients. Hospital patients in intensive care units, those suffering from chronic pulmonary or cardiac failure, and patients at bed rest with a past history of thromboembolic events all belong to the high-risk population. For these indications, the doses of LMWH are still poorly defined because of the small number of controlled therapeutic trials considering each indication. These are, however, relatively common conditions and where heparin may even be superior to those where it has been shown to be successful, as in the prophylactic treatment of general surgical patients. Two preliminary randomized double-blind studies carried out over a period of at least 10 days have given encouraging results (Dahan et al 1986, Poniewierski et al 1988).

Very recently one of the very low-molecular-weight heparin fractions was used successfully in the prevention of deep vein thrombosis in patients with hemiplegia secondary to cerebral infarction (Elias et al 1990).

The use of LMWH in pregnant women is still debated (Forestier et al 1984). One study carried out in the gravid ewe demonstrated the appearance of a dermatan sulphate type anticoagulant in the fetus which was released following enoxaparine injection but not with CY 222 (Andrew et al 1986). This is despite the fact that neither of these two preparations when radiolabelled cross the placental barrier (Andrew et al 1985).

Studies using several pharmaceutical preparations and examining transplacental passage of the AT III/LMWH complex were reported as negative (Forestier et al 1987, Omri et al 1989). Caution, however, dictates that LMWH should not be recommended during the first trimester of pregnancy. During the second or third trimester LMWH may be prescribed without haemorrhagic risk to the fetus but because of the small number of subjects studied this treatment should not be widespread. The LMWH have, however, already been used in rare isolated cases in pregnant women without notable side-effects.

In cases of thrombocytopenia occurring during treatment with standard heparin it is possible to change to LMWH (Vitoux et al 1986) when the aggregant effect of the LMWH chosen has been studied on control platelets in the presence of plasma from the patient, although this assessment is not entirely dependable (Lecrubier et al 1987). Indeed, it is not possible to guarantee that thrombocytopenia will not persist on changing to LMWH. In a small number of cases thrombocytopenia has not been corrected on the third or fourth day following changeover to LMWH despite negative in vitro aggregation studies (Horellou et al 1984). In contrast, however, thrombocytopenic events occur extremely rarely when thrombosis is treated with LMWH in the first instance. Despite these encouraging results it remains mandatory to follow the platelet count at regular intervals throughout treatment, on average every 3 days until such time as the risk of thrombocytopenia has been excluded by the results of pharmacological trials underway at present.

Finally the LMWH and their derivatives may be used in the treatment of disseminated intravascular coagulation as, theoretically, they reduce the haemorrhagic risk of treatment. There are, however, practically no studies examining this indication (Nieuwenhuis & Sixma 1986).

Haemodialysis

The LMWHs have also been used with success during extrarenal haemodialysis (Table 10.5), particularly in subjects with increased risk of haemorrhage (Schrader et al 1988). As the affinity of parietal endothelial cells for

Table 10.5 Leading trials of low-molecular-weight heparins in haemodialysis

Authors	LMWH	n	Control	n	Thrombotic events (%)		Anti-Xa Plasmatic Levels (IU/ml)
					LMWH	Control	
	Tedelparine (Fragmine®)						
Borm et al (1986)	(cross-over randomized)	10	UF	10	4 minor clots	4 minor clots	0.19–0.46
Lane et al (1986)	4000 + 750 IU/anti-Xa/h		UF 5000 + 1500 IU/h		0	0	
Ljungberg et al (1987)	5000 IU/anti-Xa bolus	11	UF (125–175% WBACT*)	11	0	0	>0.39
Schrader et al (1988)	35 IU/anti-Xa/kg bolus + 12 IU/anti-Xa/kg/h	35	UF	35	1.59	1.33	>0.5
	CY 222 (Choay, Paris)						
Renaud et al (1985)	300 IU anti-Xa/kg bolus	28	UF	28	0	0	
Hory et al (1987)	300 IU anti-Xa/kg bolus or 90 IU anti-Xa/kg + 1000 IU anti-Xa/h (cross-over)	8	UF 100 IU/kg		Higher dialyser blood loss		

*WBACT = whole blood activated clotting time.

LMWH is 20 times weaker than for standard heparin the saturatable cellular clearance is therefore negligible regardless of dose injected and clearance occurs principally through the renal route (Goudable et al 1986). It follows from this that the biological effect in patients with chronic renal failure is two times longer than in the healthy subject, a phenomenon which is not seen with standard heparin and which allows treatment to be restricted to one single dose of LMWH in the arterial circuit at the beginning of a session. Furthermore in these conditions and also in contrast to standard heparin, LMWHs cause only a mild increase in levels of platelet factor 4 and do not inhibit collagen-mediated platelet aggregation. In contrast, the blood levels of anti-Xa activity necessary to completely inhibit coagulation on the dialysis membranes varies clearly according to the investigator, but it would appear nonetheless useful to keep the blood level above or at least equal to 0.7 IU anti-Xa (Maurin & Kierdorf 1988).

Treatment of deep venous thrombosis

Recently, the use of LMWH has been proposed in the management of established deep venous thrombosis. This is based principally on clinical trials using tedelparine (Fragmin) CY 216 (Fraxiparine) and with a very low-molecular-weight heparin, CY 222 (Choay).

Two open randomized studies first compared continuous intravenous administration of 240 IU anti-Xa per 12 hours of tedelparine to an identical dose of standard heparin but this dose was associated with haemorrhagic events in two patients who had recently undergone operation. By reducing the dose to 120 IU anti-Xa per 12 hours and using venograms carried out before and after treatment it was possible to show similar activity to that of standard heparin. The APTT used for biological assessment was found to be unreliable as a monitoring test (Bratt et al 1985a).

A randomized double-blind study on 194 patients also compared intravenous administration of tedelparine over 5–10 days to that of standard heparin. The dose was adjusted to maintain a plasma level of factor anti-Xa 3–4 hours after injection between 0.3 and 0.6 IU/ml in patients at high risk of haemorrhage and between 0.4 and 0.9 IU in patients at lesser risk. The therapeutic effect was comparable in the two groups. Major bleeding occurred in 10 patients in the tedelparine treatment group whereas there were 13 haemorrhagic events in the heparin standard treatment group. The reduction in bleeding events was, however, much less than hoped for in the light of experimental animal work (Albada et al 1989). The effect of using subcutaneous administration was then studied in three comparative randomized trials (Bratt et al 1987, Anonymous 1989, Holm et al 1986). One of these was double-blind and compared non-fractionated heparin which was administered either by intravenous infusion or by subcutaneous injection (Table 10.6). The results were assessed using a Marder score (Table 10.7) and demonstrated that both tedelparine and standard heparin had equivalent effects on venography carried out in all patients before and

Table 10.6 Main therapeutic protocols in deep venous thrombosis treatment

Authors	LMWH	n	Control	n	Therapeutic plans		Biological efficacy tests	
					LMWH	UF	LMWH	UF
Bratt et al (1985a) Open-randomized (two trials)	Tedelparine (Fragmine®)	12 / 13	UF	15 / 14	240 anti-Xa IU.kg/12 h i.v. / 120 anti-Xa IU.kg/12 h i.v.	240 IU.kg/12 h i.v. / 120 IU.kg/12 h i.v.	APTT increase between 10s and 30s / APTT increase between 5s and 20s	60s <APTT<100s / 60s<APTT<100s
Holm et al (1986) (double-blind randomized)	Tedelparine (Fragmine®)	29	UF	27	W < 60 years M < 70 years 7500 anti-Xa IU s.c./12 h; W > 60 years M > 70 years 5000 anti-Xa IU s.c./12 h	W < 60 years M < 70 years 1500 IU s.c./12 h; W > 60 years M > 70 years 10 000 IU s.c./12 h	Anti-Xa level between 0.5 and 0.8 IU/ml (2.5 h after administration)	Anti-Xa level between 0.5 and 0.8 IU/ml (2.5 h after administration)
Bratt et al (1987) (open-randomized)	Tedelparine (Fragmine®)	45	UF	49	120 anti-Xa IU.kg/12 h s.c.	240 IU.kg/12 h i.v.	Anti-Xa level < 1.0 IU/ml (3–4 h after administration)	80s<APTT<120s
Duroux et al (1987) (European multicentre trial) (open-randomized)	Fraxiparine®	85	UF	81	450 U anti-Xa i.c./kg 24 h s.c.	20 IU.kg/h i.v.	Anti-Xa level > 0.5 IU/ml < 0.8 IU/ml (3 h after administration)	APTT between 1.5 and 3 times of control
Anonymous (1989) (French multicentre trial) (open-randomized)	Tedelparine (Fragmine®)	31	UF	29	100 anti-Xa IU.kg/12 h s.c.	240 IU.kg/12 h i.v. perfusion	No monitoring	Adjusted dosage (APTT or Howell time)

UF, unfractionated heparin; W, women; M, men.

Table 10.7 Deep venous thrombosis treatment efficacy results: Marder's index evolution

	Bratt et al (1985a)		Bratt et al (1987)		Holm et al (1986)		Anonymous (1989) (French multicentre trial)	
	Tedelparine (Fragmine®)	UF	Tedelparine (Fragmine®)	UF	Tedelparine (Fragmine®)	UF	Tedelparine (Fragmine®)	UF
Improve-ment	50% 77%	48%*	76%	61%	40%	48%	71%	79.3%
Un-changed condition	50% 23%	41%*	20%	33%	56%	44%	22.5%	17.3%
Aggra-vation	0	11%*	4%	6%	4%	8%	6.5%	3.4%

UF, unfractionated heparin; *, unfractionated heparin treated patients have been joined together.

after treatment. The major practical advantages, however, were that LMWH could be given subcutaneously, biological monitoring was reduced and more stable levels of anti-Xa activity could be achieved, as compared to non-fractionated heparin. The dose advised for tedelparine is of the order of 200–240 IU anti-Xa subcutaneously per 24 hours, which gives an anti-Xa activity in plasma between 0.5 and 1 IU/ml (amidolytic method) 3–4 hours following injection.

During a randomized pilot study three doses of a very low-molecular-weight heparin (CY 222) were assessed in three groups of ten patients. The doses given were 500, 750, and 1000 U anti-Xa.IC/kg per 24 hours by three subcutaneous injections.

The effectiveness was also assessed using a Marder score from venography carried out before and 7 days after treatment. The dose of 750 U anti-Xa. IC/kg per 24 hours appeared to be optimal. At this dose only the plasma anti-Xa activity was altered whereas the APTT remained normal (Elias et al 1986). This dose was used in comparison to standard heparin in an open study on 30 patients (Janvier et al 1987) and in a randomized study on 68 patients (Faivre et al 1988).

One European multicentre trial encompassing 17 centres examined 85 patients who received a fixed dose of 450 U anti-Xa.IC/kg per 24 hours of Fraxiparine in two subcutaneous injections, and on 81 patients who received initially 20 IU/kg per hour of standard heparin by continuous intravenous infusion. This dose was then adjusted according to daily measurements of the APTT or recalcification clotting time.

The changes at venography were judged using both Arnessen and Marder score before and after treatment: these demonstrated significantly greater effects with LMWH as compared to standard heparin (Duroux 1987).

Similar results were also found with enoxaparine on ten patients with proximal venous thrombosis and in whom intravenous standard heparin given during a period of 7–10 days had been shown to be ineffective. The mean dosage (0.8 ± 0.2 mg/kg per 24 hours s.c.) was adjusted in order to maintain an anti-Xa activity between 0.4 and 0.8 IU/ml throughout the treatment period, which averaged 36 days. Injections were administered by the patients themselves after departure from hospital. Although there was no significant reduction in the Arnessen score at venography, clinical improvement was seen in eight of the ten patients (Vitoux et al 1988b). According to these authors the simplicity of a single subcutaneous injection which could be administered by the patient himself and the biological stability of action had considerable advantages over conventional treatment.

The studies to date, however, need to be confirmed by new trials. They do suggest that LMWHs which were initially considered for use in the prevention of venous thromboembolic events may be equally useful in the treatment of established deep venous thrombosis. The doses required are nonetheless at least three times higher than those used in prophylaxis. This being the case, two questions remain to be answered.

1. Is there a significant reduction in haemorrhagic risk when using LMWH?
2. Should the dose of LMWH be modified according to biological monitoring using plasma anti-Xa activity?

Only studies with well-devised methodologies and examining large series of patients will be able to produce a clear response to these two questions.

In addition, will it be possible in collaboration with the general practitioner and using LMWH to reduce the hospital stay and to ease the home treatment of a patient?

The French study of Vitoux et al (1988b) and a Dutch pilot study (Bakker et al 1988) have already demonstrated that it was possible to treat patients with established deep venous thrombosis at home with at least equal success to conventional hospital treatment. As a whole, these first studies are certainly encouraging but they do require confirmation. They must define the biological surveillance parameters required. In common practice the use of LMWH must not lead to clinicians failing to make an objective diagnosis of thrombosis.

Trials in pulmonary embolus

A slightly larger dose of enoxaparine, in the region of 2–3 mg/kg per 24 hours, was used in a number of patients with pulmonary embolus and appeared to produce an identical anti-Xa amidolytic activity between 0.3 and 0.6 U anti-Xa/ml (Huet et al 1987). A very low-molecular-weight fraction (CY 222) was also given to 47 patients with acute pulmonary embolus of less than 5 days duration, by continuous intravenous infusion over 10 days. This LMWH appeared to be an effective treatment at a dose of 1000 U anti-Xa.IC/kg per 24 hours for the first 5 days followed by 750 U anti-Xa.IC/kg per 24 hours thereafter (Quilliet et al 1988).

Trials in arterial thrombosis

Studies are currently underway in the treatment of arterial thrombosis in particular myocardial infarction, in association with thrombolytic agents and also in vascular surgery.

Biological monitoring of treatment

The time of sampling is of paramount importance and is identical regardless of the indication. Sampling is carried out at the third or fourth hour following subcutaneous injection at the time of peak biological activity.

Before beginning treatment a basal platelet count should be obtained as the risk of thrombocytopaenia cannot be excluded in the absence of specific studies. Monitoring of the platelet count should be carried out again at the sixth day of treatment and then every three days for the following two weeks if treatment is continued, although the benefit of this policy has not been clearly established.

In addition, good haemostatic function must be confirmed using the prothrombin time, the APTT and by fibrinogen measurement. A normal APTT excludes the possible presence of a circulating lupus-type anticoagulant which may be a complicating factor in recurrent thrombosis.

Samples should be kept less than 4 hours at laboratory temperature. Immediately before assay they must be centrifuged at high speed at 4°C to obtain platelet free plasma. Although sampling is most often taken into a Vacutainer containing citrate solution it appears preferable and even necessary with LMWH treatment to use CTAD tubes, although this recommendation is less strict than with unfractionated heparin.

As the LMWHs induce only a weak anti-IIa activity biological monitoring cannot in any case rely on the classical monitoring tests used for standard heparin, such as the APTT and the thrombin time. Prolongation of the APTT may be seen, however, at high doses. Measurement of plasma anti-Xa activity, a marker of circulating LMWH, must be used and the assay carried out by either a colorimetric or chronometric method. Whatever the method used the first part of the assay is the same: a known excess of bovine factor Xa is incubated with the test plasma. Part of the factor Xa is neutralized by the AT III–LMWH complex present in the plasma. The assay of residual factor Xa differs according to the method used. Chronometric techniques rely on clot formation in the presence of cephalin, calcium and, for one technique, a bovine plasma fraction containing an excess of factors II, V and fibrinogen. These techniques measure the time of clot formation and may also be influenced by anti-IIa activity (Bara et al 1987b).

With colorimetric methods the results are expressed in international amidolytic anti-Xa units. Results obtained using chronometric methods are expressed in time or more strictly in anti-Xa equivalents. Defined therapeutic ranges expressed in time are awaited. In theory it does not appear legitimate to convert from time into IU anti-Xa as some of these methods may be influenced by other parameters than anti-Xa activity. Chronometric methods give in general a broader evaluation of biological activity of the heparins as they take into account to some extent the anti-IIa activity, particularly during curative treatment. With the 'Heptest' the usual values are 40–60 seconds for prophylactic treatment and 70–100 seconds for curative treatment.

Side effects

Haemorrhagic events have not been seen during the different clinical trials using recognized doses. However, it is advised that the LMWHs should not be used in conjunction with antiplatelet agents such as aspirin or ticlopidine, with non-steroidal anti-inflammatory drugs, with vitamin K antagonists or with dextran, because of the possibility of increased haemorrhagic risk. It appears that haemorrhagic risk reduction with LMWH as compared to standard heparin is not related to the anticoagulant effect but is caused by a decreased inhibition of platelet function. The very low-molecular-weight fragments in the region of 3000 daltons possess practically no anti-IIa activity, but they have only relatively weak antithrombotic activity. It would seem therefore that a minimum anti-IIa activity is necessary for expression of the antithrombotic activity of the LMWHs (Hirsh 1986).

As there have been no specific studies, the risk of thrombocytopaenia caused by LMWH cannot be ignored, and the platelet count must therefore always be followed. This risk, however, may relate to the nature of each individual LMWH as reported by Blockmans et al (1986), who studied the effects of eight LMWHs on the plasma from a patient who sustained thrombocytopaenia following standard heparin treatment. Three LMWHs induced platelet aggregation whereas five were devoid of such activity.

Allergic reactions and haematoma at the injection sites may be seen with LMWH treatment but these appear to be less frequent and less severe than with standard heparin treatment. Finally and as with non-fractionated heparin the risk of osteoporosis during long-term prophylactic treatment cannot be excluded.

Protamine reversal

The only antidote available in cases of haemorrhage related to LMWH administration is protamine, either as the chlorhydrate or sulphate. In cases of documented therapeutic overdose protamine is injected intravenously at a dose designed to take account of the time lapse between the last LMWH injection and injection of the neutralizing agent. This agent acts principally on antithrombin activity (anti-IIa activity), anti-Xa activity not being completely inhibited. Protamine appears to be effective in stopping bleeding, as was demonstrated in animals (Van Ryn-McKenna et al 1990), but significant residual anti-Xa activity remains (50–60% of the anti-Xa activity) even with very high doses of protamine (Massonet-Castel et al 1986). Preliminary studies in the human being have involved cardiac surgery with extracorporeal circulation (ECC), where it has been necessary to use an LMWH, particularly following thrombocytopenia induced by standard heparin. The administration of protamine following ECC prevented the normal bleeding always seen in the absence of neutralization (Massonet-Castel et al 1986).

In addition, the different French pharmaceutical preparations of LMWH being expressed in different units, the interrelation between milligrams, anti-Xa units of the Institute Choay and international anti-Xa units is not straightforward. This demands great care in initiating neutralization which must be carried out empirically, each preparation having its own protocol.

DERMATAN SULPHATE

This is isolated from very many tissues, particularly intestinal mucosa and vascular wall (Murata et al 1975). Dermatan sulphate, still called chondroitin sulphate B, is also present in native human plasma (Engelberg 1985) and in commercial heparin preparations (Perlin et al 1987). It is of special interest because of certain distinctive characteristics in relation to the other glycosaminoglycans; it is able selectively to inhibit thrombin without having major influence on the classical coagulation tests or on the activity of factor Xa. Its mechanism of action is specific, potentiating only heparin cofactor II alone without interaction with antithrombin III. Rare cofactor II variants have been described in association with recurrent thrombosis but the causal relationship is not generally accepted. In these cases immunoelectrophoresis in a dermatan sulphate-containing gel is abnormal (Andersson et al 1987).

Structure

Dermatan sulphate is composed of repeated disaccharide units, primarily α_1-iduronosyl-β-D-N-acetylgalactosamine-4-sulphate (Lindahl & Hook 1978). There is large inter- and intramolecular structural heterogeneity, the core structure often being hidden by additional sulphation (Suzuki et al 1976). The molecular weight is polydispersed with mean values between 25 000 and 40 000 daltons.

Anticoagulant activity

The specific anticoagulant activity of dermatan sulphate is weak in comparison to that of standard heparin. Teien et al (1976) demonstrated that, measuring the APTT in vitro, concentrations approximately 70 times higher than that of non-fractionated heparin were necessary to obtain the same anticoagulant effect. These results have recently been confirmed by Dawes et al (1989) and Toulon et al (1989) using a dermatan sulphate extract of porcine intestinal mucosa (MF 701, Mediolanum Farmaceutica, Milan). In contrast, thrombin generation in non-diluted human or rabbit plasma measured in comparison with standard heparin is inhibited in a ratio of approximately 1 : 15 (Fernandez et al 1986b) in place of 1 : 60 or 1 : 70 for the APTT (Table 10.8).

In the rabbit, after intravenous administration, anticoagulant activity as measured by the APTT is only detectable above doses of 10 mg/kg. Above this level it is proportional to the dose injected, reaching a 30% prolongation at a dose of 40 mg/kg. Under these operative conditions dermatan sulphate appears to be cleared rapidly from the circulation, as the fractional increase in anticoagulant activity seen 20 minutes following injection is just greater than half the value obtained one minute following administration (Fernandez et al 1987). Interestingly and in contrast to LMWH, where only biological activity may be measured, there is an assay for the molecule in plasma with a sensitivity limit of 0.1 µg/ml (Dupouy et al 1988).

Antithrombotic activity

The antithrombotic properties of dermatan sulphate have been studied in comparison to those of fractionated heparin in experimental models of venous thrombosis through stasis in the rabbit or following intravenous

Table 10.8 Inactivation rate of human thrombin in undiluted rabbit and human plasma after heparin or dermatan sulfate addition (incubation time 60 s)

		Human plasma	Rabbit plasma
Control	–	41	46
Heparin	0.066 µg/ml (0.1 IU)	56	52
	0.66 µg/ml (1 IU)	77	79
	6.6 µg/ml (10 IU)	81	83
Control	–	40	47
Dermatan sulphate	1 µg/ml	54	56
	10 µg/ml	73	75
	100 µg/ml	78	81

Data from Fernandez et al (1986b).

injection of carragenine in the rat. The latter induced thrombosis in the tail, the extent of which is dose dependent. With standard heparin, venous thrombosis is inhibited by 90% when induced one minute following injection. A 95% inhibition is seen with dermatan sulphate without effect on the APTT or on the thrombin time. The doses of dermatan sulphate needed to obtain an identical antithrombotic effect to that of heparin are only seven times larger, whereas to obtain the same anticoagulant effect these doses must be 50–70 times greater than those of heparin. These results suggest that other factors besides anticoagulant activity, not as yet fully identified, may be involved in the antithrombotic activity of dermatan sulphate (Desnoyers et al 1989).

In the rat, intravenous dermatan sulphate reduces the incidence of thrombosis in a dose-dependent fashion in a similar way to standard heparin in models with thrombosis created following inferior vena cava ligation (Maggi et al 1987). On the same experimental model the antithrombotic effect is still greater than 50% 16 hours after injection of a subcutaneous dose of 20 mg/kg (Morani et al 1987).

Haemorrhagic activity

In the rabbit, intravenous injection of standard heparin 20 times the antithrombotic dose leads to blood loss from standard skin incisions in the ear seven times greater than that seen in control animals who received isotonic saline. Larger doses of heparin may cause blood loss more than 30 times that seen in controls.

In contrast dermatan sulphate when administered in doses of 20 or even 40 times the antithrombotic dose does not cause blood loss greater than that seen in rabbit controls. Approximately 80 times the antithrombotic dose of dermatan sulphate is required before haemorrhagic events are seen.

These results were confirmed in the rat using different techniques. At the dose required to give maximum antithrombotic effect dermatan sulphate did not cause any change in the bleeding time, whereas heparin was associated with a significant prolongation when given in doses as low as 0.5 mg/kg.

There does not therefore seem to be any correlation between the haemorrhagic and the antithrombotic effects either of heparin or of dermatan sulphate when measured ex vivo. It does appear, however, that as for the other glycosaminoglycans it is possible with dermatan sulphate to demonstrate a correlation between the increase in blood loss seen as a function of dose and inhibition of collagen-induced platelet aggregation seen at very high doses (Fernandez et al 1986b).

Pharmacokinetics

After intravenous injection of ^{125}I-labelled dermatan sulphate in the rabbit in doses varying from 20 to 4000 μg/kg the volume of distribution, clearance and half-life of the tracer were all independent of the dose given: quantitative determinations in plasma demonstrated that approximately 90% of dermatan sulphate injected was cleared with a half-life similar to that calculated by the disappearance of radioactive tracer. The mean volume of distribution is only slightly greater than the theoretical plasma volume in the rabbit. The alpha phase of plasma distribution is less than 3 minutes, the beta phase of clearance (half-life of 10–14 minutes) corresponding to the disappearance of 90% of the dermatan sulphate injected, and the gamma phase of residual activity gives a half-life of 150–300 minutes (Dol et al 1988a). Bioavailability following subcutaneous or intramuscular administration is approximately 28% and 21%, respectively, as compared to intravenous administration, but the clearance half-life is much increased (approximately 8 hours).

The mean clearance is 8.1 ml/min in a normal animal, although bilateral nephrectomy is associated with very marked prolongation of this clearance half-life, confirming the role of the kidneys in excretion of dermatan sulphate or its metabolites.

The pharmacokinetic behaviour of dermatan sulphate is very similar to that of the LMWH previously studied using identical methods (Boneu et al 1988), and therefore very different from that of the non-fractionated heparins.

In human volunteers intravenous infusion of a dose of 0.6 mg/kg per hour of dermatan sulphate over 10 hours demonstrated a single-compartment model with a half-life of 1.28 ± 0.46 hours, a plasma clearance of 2.75 ± 0.46 litres/h and a volume of distribution of 4.92 ± 1.3 litres. Equilibrium was reached between the 3rd and 6th hour following administration, when the maximal concentration is 16.4 ± 5.7 μg/ml. As compared to basal values the APTT was prolonged by 42 ± 7%, whereas no anti-IIa or anti-Xa activity could be demonstrated using chromogenic substrate methods (Agnelli et al 1990a).

Therapeutic activity

The principal interest in dermatan sulphate as compared to heparin is in the lower frequency of haemorrhagic complications seen for an equivalent antithrombotic dose in the animal. Studies in the human have also been carried out to verify the antithrombotic activity and the absence of haemorrhagic events. At present only results from pilot studies are available. These demonstrate that, in one of the first studies examining 300 patients undergoing major thoracic or abdominal surgery, and comparing the daily administration of a single dose of 100 mg of dermatan sulphate given intramuscularly to that of three subcutaneous injections of 5000 IU non-fractionated calcium heparin, in the first 220 patients deep venous thrombosis prevention was identical in the two groups. Although haemorrhagic events were only clinically apparent in four patients out of 110 in the group treated with dermatan sulphate, this number rose to 16 patients out of 110 in the heparin treatment group (Maffei-Faccioli et al 1989). A second study carried out on 126 patients considered the effectiveness and safety of using dermatan sulphate at a dose of 600 mg by twice daily intramuscular injection as compared to placebo, in the prophylaxis of deep venous thrombosis following surgery for fractured neck of femur. The incidence of venous thrombosis both total and proximal were reduced by 41% and 52%, respectively, without haemorrhagic complications (Agnelli et al 1990b).

A single intravenous dose of 2 mg/kg of dermatan sulphate was given to patients with chronic renal failure immediately before dialysis. This demonstrated that the agent completely inhibited fibrin deposition on the dialysis membrane in 50% of cases, although some thrombotic lesions were visible in the remainder of cases (Nurmohamed et al 1989).

Higher doses in the region of 4–6 mg/kg are currently under study for this purpose.

Reversal of activity

The anticoagulant and antithrombin activity of dermatan sulphate may be reversed in vitro by protamine sulphate or by hexadimethrine bromide (Polybrene) but in human plasma Polybrene is approximately three times more active on a weight-for-weight basis (1.5 mg of polybrene inhibits 1 mg of dermatan sulphate). Both in man and animals dermatan sulphate may if necessary be completely neutralized by Polybrene provided the doses of reversing agent remain below their toxic threshold. Reversal is, however only partial with protamine sulphate (Sie et al 1989).

Hypersulphated and low-molecular-mass derivatives

Hypersulphation of dermatan has been carried out, producing two derivatives containing 2 and 3.7 sulphate groups per disaccharide unit respectively. In a purified system the catalysis of thrombin inhibition by cofactor II is increased 10 and 70 times respectively for the two derivatives. Although the anticoagulant activity measured in vitro by the APTT and thrombin clotting time is increased, neither of these two hypersulphated derivatives causes increased antithrombotic activity on stasis models of venous thrombosis. On the contrary at doses of 35, 100 and 250 μg/kg the most hypersulphated derivative did not inhibit thrombotic events (Dol et al 1988b).

The splitting of dermatan sulphate to a compound with a mean molecular weight of 4000 daltons halves the anticoagulant activity, although following single intravenous injection in the rabbit the volume of distribution is 10 times larger than that for non-fractionated dermatan sulphate. The half-life of elimination is 2–4 times longer despite a clearance of 1.4–2.3 times higher. In contrast, when administered in increasing doses from 0.1 to 1 mg/kg low-molecular-mass dermatan sulphate possesses an antithrombotic effect of only half the potency. Absorption following subcutaneous injection is fast and the bioavailability is close to 100%. One hour after subcutaneous injection of 10 mg/kg the plasma concentration is 5.6 μg/ml, the antithrombotic effect persisting for more than 4 hours. Subcutaneous injection of the same dose of non-fractionated dermatan sulphate produces a plasma concentration of 1.9 μg/ml and does not have antithrombotic activity (Dol et al 1990).

HEPARAN SULPHATE

Along with heparin and dermatan sulphate, heparan sulphate is the only other glycosaminoglycan with anticoagulant properties.

Structure

Heparan sulphate consists of the same type of monosaccharide units as standard heparin, also bound by glycosidic bridges. The molecular chains of these two compounds are, however, synthesized by different cell types. Furthermore, heparan sulphate contains a higher percentage of N-sulphated glucosamine residues, and since its extraction from different animal tissues it has become clear that its core proteins are different from standard heparin (Conrad 1989).

Anticoagulant activity

The anticoagulant activity of heparan sulphate is much weaker than that of standard heparin when measured using either the formation of thrombin/antithrombin III and thrombin/cofactor II complexes on the one hand and inhibition of prothrombin activation on the other. This anticoagulant activity is, however, slightly superior to that of dermatan sulphate (Ofosu et al 1989). When classical coagulation techniques are used, the anticoagulant activity of heparan sulphate synthesized in vitro by three different cell lines and purified by selective enzymatic degradation varies between 6 and 30 IU/mg (Piepkorn et al 1988).

Pharmacology

Because of the difficulties in extraction and purification of heparan sulphate and the difficulties in obtaining significant quantities of the compound devoid of heparin contamination, no pharmacological trials have been carried out to our knowledge examining its use in the prevention of experimental thrombosis. Recent fundamental studies, however, have demonstrated that the receptor responsible for platelet thrombospondin adhesion to Chinese hamster ovarian cells is a heparan sulphate and that this binding is dependent on the conformation of absorbed thrombospondin

(Kaesberg et al 1989). Studies have also shown that heparan sulphate presence is necessary for adhesion between primary haemopoietic progenitor cells and the cellular matrix of the marrow microenvironment (Gordon et al 1988). It would also be possible that the antithrombotic properties of the vessel wall are due more to an increase in the interaction of factor Xa or prothrombinase with AT III caused by a larger quantity of heparan being bound to the endothelial surface, than to the presence of a smaller number of heparin-like molecules with high AT III affinity (Scully et al 1988).

Metabolism

All studies examining the synthesis of heparan sulphate in cell cultures suggest that a proteoglycan heparan sulphate is continually secreted from cells and is found as a component in the extracellular matrix. This proteoglycan is then rapidly internalized and metabolized. In hepatocyte culture a part of the proteoglycan internalized is transported to the nucleus (Fedarko & Conrad 1986). The turnover of both matrix and nuclear pool is extremely rapid, with half-lives of the order of a quarter or half the cell doubling time.

Therapeutic activity

No clinical trials have been carried out with pure heparan sulphate. In contrast, a number of compounds with antithrombotic activity contain a high percentage of heparan sulphate. Its structure and anticoagulant activity predicts that its properties should be similar to those of dermatan sulphate. If extraction and purification techniques allow heparan sulphate to be obtained one day in a pure form, in industrial quantities and at an affordable cost, a new class of antithrombotic agents may appear.

THE LOW-MOLECULAR-MASS HEPARINOIDS (ORG 10172)

ORG 10172 is a mixture of different sulphated glycosaminoglycans and low-molecular-weight heparinoids extracted from porcine intestinal mucosa. The major fractions are heparan sulphate (approximately 80%), dermatan sulphate, chondroitin sulphates, and a number of low-molecular-weight heparins (Meuleman et al 1982). The molecular weight is polydispersed with a mean of 6500 daltons.

Anticoagulant activity

The specific anticoagulant activity measured by amidolytic-methods against the fourth international non-fractionated heparin standard as reference material is in the region of 8–10 U anti-Xa/mg with an anti-Xa/anti-IIa ratio greater than 20. Prolongation of the APTT is dose dependent in vitro but antithrombin activity disappears when the concentration exceeds 3 IU/ml (Ockelford et al 1985).

Antithrombotic activity and restriction of blood loss

ORG 10172 at a dose of 260 U anti-Xa/kg was compared to standard heparin at a dose producing the same plasma anti-Xa activity in 16 dogs undergoing cardiopulmonary bypass. This study examined the prevention of coagulation in the extracorporeal circuit. The results for antithrombotic activity were identical in the two groups studied, but whereas the thrombin time and the APTT were significantly prolonged in the heparin group, in the animals treated with ORG 10172 only a transitory increase in thrombin time was seen without alteration in the APTT. In addition peri- and postoperative blood loss was significantly less in the group treated with ORG 10172 (Henny et al 1985a).

When compared to standard heparin in the rat the antithrombotic and anti-Xa effects of ORG 10172 last three times as long as those of heparin for the same anti-Xa activity. In addition the half-lives of both antithrombin activity and the inhibition of thrombin generation are prolonged. The effects on the APTT and on haemorrhagic events are, however, of shorter duration than those of heparin (Hobbelen et al 1987). ORG 10172 showed itself to be effective in two models of experimental thrombosis: one induced by inferior vena cava stasis, the other in an arterio-venous shunt where the contribution from platelets is much more important. This effect was also seen with an LMWH whereas antiplatelet serum and acetylsalicylic acid only inhibited thrombus in the arterio-venous shunt (Vogel et al 1989).

Pharmacokinetics

An important feature of ORG 10172 is its prolonged half-life. A single intravenous dose of 6400 U/anti-Xa in volunteers induced only minor prolongation of the APTT. Platelet adhesion ex vivo was reduced 10 minutes after administration. The clearance half-life as measured by decay of anti-Xa activity is approximately 17.6 ± 1.1 hours and is bi-exponential (Bradbrook et al 1987). Identical results were found in elderly volunteers where the half-life was found to be 19.2 ± 6.1 hours. In contrast, however, antithrombin activity disappeared much more quickly (1.8 ± 0.6 hours), as did the inhibition of thrombin generation (6.2 ± 4.0 hours) (Stiekema et al 1989).

Clinical activity

The potential antithrombotic effects of ORG 10172 were studied in a double-blind randomized trial against placebo in 45 high-risk patients undergoing major thoracic or abdominal surgery for malignancy. Subcutaneous doses of 500, 750 or 1000 U anti-Xa were given twice daily. Deep venous thrombosis occurred in nine patients on placebo (64%), in four of 11 patients receiving the 500 U dose (36%) but no thrombosis occurred in patients who had received doses of 750 or 1000 U. Peri- and postoperative blood loss was equal in all groups: significant postoperative bleeding occurred in only one patient, who had received the 1000 U dose (Cade et al 1987).

In another series consisting of 69 general surgical patients positive radiolabelled fibrinogen tests were reduced by 75% as compared to placebo.

The antithrombotic effect of ORG 10172 was also investigated during haemodialysis in patients prone to haemorrhage (Henny et al 1983). A dose of 34.4 anti-Xa U/kg was given by a single injection before dialysis to 55 patients with terminal renal failure and produced identical results to those for standard heparin given as a continuous infusion (Henny et al 1985b). Higher doses, in the region of 4800 U anti-Xa have been used in the same situation without having a significant effect on coagulation parameters (Ireland et al 1986).

In a randomized double-blind study of patients immobilized after cerebrovascular accident, 50 patients received an intravenous bolus of 1000 U followed by two subcutaneous doses daily of 700 U, for 14 days. Venous thrombosis occurred in 4% of the treated group and 28% of the placebo group, although one severe haemorrhagic event occurred in a patient receiving ORG 10172 (Turpie et al 1987). A dose-ranging study was recently carried out for the same indication using intravenous administration over 7 days to obtain factor anti-Xa levels between 0.2 and 1 U/ml. No death, haemorrhagic event, haemorrhagic transformation of a cerebral infarct, or thrombocytopenia occurred (Biller et al 1989). Finally ORG 10172 was used to treat thrombotic problems in five patients where classical anticoagulant treatment was contraindicated because of haemorrhagic stroke.

As it possess no platelet aggregation activity in vitro ORG 10172 has been used to replace standard heparin in patients with heparin-induced thrombocytopenia (Chong et al 1987). However, when used following transurethral prostatic resection an increase in urinary blood loss was seen (Gallus et al 1987, Ten Cate et al 1987).

CONCLUSION

The discovery of LMWH 70 years after that of heparin has stimulated research on the coagulation system and on the pathophysiology of venous thrombosis. These LMWHs were born as a result of the hypotheses now questioned, concerning the role of anti-Xa activity in the prevention of venous thrombosis. The goal was for the prophylactic treatment of thrombosis with the added benefit of a diminished risk of haemorrhage. The reality today is somewhat different. Certainly these preparations, three of which are already used clinically in France, have demonstrated their good effect in prevention of postoperative venous thromboembolic events and are probably also effective in the treatment of established venous thrombosis. In contrast, however, they are not completely devoid of haemorrhagic risk and it is essential to respect the doses defined by clinical trials for each of these LMWHs.

One of the properties discovered during the first trials is their very large bioavailability, which has greatly eased their introduction into therapeutic use.

The different LMWHs all derived from standard heparin have the same therapeutic indications even if their preparation and chemical structure are different. The actual properties responsible for their clinical antithrombotic activity have still to be identified: this may allow new derivatives even more effective and possibly without haemorrhagic risk to be developed.

Within the family of glycosaminoglycans there are compounds which possess much weaker anticoagulant activity but with relatively increased antithrombotic activity and for which the risk of haemorrhage appears to be almost non-existent. Dermatan sulphate, whose clinical studies are in the preliminary stages in the prevention of venous thrombosis, during dialysis and in stroke, is one of these compounds. Its properties are probably very similar to those of heparan sulphate, whose extraction and purification remains extremely difficult, and of the heparinoid ORG 10172, which is a mixture of heparan sulphate, dermatan sulphate and LMWHs. The slower clearance of anti-Xa activity and the results from preliminary clinical trials for this latter compound suggest that it may be a potential competitor to the LMWHs.

REFERENCES

Adolf J, Knee H, Roder J D et al 1989 Prevention of thromboembolism with low molecular heparin in abdominal surgery. Dtsch Med Wochenschr 144: 48–53
Agnelli G, Borm J, Cosmi B et al 1988 Effects of standard heparin and low molecular weight heparin (KABI 2165) on fibrinolysis. Thromb Haemostasis 60: 311–313
Agnelli G, Cosmi B, Renga C et al 1990a Human pharmacokinetics and pharmacodynamics of MF 701 (dermatan sulfate) administered by continuous intravenous infusion. Fibrinolysis 4(suppl 1): 124 (Abstract)
Agnelli G, Cosmi B, Longetti M et al 1990b A randomized double blind placebo controlled trial of MF 701 (dermatan sulfate) for prevention of deep vein thrombosis (DVT) in hip fracture. Fibrinolysis 4(suppl 1): 199 (Abstract)
Aiach M, Michaud A, Balian J L et al 1983 A new molecular weight heparin derivative: in vitro and in vivo studies. Thromb Res 31: 611–622
Aiach M, Dreyfus G, Michaud A et al 1984 Low molecular weight (LMW) heparin derivatives in experimental extra-corporeal circulation (ECC). Haemostasis 14: 325–332
Albada J, Nieuwenhuis H K, Sixma J J et al 1989 Treatment of acute venous thromboembolism with low molecular weight heparin (FRAGMIN): results of a double blind randomized study. Circulation 80: 935–940
Andersson T R, Larsen M L, Abildgaard U et al 1987 Low heparin cofactor II associated with abnormal crossed immunoelectrophoresis pattern in two Norwegian families. Throm Res 47: 243–248
Andrew M, Boneu B, Cade J et al 1985 Placental transport of low molecular weight heparin in the pregnant sheep. Br J Haematol 59: 103–108

Andrew M, Ofosu F, Fernandez F et al 1986 A low molecular weight heparin alters the fetal coagulation system in the pregnant sheep. Thromb Haemostasis 55: 342–346

Andriuoli G, Mastacchi R, Barbanti M et al 1985 Comparison of the antithrombotic and haemorrhagic effects of heparin and a new low molecular weight heparin in rats. Haemostasis 15: 324–330

Anonymous 1975 Prevention of fatal postoperative pulmonary embolism by low doses of heparins: an international multicentre trial. Lancet 2: 45–51

Anonymous 1989 Traitement des thromboses veineuses profondes constituées. Etude comparative d'un fragment d'heparine de bas poids moleculaire (Fragmine®) administrée par voie sous cutanée, et de l'heparine standard administrée par voie intraveineuse continue. Etude multicentrique. Rev Med Interne 10: 375–381

Asselot C, Labat Robert J, Kern P 1989 Heparin fragments regulate collagen phenotype and fibronectin synthesis in the skin of genetically diabetic mice. Biochem Pharmacol 38: 895–899

Baird R J 1989 The story of heparin, as told by sketches from the lives of William Howell, Jay McLean, Charles Best and Gordon Murray. J Vasc Surg 11: 4–18

Bakker M, Dekker P J, Knot E A, Van Bergen P F, Jonker J J 1988 Home treatment for deep venous thrombosis with low molecular weight heparin. Lancet 2: 1142

Bara L, Samama M M 1986 The need for standardization of low molecular weight heparin (LMWH). Thromb Haemostasis 56: 418

Bara L, Samama M M 1988 Pharmacokinetics of low molecular weight heparins. Acta Clin Scand Suppl 543: 65–72

Bara L, Kher A, Gramond G et al 1984 Comparative pharmacokinetics of low molecular weight heparin administered intravenously and subcutaneously. VIIIth Intern Congress on Thrombosis, Istanbul: 311 (Abstract)

Bara L, Billaud E, Gramond G et al 1985 Comparative pharmacokinetics of low molecular weight heparin (PK 10169) and unfractionated heparin after intravenous and subcutaneous administration. Thromb Res 39: 631–636

Bara L, Trillou M, Mardiguian J et al 1986 Comparison of antithrombotic activity of two heparin fragments PK 10169 (MW 5 000) and EMT 680 (MW 2 500) and unfractionated heparin in a rabbit experimental thrombosis model. Relative importance of systemic anti Xa and anti IIa activities. Nouv Rev F Haematol 25: 355–358

Bara L, Combe-Tamzali S, Conard J et al 1987a Modifications biologiques induites par 3 héparines de bas poids moléculaire (PK 10169, KABI 2165 et CY 216) comparées à l'héparine non-fractionnée, injectées par voie sous-cutanée chez le volontaire sain en chirurgie générale, et chez le sujet âgé en médecine. J Mal Vascul 12: 78–84

Bara L, Combe-Tamzali S, Conard J et al 1987b Laboratory monitoring of a low molecular weight heparin (enoxaparine) with a new clotting test (Heptest). Haemostasis 17: 127–133

Barre J, Pfister G, Potron G et al 1987 Efficacité et tolérance comparée du KABI 2165 et de l'héparine standard dans la prévention des thromboses veineuses profondes au cours des prothèses totales de hanche. J Mal Vascul 12: 90–95

Barrowcliffe T W 1986 Lipolytic activities of low molecular weight heparins. Thromb Res 42: 583–584

Barrowcliffe T W, Curtis A D, Tomlinson T P et al 1985 Standardization of low molecular weight heparins: a collaborative study. Thromb Haemostasis 54: 675–679

Barrowcliffe T W, Curtis A D, Johnson E A et al 1988a An international standard for low molecular weight heparin. Thromb Haemostasis 60: 1–7

Barrowcliffe T W, Menton R E, Gray E et al 1988b Heparin and bleeding: an association with lipase release. Thromb Haemostasis 60: 434–436

Barzu T, Molho P, Tobelem G et al 1985 Binding and endocytosis of heparin by human endothelial cells in culture. Biochem Biophys Acta 845: 196–203

Beguin S, Lindhout T, Hemker C 1988 The mode of action of heparin in plasma. Thromb Haemostasis 60: 457–462

Bender N, Seidl C, Weichert W et al 1988 Evaluation of the biological effects of low molecular weight heparins. Haemostasis 18(suppl 3): 23–32

Bendetowicz A V, Bara L, Samama M 1990 The inhibition of intrinsic prothrombinase and its generation by heparin and four derivatives in prothrombin poor plasma. Thromb Res 58: 445–454

Bergqvist D, Nilsson B, Hedner U et al 1985 The effect of heparin fragments of different molecular weights on experimental thrombosis and haemostasis. Thromb Res 38: 589–601

Bergqvist D, Burmark U S, Frisell J et al 1986 Low molecular weight heparin once daily compared with conventional low-dose heparin twice daily: a prospective double blind multicentre trial on prevention of postoperative thrombosis. Br J Surg 73: 204–208

Bergqvist D, Matzsch T, Burmark U S et al 1988 Low molecular weight heparin given the evening before surgery compared with conventional low dose heparin in prevention of thrombosis. Br J Surg 75: 888–891

Biller J, Massey E W, Marler J R et al 1989 A dose escalation study of ORG 10172 (low molecular weight heparinoid) in stroke. Neurology 39: 262–265

Blockmans D, Bounameaux H, Vermylen J et al 1986 Heparin induced thrombocytopenia: platelet aggregation studies in the presence of heparin fractions or semi-synthetic analogues of various molecular weight and anticoagulant activities. Thromb Haemostasis 55: 90–93

Boneu B, Buchanan M R, Cade M R et al 1985 Effects of heparin, its low molecular weight fractions and other glycosaminoglycans on thrombus growth in vivo. Thromb Res 40: 81–89

Boneu B, Buchanan M R, Caranobe C et al 1987 The disappearance of a low molecular weight fraction (CY 216) differs from standard heparin in rabbits. Thromb Res 46: 845–853

Boneu B, Caranobe C, Cadroy Y et al 1988 Pharmacokinetic studies of standard unfractionated heparin and low molecular weight heparins in the rabbit. Semin Thromb Haemostasis 14: 18–27

Borm J J, Krediet R, Sturk A et al 1986 Heparin versus low molecular weight heparin Kabi 2165 in chronic hemodialysis patients: a randomized cross over study. Haemostasis 16(suppl 2): 59–68

Bradbrook I D, Magnani H N, Moelker H C et al 1987 ORG 10172: a low molecular weight heparinoid anticoagulant with a long half life in man. Br J Clin Pharmacol 23: 667–675

Bratt G, Tornebohm E, Granqvist S et al 1985a A comparison between low molecular weight heparin (Kabi 2165) and standard heparin in the intravenous treatment of deep vein thrombosis. Thromb Haemostasis 54: 813–817

Bratt G, Tornebohm E, Lockner D et al 1985b A human pharmacological study comparing conventional heparin and a low molecular weight heparin fragment. Thromb Haemostasis 53: 208–211

Bratt G, Tornebohm E, Widlund L et al 1986 Low molecular weight heparin (KABI 2165, FRAGMIN): pharmacokinetics after intravenous and subcutaneous administration in human volunteers. Thromb Res 42: 613–620

Bratt G, Aberg W, Tornebohm E et al 1987 Kabi 2165 in the treatment of deep venous thrombosis (DVT) of the leg. Thromb Res (suppl VII): 24

Briant L, Caranobe C, Saivin S et al 1989 Unfractionated heparin and CY 216: pharmacokinetics and bioavailabilities of the anti-factor Xa and IIa. Effects after intravenous and subcutaneous injection in rabbits. Thromb Haemostasis 61: 348–353

Cade J F, Wood M, Magnani H N et al 1987 Early clinical experience of a new heparinoid ORG 10172 in prevention of deep venous thrombosis. Thromb Res 45: 497–503

Cadroy Y 1988 In vivo mechanisms of thrombus formation: studies using a primate model. Thèse Université Paul Sabatier, Toulouse, France

Caen J P 1988 A randomized double blind study between a low molecular weight heparin (KABI 2165) and standard heparin in the prevention of deep vein thrombosis in general surgery: a French multicenter trial. Thromb Haemostasis 59: 216–220

Caranobe C, Barret A, Gabaig A M et al 1985 Disappearance of circulating anti Xa activity after intravenous injection of standard heparin and a low molecular weight heparin (CY 216) in normal and nephrectomized rabbits. Thromb Res 40: 129–133

Carter C J, Kelton J G, Hirsh J et al 1982 The relationship between the haemorrhagic properties of low molecular weight heparin in rabbits. Blood 59: 1239–1245

Chiapuzzo E, Orengo G B, Ottria G et al 1988 The use of low molecular weight heparins for postsurgical deep vein thrombosis prevention in orthopaedic patients. J Int Med Res 16: 359–366

Choay J, Petitou M 1986 The chemistry of heparin: a way to understand its mode of action. Med J Aus 144(HS): 7–10

Choay J, Petitou M, Lormeau J C et al 1983 Structure activity relationship in heparin: a synthetic pentasaccharide with high affinity for antithrombin III, and eliciting high anti-factor Xa activity. Biochem Biophys Res Commun 116: 492–499

Chong B H, Ismail F, Cade J et al 1987 Heparin-induced thrombocytopenia: in vitro studies with low molecular weight heparinoid ORG 10172. Thromb Haemostasis 58: 308 (Abstract 1127)

Collins R, Scrimgeour A, Yusuf S et al 1988 Reduction in fatal pulmonary embolism and venous thrombosis by perioperative administration of subcutaneous heparin. N Engl J Med 318: 1162–1173

Conrad H E 1989 Structure of heparan sulfate and dermatan sulfate. Ann NY Acad Sci 556: 18–28

Dahan D, Houlbert D, Caulin C et al 1986 Prevention of deep vein thrombosis in elderly medical in-patients by a low molecular weight heparin: a randomized double-blind trial. Haemostasis 16: 159–164

Dawes J, Hodson B A, McGregor I R et al 1989 Pharmacokinetics and biological activities of dermatan sulfate (Mediolanum MF 701) in healthy volunteers. Ann NY Acad Sci 556: 292–303

Dechavanne M, Ville D, Berruyer M et al 1989 Randomized trial of a low molecular weight heparin (KABI 2165) versus adjusted dose subcutaneous standard heparin in the prophylaxis of deep vein thrombosis after elective hip surgery. Haemostasis 19: 5–12

Desnoyers P, Bara L, Samama M 1989 Dermatane sulfate et prévention des thromboses veineuses expérimentales. Pathol Biol 37: 759–767

Dol F, Houin G, Dupouy D et al 1988a Pharmacokinetics of dermatan sulfate in the rabbit after intravenous injection. Thromb Haemostasis 59: 255–258

Dol F, Caranobe C, Dupouy D et al 1988b Effects of increased sulfation of dermatan sulfate on its in vitro and in vivo pharmacological properties. Thromb Res 52: 153–164

Dol F, Petitou M, Lormeau J C et al 1990 Pharmacological properties of a low molecular weight dermatan sulfate: comparison with unfractionated dermatan sulfate. J Lab Clin Med 115: 43–51

Doutremepuich C, Bousquet F, Gestreau G L et al 1987 Comparative study on the effects of a low molecular weight heparin (CY 216) and standard heparin in low dosage on experimental venous thrombosis. Haemostasis 17: 201–205

Doutremepuich C, Toulemonde F, Doutremepuich F et al 1988 The tPA like activity induced by heparin and a heparin fragment binds on experimental thrombus. Thromb Res 50: 335–338

Dupouy D, Sie P, Boneu B 1988 A simple method to measure dermatan sulphate at sub-microgram concentrations in plasma. Thromb Haemostasis 60: 236–239

Duroux P 1987 Traitement curatif des thromboses veineuses profondes (TVP): Fraxiparine® versus heparine non fractionnée (HNF) Premier Symposium International, Cité des Sciences, Paris

Elias A, Lecorff G, Bouvier J L et al 1986 Treatment of deep vein thrombosis by a very low molecular weight heparin (CY 222): a dose range study. Thromb Res 162(suppl VI): 82

Elias A, Milandre L, Lagrange G et al 1990 Prevention des thromboses veineuses profondes des membres inférieurs par une fraction d'heparine de très bas poids moléculaire (CY 222) chez des patients porteurs d'une hémiplégie secondaire à un infarctus cérébral: étude pilote randomisée (30 patients). Mouvement Ther 11: 95–98

Encke A, Breddin K 1988 Comparison of a low molecular weight heparin and unfractionated heparin for the prevention of deep vein thrombosis in patients undergoing abdominal surgery. The European Fraxiparin Study (EFS) Group. Br J Surg 75: 1058–1063

Engelberg H 1985 Endogenous anticoagulant activity in native human plasma. Thromb Haemostasis 54: 292 (Abstract)

Eriksson B I, Zachrisson B E, Teger-Nilsson A C et al 1988 Thrombosis prophylaxis with low molecular weight heparin in total hip replacement. Br J Surg 75: 1053–1057

Faivre R, Neuhart Y, Kieffer Y et al 1988 Un nouveau traitement des thromboses veineuses profondes: les fractions d'heparine de bas poids moléculaire. Etude randomisée. Presse Med 17: 197–200

Fareed J, Walenga J M, Hoppensteadt D A et al 1985 Studies on the profibrinolytic actions of heparin and its fractions. Semin Thromb Hemostasis 11: 199–207

Fareed J, Hoppensteadt D A, Walenga J M et al 1988 Validity of the newly established low molecular weight heparin standard in cross referencing low molecular weight heparins. Haemostasis 3(suppl): 33–47

Fedarko N S, Conrad H E 1986 A unique heparan sulfate in the nuclei of hepatocytes: structural changes with the growth state of the cells. J Cell Biol 102: 587–599

Fernandez F, Nguyen P, Van Ryn J et al 1986a Haemorrhagic doses of heparin and other glycosaminoglycans induce a platelet defect. Thromb Res 43: 491–495

Fernandez F, Van Ryn J, Ofosu F A et al 1986b The haemorrhagic and antithrombotic effects of dermatan sulfate. Br J Haematol 64: 309–317

Fernandez F, Buchanan M R, Hirsh J et al 1987 Catalysis of thrombin inhibition provides an index for estimating the antithrombotic potential of glycosaminoglycans in rabbit. Thromb Haemostasis 57: 286–293

Follea G, Laville M, Pozet N et al 1986 Pharmacokinetic studies of standard heparin and low molecular weight heparin in patients with chronic renal failure. Haemostasis 16: 147–151

Forestier F, Daffos F, Capella-Pavlovsky M 1984 Low molecular weight heparin (PK 10169) does not cross the placenta during the second trimester of pregnancy: study by direct fetal blood sampling under ultrasound. Thromb Res 34: 557–560

Forestier F, Daffos F, Rainaut M et al 1987 Low molecular weight heparin (CY 216) does not cross the placenta during the third trimester of pregnancy. Thromb Haemostasis 57: 234

Frydman A M, Bara L, Le Roux Y et al 1988 The antithrombotic activity and pharmacokinetics of Enoxaparine, a low molecular weight heparin, in humans given single subcutaneous doses of 20 to 80 mg. J Clin Pharmacol 28: 609–618

Gallus A, Murphy W, Nacey J et al 1987 ORG 10172 causes increased urinary bleeding after transurethral prostatectomy (TURP). Thromb Haemostasis 58: 440 (Abstract)

Gordon M Y, Riley G P, Clarke D 1988 Heparan sulfate is necessary for adhesive interactions between human early hemopoietic progenitor cells and the extracellular matrix of the marrow microenvironment. Leukemia 2: 804–809

Goudable C, Ton-That H, Damani A et al 1986 Low molecular weight heparin half-life is prolonged in haemodialysed patients. Thromb Res 43: 1–5

Gray E, Bengtsson-Olivecrona G, Barrowcliffe T W 1987 Anti Xa activity of human hepatic triglyceride lipase. J Lab Clin Med 109: 653–659

Grimaudo V, Omri A, Kruithof E K O et al 1988 Fibrinolytic and anticoagulant activity after a single subcutaneous administration of a low dose of heparin or a low molecular weight heparin dihydroergotamine combination. Thromb Haemostasis 59: 388–391

Guizzardi S, Mastachi R, Govoni P et al 1987 Pharmacokinetics and organ distribution in rats of a low molecular weight heparin. Arzneim Forsch (Drug Res) 37: 1281–1283

Hemker H C 1989 A standard for low molecular weight heparin? Haemostasis 1: 1–4

Hemker H C, Willems G H, Beguin S A 1986 A computer assisted method to obtain the prothrombin activation velocity in whole plasma independent of thrombin decay processes. Thromb Haemostasis 56: 9–17

Henny C P, Ten Cate H, Ten Cate J W et al 1983 Use of new heparinoid as anticoagulant during acute haemodialysis of patients with bleeding complications. Lancet 1: 890–893

Henny C P, Ten Cate H, Ten Cate J W et al 1985a A randomized blind study comparing standard heparin and a new low molecular weight heparinoid in cardiopulmonary bypass surgery in dogs. J Lab Clin Med 106: 187–196

Henny C P, Ten Cate H, Surachno S et al 1985b The effectiveness of a low molecular weight heparinoid in chronic intermittent haemodialysis. Thromb Haemostasis 54: 460–462

Hirsh J 1986 In vitro effects of low molecular weight heparin on experimental thrombosis and bleeding. Haemostasis 16: 82–86

Hobbelen P M, Vogel G M, Meuleman D G 1987 Time courses of the antithrombotic effects, bleeding enhancing effects and interactions with factors Xa and thrombin after administration of low molecular weight heparinoid ORG 10172 or heparin to rats. Thromb Res 48: 549–558

Holm H A, Ly B, Handeland G F et al 1986 Subcutaneous heparin treatment of deep venous thrombosis: a comparison of unfractionated and low molecular weight heparin. Haemostasis 16(suppl 2): 30–37

Holmer E, Kurachi K, Söderström G 1981 The molecular weight dependence of the rate enhancing effect of heparin on the inhibition of thrombin, factor Xa, factor XIa, factor XIIa and kallikrein by antithrombin. Biochem J 193: 395–400

Horellou M H, Conard J, Lecrubier C et al 1984 Persistent heparin induced thrombocytopenia despite therapy with low molecular weight heparin. Thromb Haemostasis 51: 134–135

Hory B, Cachoux A, Saunier F et al 1987 Etude comparative de l'heparine et d'une heparine de très faible masse moléculaire en hémodialyse, dans l'insuffisance rénale chronique. Presse Med 16: 955–958

Huet Y, Gouault-Heilmann M, Contant G et al 1987 Treatment of acute pulmonary embolism by low molecular weight heparin fraction: a preliminary study. Intensive Care Med 13: 126–130

Ireland H, Lane D A, Flynn A et al 1986 The anticoagulant effect of heparinoid ORG 10172 during haemodialysis: an objective assessment. Thromb Haemostasis 55: 271–275

Janvier G, Winnock S, Dugrais G et al 1987 Treatment of deep venous thrombosis with a very low molecular weight heparin fragment (CY 222). Haemostasis 7: 49–58

Johnson E A, Kirkwood T B L, Stirling Y et al 1976 Four heparin preparations anti Xa potentiating effect of heparin after subcutaneous injection. Thromb Haemostasis 35: 586–591

Kaesberg P R, Ershler W B, Esko J D et al 1989 Chinese hamster ovary cell adhesion to human platelet thrombospondin is dependent on cell surface heparan sulfate proteoglycan. J Clin Invest 83: 994–1001

Kakkar V V 1984 Prevention of post operative venous thromboembolism by a new low molecular weight heparin fraction. Nouv Rev Fr Hématol 26: 277–282

Kakkar V V, Murray W J 1985 Efficacy and safety of low molecular weight heparin (CY 216) in preventing postoperative venous thromboembolism: a cooperative study. Br J Surg 72: 786–791

Keller K M, Keller J M, Kuhn K 1986 The C-terminus of type I collagen is a major binding site for heparin. Biochem Biophys Acta 882: 1–5

Koller M, Schoch U, Buchmann P et al 1986 Low molecular weight heparin (KABI 2165) as thromboprophylaxis in elective visceral surgery: a randomized double blind study versus unfractionated heparin. Thromb Haemostasis 56: 243–246

Lane D A 1989 Heparin binding and neutralizing proteins. In: Lane D A, Lindahl U (eds) Heparin, chemical and biological properties, clinical applications. Edward Arnold, London, pp 363–386

Lane D A, Denton J, Flynn A M et al 1984 Anticoagulant activities of heparin oligosaccharides and their neutralization by platelet factor 4. Biochem J 218: 725–732

Lane D A, Flynn A, Ireland H et al 1986 On the evaluation of heparin and low molecular weight heparin in haemodialysis for chronic renal failure. Haemostasis 16(suppl 2): 38–47

Lawler J, Hynes R O 1987 The structural organization of the thrombospondin molecule. Semin Thromb Haemostasis 13: 245–254

Lecrubier C, Lecompte T, Potevin F et al 1987 Tests d'agrégation plaquettaire dans 26 cas de thrombopénies induites par l'héparine. J Mal Vascul 12: 128–132

Levine M N, Hirsh J 1988 An overview of clinical trials of low molecular weight heparin fractions. Acta Chir Scand 543(suppl): 73–79

Levine M N, Planes A, Hirsh J et al 1989 The relationship between anti-factor Xa level and clinical outcome in patients receiving Enoxaparine, a low molecular weight heparin to prevent deep vein thrombosis after hip replacement. Thromb Haemostasis 62: 940–944

Lindahl U, Hook M 1978 Glycosaminoglycans and their binding to biological macromolecules. Ann Rev Biochem 47: 385–417

Ljungberg B, Blomback M, Johnsson H et al 1987 A single dose of a low molecular weight heparin fragment for anticoagulation during haemodialysis. Clin Nephrol 27: 31–35

Loscalzo J, Melnick B, Handin R I 1985 The interaction of platelet factor four and glycosaminoglycans. Arch Biochem Biophys 240: 446–455

Maffei-Faccioli A, Prandoni P, Meduri F et al 1989 A pilot study of dermatan sulfate in the prevention of postoperative deep venous thrombosis (DVT). Thromb Haemostasis 62: 397 (Abstract)

Maggi A, Abbadini M, Pagella P G et al 1987 Antithrombotic properties of dermatan sulfate in a rat venous thrombosis model. Haemostasis 17: 329–335

Massonet-Castel S, Pelissier E, Bara L et al 1986 Partial reversal of low molecular weight heparin (PK 10169) anti Xa activity by protamine sulfate: in vitro and in vivo study during cardiac surgery with extracorporeal circulation. Haemostasis 16: 139–146

Matzch T, Bergqvist D, Hedner U et al 1987 Effect of an enzymatically depolymerized heparin as compared with conventional heparin in healthy volunteers. Thromb Haemostasis 57: 97–101

Matzsch T, Bergqvist D, Fredin H et al 1988 Safety and efficacy of a low molecular weight heparin (Logiparin) versus dextran as prophylaxis against thrombosis after total hip replacement. Acta Chir Scand 154(suppl 543): 80–84

Maurin N, Kierdorf H 1988 A low molecular weight heparin in hemodialysis. Klin Wochenschr 66: 246–249

Mestre M, Clairefond P, Mardiguian J et al 1985 Comparative effects of heparin and PK 10169, a low molecular weight fraction, in a canine model of arterial thrombosis. Thromb Res 38: 389–399

Meuleman D G, Hobbelen P M J, Van Dedem G et al 1982 A novel antithrombotic heparinoid (ORG 10172) devoid of bleeding inducing capacity: a survey of its pharmacological properties in experimental animal models. Thromb Res 27: 353–363

Millot F, Bara L, Etienne J et al 1987 Activités lipolytique et anticoagulante de l'héparine et d'un de ses dérivés de faible poids moléculaire. Nouv Rev Fr Haematol 29: 397–400

Monkovic D D, Tracy P B 1990 Activation of human factor V by factor Xa and thrombin. Biochemistry 29: 1118–1128

Morani A, Gianese F, Bianchini F 1987 Kinetics of experimental antithrombotic activity of MF 701, dermatan sulfate. Thromb Haemostasis 58: 124 (Abstract 445)

Murata K, Nakazawa K, Hamai A 1975 Distribution of acidic glycosaminoglycans in the intima, media and adventitia of bovine aorta, and their anticoagulant properties. Atherosclerosis 21: 93–103

Nieuwenhuis H K, Sixma J J 1986 Treatment of disseminated intravascular coagulation in acute promyelocytic leukemia with low molecular weight heparinoid ORG 10172. Cancer 58: 761–764

Nurmohamed M T, Hoek J A, Ten Cate J W et al 1989 Coagulation studies with dermatan sulfate (DS) in six chronic hemodialysis patients. Thromb Haemostasis   62: 1537 (Abstract)

Ockelford P A, Carter C J, Hirsh J 1985 In vitro activity of a new heparinoid. Pathology 17: 78–81

Ockelford P A, Patterson J, Johns A S 1989 A double blind randomized placebo controlled trial of thromboprophylaxis in major elective general surgery using once daily injection of a low molecular weight heparin fragment (Fragmin). Thromb Haemostasis 62: 1046–1049

Ofosu F A, Fernandez F, Anvari N et al 1988a Further studies on the mechanism for the antithrombotic effects of sulfated polysaccharides in rabbits. Thromb Haemostasis 60: 182–192

Ofosu F A, Smith L M, Anvari N et al 1988b An approach to assigning in vitro potency to unfractionated and low molecular weight heparins based on the inhibition of prothrombin activation and catalysis of thrombin inhibition. Thromb Haemostasis 60: 193–198

Ofosu F A, Buchanan M R, Anvari N et al 1989 Plasma anticoagulant mechanisms of heparin, heparan sulfate and dermatan sulfate. Ann NY Acad Sci 556: 123–131

Omri A, Delaloye J F, Andersen H et al 1989 Low molecular weight heparin NOVO (LHN-1) does not cross the placenta during the second trimester of pregnancy. Thromb Haemostasis 61: 55–56

Palm M, Mattsson C H 1987 Pharmacokinetics of heparin and low molecular weight heparin fragment (Fragmin) in rabbits with impaired renal or metabolic clearance. Thromb Haemostasis 58: 932–935

Perlin A S, Sauriol F, Cooper B et al 1987 Dermatan sulfate in pharmaceutical heparins. Thromb Haemostasis 58: 792

Peterson C B, Morgan W T, Blackburn M N et al 1987 Histidine-rich glycoprotein modulation of the anticoagulant activity of heparin. J Biol Chem 262: 7567–7574

Pezzuoli G, Neri-Serneri G G, Settembrini P et al 1989 Prophylaxis of fatal pulmonary embolism in general surgery, using low molecular weight heparin CY 216: a multicentre, double-blind, randomized controlled clinical trial versus placebo (STEP). Int Surg 74: 205–210

Piepkorn M, Hovingh P, Hentschel W M 1988 Isolation of heparan sulfates with antithrombin III affinity and anticoagulant potency from BALB/c 3T3, B16 F 10 melanoma, and cutaneous fibrosarcoma cell lines. Biochem Biophys Res Commun 151: 327–332

Planes A, Vochelle N, Mazzas F et al 1988 Prevention of post operative venous thrombosis: a randomized trial comparing unfractionated heparin with low molecular weight heparin in patients undergoing total hip replacement. Thromb Haemostasis 60: 407–410

Poniewierski M, Barthels M, Kuhn M et al 1988 Efficacy of low molecular weight heparin (Fragmin) for thromboprophylaxis in medical patients: a randomized double blind trial. Med Klin 83: 241–245

Potron G M, Choisy H, Droulle C L et al 1989 Suivi prospectif post-marketing de la Fraxiparine à Reims. In: Breddin K, Fareed J, Samama M (eds) Fraxiparine: Premier Symposium International. Données analytiques, structurales, pharmacologiques et cliniques. Schattauer, Stuttgart, pp 161–170

Preissner K T, Heimburger N, Anders E et al 1986 Physicochemical, immunochemical and functional comparison of human-S protein and vitronectin: evidence for the identity of both plasma proteins. Biochem Biophys Res Commun 134: 951–956

Quilliet L, Charbonnier B, Delahousse B et al 1988 Traitement des embolies pulmonaires aiguës par une heparine de bas poids moléculaire par voie intraveineuse: recherche de la posologie optimale. Arch Mal Coeur 81: 1219–1225

Renaud H, Moriniere P, Dieval J et al 1985 Low molecular weight heparin in haemodialysis and haemofiltration: comparison with unfractionated heparin. Proc Eur Dial Transplant Assoc Eur Ren Assoc 21: 276–280

Rostin M, Montastruc J L, Houin G et al 1990 Pharmacodynamics of CY 216 in healthy volunteers: inter-individual variations. Fundam Clin Pharmacol 4: 17–23

Salzman E W, Rosenberg R, Smith M et al 1980 Effect of heparin and heparin fractions on platelet aggregation. J Clin Invest 65: 64–73

Samama M M, Bernard P, Bonnardot J P et al 1988 Low molecular weight heparin compared with unfractionated heparin in prevention of postoperative thrombosis. Br J Surg 75: 128–131

Samama M M, Boissel J P, Combe Tamzali S et al 1989 Clinical studies with low molecular weight heparin in the prevention and treatment of venous thromboembolism. Ann Acad Med NY 556: 386–405

Sandset P M, Abildgaard U, Larsen M L 1988 Heparin induces release of extrinsic coagulation pathway inhibitor (EPI). Thromb Res 50: 803–813

Schrader J, Stibbe W, Armstrong V W et al 1988 Comparison of low molecular weight heparin to standard heparin in hemodialysis/hemofiltration. Kidney Int 33: 890–896

Scully M F, Ellis V, Kakkar V V 1988 Heparan sulfate with no affinity for antithrombin III, and the control of haemostasis. FEBS Lett 241: 11–14

Sie P, Dupouy D, Caranobe C et al 1989 Neutralization of dermatan sulfate in vitro and in vivo by protamine sulfate and polybrene. Thromb Haemostasis 62: 1393 (Abstract)

Stiekema J C, Wijnand H P, Van Dinther T G et al 1989 Safety and pharmacokinetics of the low molecular weight heparinoid ORG 10172 administered to healthy elderly volunteers. Br J Clin Pharmacol 27: 39–48

Suzuki S, Suzuki S, Nakamura N et al 1976 The heterogenicity of dermatan sulfate and heparan sulfate in rat liver and a shift in the glycosaminoglycans content in carbon tetrachloride damaged liver. Biochem Biophys Acta 428: 166–181

Suzuki S, Pierschbacher M D, Hayman E G et al 1984 Domain structure of vitronectin: alignment of active sites. J Biol Chem 259: 15307–15314

Teien A, Abildgaard U, Hook M 1976 The anticoagulant effect of heparan sulfate and dermatan sulfate. Thromb Res 8: 859–867

Ten Cate H, Henny C P, Ten Cate J W et al 1987 Randomized double blind, placebo controlled safety study of a low molecular weight heparinoid in patients undergoing transurethral resection of the prostate. Thromb Haemostasis 57: 92–96

Tollefsen D M, Majerus D W, Blank M K 1982 Heparin cofactor II. Purification and properties of thrombin in human plasma. J Biol Chem 257: 2162–2169

Toulon P, Aiach M, Gianese F 1989 In vitro study of a new potential antithrombotic drug MF 701 (dermatan sulfate). Ann NY Acad Sci 556: 486–488

Turpie A G, Levine M N, Hirsh J et al 1986 A randomized controlled trial of a low molecular weight heparin (enoxaparin) to prevent deep vein thrombosis in patients undergoing elective hip surgery. N Engl J Med 315: 925–929

Turpie A G, Levine M N, Hirsh J et al 1987 Double blind randomized trial of ORG 10172, low molecular weight heparinoid, in prevention of deep vein thrombosis in thrombotic stroke. Lancet 1: 523–526

Vairel E G, Brouty-Boye H, Toulemonde F et al 1983 Heparin and a low molecular weight fraction enhances thrombolysis and by this pathway exercises a protective effect against thrombosis. Thromb Res 30: 219–224

Van Ryn-McKenna J, Cai L, Ofosu F A et al 1990 Neutralization of enoxaparine induced bleeding by protamine sulfate. Thromb Haemostasis 63: 271–274

Vinazzer H, Stemberger A, Haas S et al 1982 Influence of heparin, of different heparin fractions and a low molecular weight heparin like substance on the mechanism of fibrinolysis. Thromb Res 27: 341–352

Vitoux J F, Mathieu J F, Roncato M et al 1986 Heparin associated thrombocytopenia: treatment with low molecular weight heparin. Thromb Haemostasis 55: 37–39

Vitoux J F, Aiach M, Roncato M et al 1988a Should thromboprophylactic dosage of low molecular weight heparin be adapted to patient's weight? Thromb Haemostasis 59: 120 (Letter)

Vitoux J F, Fiessinger J N, Roncato M et al 1988b Long term treatment of acute deep venous thrombosis with low molecular weight heparin derivative. JAMA 259: 1180–1181

Vogel G M, Meuleman A G, Bourgondien F G et al 1989 Comparison of two experimental thrombosis models in rats: effects of four glycosaminoglycans. Thromb Res 54: 399–410

Walenga J M, Fareed J, Petitou M et al 1986 Intravenous antithrombotic activity of a synthetic heparin polysaccharide in human serum induced thrombosis model. Thromb Res 43: 243–248

Weisgraber K H, Rall S C Jr, Mahley R W et al 1986 Human apolipoprotein E: determination of the heparin binding sites of apolipoprotein E_3. J Biol Chem 261: 2068

11

Hirudo medicinalis and hirudin

B. Hoet   P. Close   J. Vermylen   M. Verstraete

Hirudin is produced by the salivary glands of medicinal leeches. During leeching it is secreted into the sucked blood. Without anticoagulation the blood flow would cease due to clotting and the leeches would be prevented from further sucking. It was Haycraft (1884), working in Schmiedeberg's pharmacological laboratory in Strasbourg, who discovered the anticoagulant property present in leeches. In the first studies aqueous extracts of the head of leeches were used containing only minute amounts of the active principle. Its protein nature was recognized by Markwardt (1955), who also described the selective thrombin inhibitory property of the polypeptide. The name was coined by Jacoby in 1904.

With advanced methods of peptide isolation and genetic engineering, cloning and expression of a DNA coding for hirudin has been obtained in *Escherichia coli*, yeast, *Bacillus subtilis* and other systems (Bergmann et al 1986, Dodt et al 1986, Fortkamp et al 1986, Harvey et al 1986, Courtney et al 1987, 1989, Meyhack et al 1987, Roitsch et al 1987, Tripier 1987, Johnson et al 1989). A comparison of different natural hirudin extracts and recombinant hirudins has recently been reported (Fink 1989). At least 12 commercial sources are reported to provide natural or recombinant hirudin (Fareed et al 1989).

BIOLOGICAL PROPERTIES

Natural hirudin is a potent inhibitor of human α-thrombin. It forms an equimolar complex with a very low dissociation constant (2×10^{-14} M; Stone & Hofsteenge 1986). The formed complex is very stable in the physiological pH range but can be dissociated by acidification or heating whereby thrombin is denatured and hirudin released in its active form (Baskova et al 1983).

The antithrombin activity of hirudin corresponds to a 1 : 1 reaction calculated by means of molecular weight. The activity of hirudin can be measured in antithrombin units (AT-U): 1 AT-U is the amount of hirudin that neutralizes one international unit of thrombin (Markwardt 1958). One microgram of pure hirudin inhibits about 5 μg of human thrombin. Pure hirudin contains approximately 10^4 AT-U/mg protein.

Furthermore, hirudin is specific for α-thrombin as prothrombin activated with the non-enzymatic protein staphylocoagulase (resulting in an activity of 20% in comparison to α-thrombin) is not blocked by hirudin (Kawabata et al 1986). The same holds for snake venoms, such as batroxobin, which catalyse the release of fibrinopeptides of fibrinogen (Walsmann & Markwardt 1981). It is interesting to note that endothelial thrombomodulin prevents the interaction between hirudin and thrombin (Stone & Hofsteenge 1986).

Hirudin exhibits a selectivity of greater than four orders of magnitude for thrombin, over all other proteolytic enzymes tested (Bagdy et al 1976, Markwardt 1970). CGP 39393, a recombinant desulphate HV1 type hirudin (see below), has no effect on the digestive enzymes trypsin and chymotrypsin (at 12 μM), on the coagulation enzymes factor Xa, kallikrein or plasmin (at 22 μM), or on any of the elements of the complement pathway (Talbot 1989).

Hirudin not only prevents fibrinogen conversion to fibrin by immediate blocking of any thrombin generated but also inhibits the thrombin-catalysed activation of factors V, VIII, XIII and thrombin-induced platelet activation (Markwardt et al 1983, Kaiser & Markwardt 1986). In particular, hirudin is significantly more potent than unfractionated heparin in preventing thrombin activation of factor VIII (Gray et al 1989, Pieters et al 1989).

By instantaneous inhibition of the small amount of thrombin generated after activation of the clotting system, the autocatalytic reaction that would otherwise lead to the accelerated generation of further thrombin is prevented. In fact, thrombin generation is remarkably amplified (280 000-fold; Mann et al 1985) by formation of the prothrombinase complex produced by the binding of factors Va, Xa and Ca^{2+} to the phospholipid of the platelet membrane. Thus, hirudin suppresses this feedback effect of thrombin.

Effect on clotting times in vitro

Both hirudin and heparin inhibit the coagulation of human or rat plasma, irrespective of whether it is induced by the intrinsic (activated partial thromboplastin time, APTT) or extrinsic (prothrombin time, PT) route or directly by thrombin (thrombin time, TT) (Talbot 1989, Walsman & Markwardt 1981).

The profile of a recombinant hirudin such as CGP 39393 resembles that of natural leech hirudin when examined with respect to its in vitro clotting activity. The TT is the most sensitive measurement for hirudin since a concentration of 0.005 μM doubles the clotting time. This method critically depends on the thrombin concentration used and the stability of thrombin in solution. Although both these drawbacks can be overcome, they do limit the clinical application of this test.

The PT measurement is the least sensitive to hirudin since a concentration of 1.14 μM is required to double the clotting time and this method is not considered to be sensitive enough. The APTT is doubled by 0.08 μM hirudin and since this is the method routinely used to monitor heparin therapy in man this method was selected in most studies and for comparative work.

Comparison of the effects of hirudins which directly inhibit thrombin, with those of heparin which indirectly (via antithrombin III) inhibit several enzymes in the coagulation pathway, show that by increasing the hirudin concentration it is possible to attain controlled anticoagulation to a level five times higher than the control APTT, before reaching an uncoagulable state. This differs from the results found with heparin where, at levels of anticoagulation required in clinical use (1.5–2 × control APTT), the dose–response curve is undesirably steep (Fig. 11.1).

Effect on platelet aggregation

Hirudin inhibits human platelet aggregation induced by thrombin, presumably by virtue of its affinity for the enzyme, although more hirudin seems to be needed than for inhibition of clotting (Hoffmann & Markwardt 1984). It is the strongest inhibitor of thrombin-induced serotonin secretion

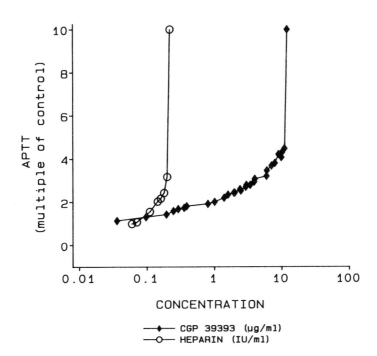

Fig. 11.1 Effect of desulphatohirudin and heparin on the APTT in vitro. (Courtesy of R.B. Wallis.)

(Markwardt et al 1983). It has little effect on platelet aggregation induced by other agents than thrombin (ADP, collagen, arachidonic acid and PAF) at concentrations more than two orders of magnitude higher than those that inhibit thrombin-induced aggregation. The minor effects observed exhibit no concentration dependence (Glusa & Urban 1988, Talbot et al 1989a, b). However, hirudin-induced inhibition of thrombin generated during platelet aggregation results in a marked decrease in platelet sensitivity to arachidonic acid, epinephrine and heparin in vitro (Brace et al 1989).

These data serve to highlight the importance of thrombin in platelet aggregation and the specificity of the effect of hirudin on platelet aggregation in contrast to the diverse and ill-understood actions of heparin on platelet aggregation (Saba et al 1984, de Prost 1986).

Moreover, thrombin promotes the stabilization of platelet aggregation by cleaving fibrinogen to fibrin and by activation of factor XIII, which cross-links fibrin. This action is also inhibited by hirudin.

Effect on other cells

Thrombin also stimulates the proliferation of endothelial cells (Yeo & Detwiler 1985), neuroblastoma cells (Snider 1986) and fibroblasts (Perdue et al 1981, van Obberghen-Schilling & Perez-Rodriquez 1982). Hirudin appears to be a specific antagonist of these effects of thrombin on other cells (Walsmann 1988).

The contractile response of vascular smooth muscle (rabbit aorta ring, pig coronary artery) to thrombin is also inhibited by hirudin, although higher concentrations are required than for the inhibition of fibrinogen conversion (Glusa & Wolfram 1988).

STRUCTURE AND FUNCTIONAL DOMAINS OF HIRUDIN

The complete primary and secondary structure of the natural hirudin molecule has been described (Petersen et al 1976, Dodt 1984, Dodt et al 1984, 1985) (Fig. 11.2). It contains 64–66 amino acids and its molecular weight is about 7000 daltons.

The N-terminal moiety (residues 1–39) is stabilized by three disulphide bridges. The C-terminal moiety (residues 40–65) is highly acidic: the last nine C-terminal residues contain 4 Glu and one Tyr residues. This Tyr residue in position 63 is sulphated. Recombinant hirudins do not contain this sulphation of Tyr[63]. Desulphation of the Tyr[63] of natural hirudin leads to a six-fold (Dodt et al 1988) to ten-fold (Stone & Hofsteenge 1986) increase in dissociation constant and a two-fold loss in potency (Chang 1983) without any change in the specificity of the thrombin–hirudin action.

The three-dimensional structure of hirudin in solution has been elucidated by nuclear magnetic resonance techniques (Sukumaran et al 1987, Clore et al 1987). Hirudin is composed of three domains: a central core made up

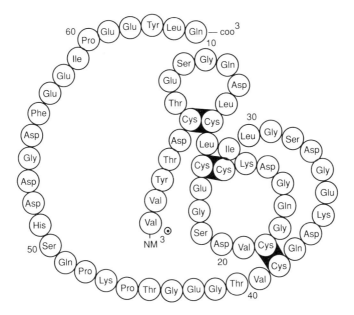

Fig. 11.2 Structure of desulphatohirudin. (Reproduced with permission from M. Talbot. Biology of recombinant hirudin (CGP 39393): a new prospect in the treatment of thrombosis. Semin Thromb Hemost 1989, 15: 293–301.)

of residues 3–30, 37–46 and 56–57 containing β-pleated sheets stabilized by the three disulphide bridges; a protruding 'finger' (residues 31–36) consisting of the tip of an antiparallel β-sheet; and an exposed loop (residues 47–55). The structure of the C-terminal end (residues 57–65) is too mobile to be determined by nuclear magnetic resonance.

Bagdy et al (1976), isolating hirudin from whole leeches instead of leech heads, concluded that their preparations contained hirudin with 2 Val (later called HV1) on the N-terminal end of the molecule whereas Ile-Thr was reported earlier (later called HV2) (Markwardt 1970, Markwardt & Walsmann 1967).

Later on, Baskova et al (1983) even discovered an inactive form in leech bodies called 'pseudohirudin' with a Val-Val N-terminal end and 20 amino acids less, assuming that pseudohirudin was an inactive cleavage product of original hirudin.

Different hirudins thus seem to be present in different parts of the leech body. Several other 'isoinhibitors' (Tripier 1987, 1988) have actually been isolated leading to a complex classification (Dodt et al 1986, Harvey et al 1986, Tripier 1987, 1988, Scharf et al 1989). These 20 different hirudins have an overall homology of 66%.

None of these hirudins contain Arg, Trp or Met, but a large amount of Glu and Asp are found. The Cys residues are consistent. Three Lys are present in most, but not all, hirudin forms. Two different constant N-termini are found (Val-Val or Ile-Thr).

The non-covalent complex formation between thrombin and hirudin is stoichiometric and tight. Based on kinetic analysis of hirudin–thrombin interaction, two binding sites in complex formation have been delineated: a low-affinity site, which does not impair thrombin-catalysed hydrolysis of small substrates, and a high-affinity site binding to or near the catalytic site of the enzyme (Stone & Hofsteenge 1986, Villanueva et al 1987). All catalytic functions of thrombin (i.e. procoagulant, proteolytic, amidolytic and esterolitic) are blocked (Stone & Hofsteenge 1986). The dissociation constant of hirudin was found to be 20 fM at an ionic strength of 0.125 M but this was markedly dependent on the ionic strength of the assay (it was increased 20-fold when the ionic strength was increased from 0.1 M to 0.4 M). Other authors, however, found an apparent K_i of about three orders of magnitude higher (Fenton 1981, 1989, Walsmann & Markwardt 1981) but this K_i was an underestimate of the true K_i because Michaelis–Menten kinetics are not valid under the reported conditions in which the concentration of inhibitor was similar to that of the enzyme.

Stone et al (1987) showed that thrombin whose active site is blocked with diisopropyl phosphate is still capable of forming a complex with hirudin. The same author also demonstrated that the active-site binding of thrombin is not essential. Hirudin, nevertheless, binds to this region of thrombin as evidenced by the fact that it is a competitive inhibitor with respect to tripeptidyl p-nitroanilide substrates (Stone & Hofsteenge 1986).

Thus, in order to compare hirudin with the serine protease inhibitor families several digestions and mutations of the inhibitor have been performed (Chang 1983, Braun et al 1988, Dodt et al 1988, Degryse et al 1989).

Serine protease inhibitors generally present themselves as a pseudo-substrate to the target protease (Carrell et al 1987, for review). The region around Lys[47] (residues 40–48) is very similar to the sequence of the binding site for thrombin on prothrombin (residues 149–157) (Petersen et al 1976). The last two residues of this domain in prothrombin are Arg-Ser, the cleaving site of thrombin. These are replaced by Lys-Pro in hirudin, which resembles a P_1P_2 reactive centre of a serine protease inhibitor (Blombäck et al 1977). In this model Lys[47] would fit into the Arg site pocket of thrombin (containing Gln[192]) adjacent to its active site. But the Lys[47]-Pro[48] peptide bond does not present a free amino group to the His[57] of the charge relay system of thrombin and hence would not be hydrolysed. Moreover, Lys-Pro bonds are usually resistant to proteolysis, and thrombin usually cleaves adjacent to Arg residues (Blombäck et al 1977, Mann & Lundblad 1982).

Point mutation of the Lys[47] residue to Glu (Braun et al 1988) or to Ile or Gln (Dodt et al 1988) have led to a small increase in the K_i but certainly not to the drastic increase expected in the case of a classic serine protease inhibitor. Mutation of the three other basic residues of hirudin (Lys[27] and

Lys[36] to Glu, Gln or Ile and His[51] to Glu, Leu or Asp; Braun et al 1988, Dodt et al 1988) have not led to any significant increase in K_i although Lys[36] is situated in the protruding finger domain (residues 31–36) that could be available for intermolecular reaction (Clore et al 1987).

Moreover, none of the three Lys is conserved in the 20 hirudin variants known. Degryse et al (1989) mutated the hirudin variant HV2 containing an Asn in position 47 to HV2 Lys[47] and HV2 Arg[47]. The dissociation constants of these hirudins decreased only five-fold and six-fold respectively. However, HV2 Lys[47] was also tested in a rabbit Wessler model (Buchanan et al 1985) in which it proved to be 100 times more potent than HV2. The same authors also showed that mutation of Lys[35] to Thr in HV2 and in HV2 Lys[47] did not improve the dissociation constant. These results indicate that, although the structure around Lys[47] plays a role in the activity of hirudin on thrombin, it is not the major binding site of hirudin.

Clore et al (1987) showed that the ε-amino group of Lys[47] is involved in an electrostatic interaction with backbone carboxyl oxygen atoms. The disruption of these interactions by mutation of Lys[47] could result in minor alterations in the tertiary structure of the molecule and thus be responsible for the small increase in the dissociation constant.

Stone & Hofsteenge (1986) also suggested that ionic interaction may be involved in the formation of the complex by showing the influence of ionic strength on the thrombin–hirudin interaction. Moreover, a region of thrombin (residues 62–73), rich in positively charged residues, is important for its interaction with hirudin (Stone et al 1987, Noe et al 1988). As the C-terminal region of hirudin is highly negatively charged, it could be involved in the putative ionic interaction.

Removal of the last seven acidic C-terminal amino acids of natural hirudin resulted in a concomitant loss of at least 90% hirudin inhibition activity and removal of the last 22 C-terminal amino acids causes nearly quantitative abolishment of hirudin inhibition activity (Chang 1983). Other authors mention diminished activity of recombinant desulphate hirudin when one or two of the last residues are deleted (Grossenbacher et al 1987, Riehl-Bellon et al 1989) or the nine last residues (Degryse et al 1989).

Point mutations on the 4 Glu residues of recombinant desulphatohirudin to Gln residues (Braun et al 1988) presented an increase in the dissociation constant proportional to the amount of Glu residues mutated. Mutation of Glu[61] and Glu[62] caused, respectively, a 1.6- and 2.3-fold increase in the dissociation constant; double mutation of Glu[57] and Glu[58] leads to a ten-fold increase in dissociation constant; triple (Glu[57], Glu[58] and Glu[62]) and quadruple (Glu[57], Glu[58], Glu[61] and Glu[62]) mutants have a 37- and 61-fold higher dissociation constant, respectively.

It is nevertheless worthwhile to note that mutations of Glu[57] could lead to conformational changes due to the involvement of Glu[57] in an electrostatic interaction with Ser[9] in the central core of hirudin (Clore et al 1987).

Small synthetic fragments, corresponding to the C-terminus of hirudin, inhibit the clotting activity and the release of fibrinopeptide A by thrombin (Hir 45–65; Krstenansky et al 1987, 1988; and Hir 53–64 being the smallest hirudin fragments still showing maximal anticoagulant activity, Maraganore et al 1989) but these fragments did not inhibit the hydrolysis of tripeptidyl p-nitroanilide substrates by thrombin, showing that these hirudin derivatives block the fibrinogenolytic activity of thrombin via interaction at a non-catalytic site. Binding studies revealed a single binding site for Hir 45–65 on thrombin, with a dissociation constant of 10^{-5} M (Krstenansky & Mao 1987). In particular Phe[56], Glu[57], Ile[59], Pro[60] and Leu[64] are the most critical residues of this region (Krstenansky et al 1987).

An interesting feature from this viewpoint is presented by the structural similarities between the C-terminal end of hirudin and fibrinopeptides A and B (Chang 1989).

For example, Phe[56] (conserved in all hirudin variants sequenced so far; Mao et al 1988, Scharf et al 1989) is aligned with Phe[8] of fibrinopeptide A which is conserved in virtually all species (Blombäck 1967) and has been shown to be important for fibrinopeptide A release by thrombin (Meinwald et al 1980, Marsh et al 1985).

It should moreover be noted that thrombomodulin is able to compete for the binding of thrombin with hirudin (Hofsteenge et al 1986). Binding of thrombomodulin to thrombin also inhibits the clotting activity and does not inhibit the hydrolysis of tripeptidyl p-nitroaniline substrates (Jakubowski et al 1986).

Resulphation of Tyr[11] of Hir 53–64 (corresponding to Tyr[63] in natural hirudin) leads to a ten-fold decrease in the dissociation constant (Maraganore et al 1989) which corresponds to the increase in the dissociation constant resulting from the desulphation of natural hirudin (Dodt et al 1988, Stone & Hofsteenge 1986). This product prolongs the clotting times and inhibits platelet aggregation induced by thrombin, in the same way as natural hirudin.

Hirudin and resulphated Hir 53–64 exhibit a relatively small difference in inhibition of the action of thrombin on coagulation and platelet activation and, thus, it is likely that the interaction of hirudin with a non-catalytic site in thrombin defines a predominant component of physiologically relevant antithrombin activities.

Nevertheless, the secondary and tertiary structure of hirudin are basic for its antithrombin function which is lost during reduction of the disulphide bridges. This issue was studied by Tertrin et al (1967), who found that even partial reduction and alkylation, carried out with 5–20 molar excess of dithiothreitol over protein disulphide content in the absence of denaturants, affects only two disulphides in hirudin and is accompanied by a considerable decrease in biological activity. More disulphide bonds could be cleaved in the presence of 8 M urea leading to the complete reduction and alkylation of the disulphide bonds in hirudin, and also to an additional decrease but not complete abolition of the biological activity.

Recently the contribution of the N-terminal region ‹
interaction with thrombin was studied. Most of the hiru‹
either Val-Val or Ile-Thr as their N-terminal region (excep
Thr and one Thr; Tripier 1987). Those are all hydroph
with branched side chains. An eight-residue N-terminal
antithrombin activity (Fortkamp et al 1986), and ano'
form produced by *E. coli* contains an extra N-terminal metniony1 ....___,
presenting a reduced affinity for thrombin (Loison et al 1988, Wallace et al
1989).

Replacement of the two N-terminal Val residues of recombinant
desulphatohirudin by polar groups caused a marked decrease in binding
energy whereas conservative replacements by other hydrophobic groups,
resulted in only moderate changes in strength of inhibition (Wallace et al
1989).

PHARMACOKINETIC STUDIES IN ANIMALS

After intravenous bolus administration of 1 and 0.5 mg/kg of natural
hirudin in rats, rabbits and dogs, values of 10–15 minutes for the distribution
and 50–65 minutes for the elimination half-lives were obtained (Markwardt
et al 1982). Similar values were found with recombinant desulphatohirudin
in rats and dogs (Grossenbacher et al 1987, Markwardt 1989, Markwardt
et al 1989, Meyhack et al 1987). The pharmacokinetic data can best be
described by an open two-compartment model with first-order kinetics.

In nephrectomized dogs about 80% of an intravenously administered
recombinant hirudin was distributed into extravascular compartments within
60 minutes. After this distribution phase the blood levels of hirudin remained
nearly constant for at least 4 hours (Nowak et al 1988), showing nearly
complete renal excretion of hirudin.

After intravenous (and also subcutaneous) administration of natural
hirudin or recombinant desulphated hirudin the pharmacokinetic data in
dogs (Nowak et al 1988) and rats (Markwardt et al 1988a, 1989) are
similar. Only the renal excretion is increased by 20–25% with recombinant
hirudin, presumably due to the absence of sulphation on Tyr^{63} (Nowak
et al 1988).

Following intravenous injection, radioactively labelled recombinant [^{125}I]
iododesulphatohirudin is uniformly distributed in all organs, but the peak
radioactivity in the kidneys reflects extensive renal excretion (Richter et al
1986, 1988). The renal clearance of hirudin approximates the creatinine
clearance, which suggests a glomerular filtration. Seventy-five per cent of
the injected dose of hirudin (i.v. or s.c.) is recovered unchanged in the urine
1 hour after administration and 95% after 5 hours (Markwardt et al 1988a).
Natural (sulphated) or recombinant (non-sulphated) hirudin preparations,
given to dogs, were isolated from urine and compared with the administered
preparation by reversed-phase high-performance liquid chromatography,

no acid sequence and composition analysis (Henschen et al 1987, 1988). It was shown that the hirudins were excreted in unmodified form.

In the case of recombinant hirudin infusion in the dog, plateau values were reached within 30–60 minutes (Markwardt et al 1989).

Natural hirudin and recombinant desulphated hirudin are nearly completely absorbed after subcutaneous administration in rats, rabbits and dogs. Peak plasma hirudin levels are reached after 1–2 hours and the apparent elimination half-lives are between 1.9 and 5.7 hours (Nowak & Markwardt 1987, Markwardt et al 1984, 1987, 1988a, Richter et al 1988).

There is some absorption of recombinant hirudin after intratracheal instillation in rats with an elimination half-life of about 3.3 hours (Markwardt et al 1988a). Rectal or intraduodenal administration of either natural or recombinant hirudin in dogs did not generate detectable plasma levels of either compound (Markwardt et al 1987, 1988a).

Hirudin does not seem to pass through the blood–brain barrier but there is slight transfer through the placenta in rabbits (Markwardt et al 1988a).

IN VIVO STUDIES WITH HIRUDIN

Effects on clotting times ex vivo

The doses of desulphatohirudin required in rats to double the APTT are 0.1 mg/kg i.v. and 2 mg/kg s.c. (Talbot 1989, Ambler et al 1989, using CGP 39393). Comparison of the dose–response curves for desulphated hirudin and heparin, based on ex vivo coagulation (APTT), indicates that irrespective of the route of administration (i.v. or s.c.), desulphatohirudin controls the degree of anticoagulation (i.e. maintains linearity) over a greater concentration range than heparin before reaching the incoagulable state. The duration of action of desulphatohirudin and of heparin was determined by APTT after both intravenous and subcutaneous administration in rats. Doses of each were chosen to give 2.0–3.5 times the control APTT levels, namely 0.3 mg/kg i.v. and 3 mg/kg s.c. for CGP 39393 and 30 IU/kg i.v. and 300 IU/kg s.c. for heparin.

After intravenous administration the time course of desulphatohirudin (0.3 mg/kg) appears to be biphasic; after an initial peak APTT decreases but remains elevated for 60 minutes after administration. Intravenous heparin (30 IU/kg) shows a very similar profile in this respect.

When given by intravenous infusion to rats for up to 30 minutes, desulphatohirudin caused a dose-related increase in APTT. An approximate doubling of control APTT was achieved at 12.50 μg/kg per minute (750 μg/kg per hour).

After subcutaneous administration desulphatohirudin (3 mg/kg) rapidly achieves an elevation of APTT which reaches a plateau after 15 minutes and lasts for approximately 2–4 hours. APTT returns to the control level by 4 hours. This contrasts with a much slower onset of the effect of heparin

(300 IU/kg) when administered by this route. The longer duration of action of heparin may be due to slower absorption from the subcutaneous injection site.

Antithrombotic effect in a venous thrombosis model in rat

The effects of natural hirudin, desulphatohirudin and heparin on venous thrombosis were determined in the rat (Markwardt et al 1982, 1989, Talbot et al 1989a, b). Systemic hypercoagulability was induced by i.v. thromboplastin C (Dade; 20 μl/kg) or activated human serum administration prior to the production of stasis in the inferior vena cava by ligation. After 10 minutes the vessel was removed and the thrombus withdrawn, rinsed with citrate and weighed. Results were calculated in percentage difference in thrombus weight between placebo- and drug-tested animals.

Desulphatohirudin demonstrates a potent antithrombotic action with a steep dose–response curve in this model, with an ID_{50} of 0.01 mg/kg i.v. and 0.45 mg/kg s.c. and total inhibition at 0.03 mg/kg i.v. and 1.0 mg/kg s.c. (Talbot et al 1989a, b; using CGP 39393). Other authors obtained essentially the same results with recombinant (also CGP 39393) and natural hirudin (Markwardt et al 1982, 1989). Heparin and low-molecular-weight heparin are also very potent in this model, with an ID_{50} of 3.0 IU/kg i.v. and 110 IU/kg s.c. for heparin and similar doses for low-molecular-weight heparin (Ambler et al 1989).

Antithrombotic effect in a shunt thrombosis model in rat

The antithrombotic effects of desulphatohirudin and standard heparin were determined by a modification of the arteriovenous shunt thrombosis model of Smith & White (1982). An extracorporeal shunt made of polystyrene tubing was implanted between the carotid artery and jugular vein of the anaesthetized rat. Thrombus formation was measured either by weight of the thrombus formed on a cotton thread inserted in the shunt (Talbot et al 1989a, b) or by measuring the fall in temperature on the tubing (Markwardt et al 1982, 1989). A spontaneous occlusion is seen within a few minutes under normal conditions.

Desulphatohirudin is a potent antithrombotic agent which inhibits thrombus formation completely in this model. A dose of 0.3 mg/kg i.v. or 1 mg/kg s.c. inhibits thrombus formation in the rat by approximately 50%. This compares with 200 IU/kg s.c. heparin. Total inhibition was obtained with 2 mg/kg i.v. or 10 mg/kg s.c. desulphatohirudin (CGP 39393, Talbot et al 1989a, b).

Natural hirudin in intravenous bolus (Markwardt et al 1982) and recombinant desulphatohirudin (CGP 39393) in intravenous bolus, subcutaneous injection (Talbot et al 1989a) and in infusion (Markwardt et al 1989) were tested in this model. Total inhibition of thrombus formation was achieved at more than 50 AT-U/ml plasma for natural hirudin, 3 mg/kg for intravenous bolus or 10 mg/kg for subcutaneous administration and 40 μg/kg per minute for infusion. Fifty per cent of thrombus formation was achieved with 0.3 mg/kg i.v. or 1 mg/kg s.c.

In the shunt thrombosis model in the rat, an intravenous bolus dose of desulphatohirudin, followed by intravenous infusion to maintain a plateau level of two times the control APTT over the period of thrombus formation, resulted in 71% inhibition of thrombus weight. Almost total inhibition was achieved at a plateau level of three times the control APTT. In contrast, similar administration of unfractionated heparin, producing a plateau of approximately two times the control APTT, caused only 50% inhibition of thrombus weight. An increase in APTT of more than 15-fold was required to inhibit thrombus weight by more than 80%. Using a low-molecular-weight heparin (Fragmin, KabiVitrum), over 90% inhibition was achieved at three times the control APTT (Ambler et al 1989).

It is interesting to note that the surface of the control thrombi appeared homogeneously red under the microscope, whereas the surface of the thrombi formed in the presence of hirudin showed large white areas, indicating the prevalence of platelet material (Markwardt et al 1982).

Microthrombosis, experimental disseminated intravascular coagulation

In the treatment of disseminated intravascular coagulation (DIC) a relatively slight effect of heparin has been observed by several authors (Colman et al 1972, Braunstein & Eurenius 1976, Ishikawa et al 1979, Lasch & Heene 1975). This is to be linked to the consumption of antithrombin III during DIC. The action of natural hirudin on DIC was first demonstrated in an endotoxin-induced generalized Schwartzman reaction in rabbits by Ishikawa et al (1980) in which an inhibition of glomerular microthrombosis, renal failure, fibrinogen fall and platelet count drop was observed.

Natural hirudin was compared to heparin, in an equi-effective dose as measured by in vitro clotting tests, in a thrombin-induced DIC model in rats. By using iodine-labelled fibrinogen (Markwardt et al 1977) and measuring the radioactivity of liver, spleen, suprarenals, lungs and kidneys they also found only a slight effect of heparin and a clear effect of hirudin.

Infusion of tissue thromboplastin also induces microthrombosis with accumulation of fibrinogen and platelets in the lung capillaries. This could be studied by labelling fibrinogen with iodine and platelets with indium. Desulphatohirudin infusion, started 60 minutes prior to the beginning of the tissue thromboplastin administration, inhibited fibrin deposition at doses higher than 1.5 μg/kg per minute and platelet deposition at doses higher than 65 μg/kg per minute (Markwardt et al 1989).

Antithrombotic effect in an arterial thrombosis model in rat

To prevent electrically induced arterial thrombosis in rats five-fold higher doses of hirudin are required than needed to prevent venous stasis thrombosis (Markwardt et al 1982, 1989). At 10 mg/kg desulphatohirudin s.c., thrombus development is inhibited by more than 70% with an associated APTT value of less than four times the control, whereas heparin and low-molecular-weight heparin, at doses of 600 IU/kg s.c. and 10 mg/kg s.c., respectively, giving over ten times the control APTT, were inactive in this model (Talbot et al 1989a, b).

Hirudin and bleeding time

One of the drawbacks of heparin is that at doses at which an effective protection against thrombosis is obtained haemostasis also is impaired, with the associated risk of bleeding (Brace & Fareed 1985, Hirsh 1984, Salzman et al 1980).

Kaiser & Markwardt (1986) compared the prolongation of the bleeding time in rats and mice after transection of the tail (mainly dependent on coagulation; Dejana et al 1982) and after standardization longitudinal incision of the tail basis (mainly influenced by platelet number and function; Dejana et al 1982). After transection of the tail hirudin and heparin prolonged the bleeding time in a dose-dependent manner; after the standardized longitudinal incision heparin caused a much more prolonged bleeding time than hirudin.

Markwardt et al (1989) showed that the rat tail bleeding time performed by a standardized incision of the rat tail was prolonged depending on the dose of recombinant desulphatohirudin administered but that this prolongation was only pronounced at relatively high doses (>60 μg/kg per minute) at which the antithrombotic effect was already completely achieved in all models tested (venous thrombosis, arterial thrombosis, shunt thrombosis and microthrombosis).

It is most interesting to note that the dose of hirudin required for inhibition of thrombosis dependent on coagulation (venous stasis, fibrin deposition in experimental DIC) is ten times lower than the dose required to inhibit platelet aggregation-dependent thrombosis (arterial thrombosis and platelet deposition in experimental DIC (Markwardt et al 1989)) (Fig. 11.3).

An even 100 times higher dose of hirudin is required to prolong the bleeding time as compared to the inhibition of venous thrombosis (Markwardt et al 1989) (Fig. 11.3), presumably because hirudin does not affect the ADP- and collagen-induced platelet responses and because the presence of hirudin does not prevent platelets from adhering to the subendothelium of rabbit aorta as heparin does (Glusa & Urban 1988, Glusa & Wolfram 1988).

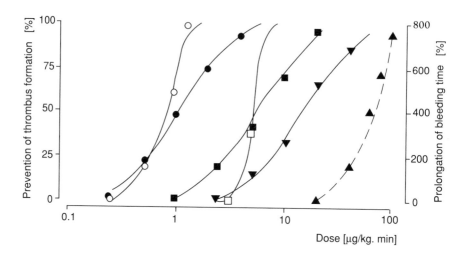

Fig. 11.3 Comparison of antithrombotic and bleeding effects of recombinant hirudin in rats. ●: venous thrombosis, ■: arterial thrombosis, ○: microthrombosis (fibrin deposits), □: microthrombosis (platelet aggregates), ▼: arterio-venous shunt thrombosis, ▲: bleeding time. (Reproduced with permission from Markwardt et al, Thromb Res 1989, 54: 377–388.)

Using another recombinant form of hirudin (HV2-Lys[47]) Maffrand et al (1989) also showed a clear inhibition of a venous stasis-induced thrombosis and a prolongation of the bleeding time. The ED_{50} to prolong the bleeding time was 280 times higher than the ED_{50} against venous thrombosis.

Thus, clinically, the required dosage of hirudin will depend on the degree of thrombin generation encountered in the clinical situation. For example, the predicted dose for anticoagulation in extracorporeal circulations or prevention of arterial thrombosis is likely to be significantly greater than that needed for the prophylaxis of deep venous thrombosis.

Comparison of heparin and desulphatohirudin in the development of acute platelet thrombus deposition during angioplasty in pigs

Carotid angioplasty was performed in 55 anaesthetized pigs randomized to one of six heparin dosages (heparin boluses of 35, 50, 100, 150, 200 or 250 units/kg followed by a continuous infusion of 35, 50, 100, 150, 200 or 250 units/kg per hour, respectively). A further five pigs received a bolus of 1 mg desulphatohirudin/kg followed by an infusion of 1 mg/kg per hour (Heras et al 1989). Bilateral carotid angioplasty was performed 20 minutes after starting the infusion and the pigs were sacrificed 1 hour after the procedure.

Platelet and fibrinogen deposition in deeply injured arteries was studied. A regression analysis showed a negative correlation of the log of platelet deposition in deeply injured arteries, with administered total units of heparin and with heparin concentration. But the lowest platelet and fibrinogen deposition was observed in the hirudin-treated group. The amount of deeply injured arterial segments covered with mural thrombus decreased from 72% of all the deeply injured arterial segments in the lowest heparin group to 10% in the highest heparin group and to 0% in the animals treated with hirudin. APTT were 2.5–3.5 times those of the control basal values in the hirudin group and in the lowest dose heparin group (35 units/kg) but, of course, longer at higher heparin doses.

Thus, hirudin at a dose prolonging activated partial thromboplastin to the same extent as 35 U heparin/kg resulted in a most effective prevention of thrombosis in this model (even more so than with 250 U heparin/kg) while heparin in this dose had a limited effect.

Prevention of experimental coronary thrombosis by hirudin

Natural hirudin administered subcutaneously in rats was able to prevent in a dose-dependent way coronary thrombosis (doses of 0.25, 0.5 and 1.0 mg/kg) (Bucha et al 1988), as monitored by the extent of the infarct size. The most pronounced antithrombotic effect of hirudin in this model was related to plasma concentrations of between 0.20 and 0.35 μg hirudin/ml.

Comparison of the inhibition of coagulation activation by heparin and desulphatohirudin during recombinant tissue-type plasminogen activator-induced thrombolysis

Thrombin bound to a fibrin clot remains active and is poorly accessible to antithrombin III. During fibrinolysis, as successive fibrin layers are removed, these inaccessible molecules of thrombin are exposed to the surface of the residual clot and possibly contribute to the occurrence of coagulation during thrombolytic therapy, that is poorly controlled by heparin. The TIMI-I study, for example, showed a very high reocclusion rate after short-term recombinant tissue-type plasminogen activator administration despite early heparinization (Williams et al 1986). Hirudin has been shown, in vitro, to inhibit efficiently the fibrinogenolytic activity of fibrin-bound thrombin, whereas heparin at the same antithrombotic dose did not have this effect (Mirshahi et al 1989).

TOXICOLOGY AND IMMUNOGENICITY

Toxicology studies

The acute toxicology of a bolus intravenous dose of desulphatohirudin was studied in rats (50 mg/kg) and no adverse effect was noted.

Subchronic toxicity of recombinant hirudin (Genbiotec) has also been studied in rats. After daily subcutaneous administration of 1 mg/kg over 4 weeks there was no indication of treatment-related effects and haemorrhagic complications did not occur. No antibodies were detected against the hirudin used (Klöcking et al 1988).

Immunological response to hirudin

Hirudin, being a protein produced by the leech *Hirudo medicinalis*, has the theoretical potential to elicit an immunological response and/or allergic reaction, including systemic anaphylaxis in man.

An absence of immune or allergic reactions in experimental studies (Klöcking et al 1988, Seemüller et al 1986) and man (Markwardt et al 1984, Bichler et al 1988) was noted.

Biweekly intravenous injection in rabbits (Spinner et al 1988) and several intravenous injections of either natural or recombinant hirudin in baboons (Bichler et al 1990) did not induce immune reactions. Only two of 11 sheep subjected to an immunization protocol produced precipitating, hirudin-specific antibodies (Spinner et al 1986).

HUMAN PHARMACOKINETIC STUDIES WITH NATURAL HIRUDIN

Natural hirudin has been injected intravenously (bolus of 1000 AT-U/kg) or subcutaneously (1000 AT-U/kg) in six healthy volunteers (Markwardt et al 1984). After intravenous administration, the half-life of distribution was 0.15 ± 0.06 hours and of elimination 0.84 ± 0.19 hours. The volume of distribution was 12.9 ± 2.8 litres; total systemic clearance was 230 ± 98 ml/min, and renal clearance 99.6 ± 63.2 ml/min following first-order elimination kinetics. In another study in 12 human volunteers the half-life of natural hirudin was 65 minutes after intravenous injection (Bichler et al 1989).

After subcutaneous injection of natural hirudin its level in blood increased within 60 minutes and reached plateau values in plasma at 0.5 AT-U/ml. The elimination half-life was 0.64 ± 0.33 hours. The subcutaneous bioavailability is 36% (Markwardt et al 1984). A more recent study gives a half-life of 100 minutes after subcutaneous injection of natural hirudin (Bichler et al 1989).

HIRUDIN ACTIVITY IN MAN

Clotting assays performed in tolerability studies correlate closely with the hirudin concentration: the activated partial thromboplastin time appeared to be the most reliable test to estimate the actual inhibitory concentration in the plasma (Markwardt et al 1984, 1988b, Bichler et al 1988).

A preliminary therapeutic study was performed in patients with subacute DIC. After subcutaneous administration of 0.1 mg/kg at 8-hourly intervals, plasma levels of 0.05–0.1 μg/ml were obtained, resulting in a normalization of fibrinogen levels and platelet counts and a disappearance of fibrin monomer complexes and degradation products (Vogel & Markwardt 1987, 1988).

Neutralization of hirudin

Hirudin being a specific and potent inhibitor of thrombin, it is desirable to have an antidote available for reversal of its biological effects. Protamine sulphate, which neutralizes heparin, does not affect hirudin.

The haemorrhagic effect of recombinant hirudin is markedly reduced in a concentration-dependent manner by addition of increasing concentrations of a prothrombin complex concentrate at a 2.0 mg/kg dosage of hirudin, administered intravenously in rabbits; an increase in blood loss was produced that was approximately four-fold higher than the baseline value. When FEIBA as a source of prothrombin complex was administered 5 minutes after hirudin by a 25 U/kg slow infusion, a 50% reduction from the original bleeding response was obtained (Walenga et al 1989). This suggests that prothrombin complex concentrates may be useful in reversing the haemorrhagic effect of hirudin.

Three monoclonal antibodies (IgG, kappa) against hirudin have been obtained and characterized (Spinner et al 1986). They were detected towards continuous overlapping epitopes that are likely to be located in the C-terminal region of the protein. One of the monoclonal antibodies interferes with the interaction of hirudin with α-thrombin. Whether monoclonal or polyclonal antibodies against hirudin or inactivated thrombin could be used to neutralize hirudin in vivo is still to be carefully evaluated.

CONCLUSION

Hirudin is a most potent and selective inhibitor of thrombin, the pivotal enzyme in the coagulation process. Recombinant hirudin can now be produced through biotechnology in liberal amounts. One of the advantages of hirudin over heparin is that it does have minor direct effects on platelets and acts independently of antithrombin III and without interference of platelet factor 4. These characteristics render hirudin an attractive alternative to heparin, provided inhibition of protein C activation and of the release of tissue plasminogen activator are not major drawbacks. While the odds are in favour of predicting that bleeding will less readily occur with hirudin than with heparin at antithrombotic blood levels, this hope is still to be substantiated in comparative clinical trials.

REFERENCES

Ambler J, Butler K D, Kerry P et al 1989 Thrombosis pharmacology of CGP 39393 in infusion studies: comparisons with heparin and fragmin. Circulation 80: 316 (abstract)

Bagdy D, Barabas E, Graf L, Peterson T E, Magnusson S 1976 Hirudin. In: Lorand L (ed) Methods in enzymology, vol 45: proteolytic enzymes. Academic Press, New York, pp 669–678

Baskova I P, Cherkesova D U, Mosolov V V 1983 Hirudin from leech heads and whole leeches and 'pseudo-hirudin' from leech bodies. Thromb Res 30: 459–467

Bergmann C, Dodt J, Köhler S, Fink E, Gassen H G 1986 Chemical synthesis and expression of a gene coding for hirudin, the thrombin-specific inhibitor from the leech *Hirudo medicinalis*. Biol Chem Hoppe-Seyler 367: 731–740.

Bichler J, Fichtl B, Siebeck J, Fritz H 1988 Pharmacokinetics and pharmacodynamics of hirudin in man after single subcutaneous and intravenous bolus administrations. Drug Res 38: 704–710

Bichler J, Siebeck M, Fichtl B, Fritz H 1989 Pharmacokinetics, effect on clotting parameters and assessment of the immunoallergic potential of hirudin in man after single subcutaneous and intravenous bolus administration. Thromb Haemostasis 62(suppl 1): 533 (Abstract)

Bichler J, Gemmerli R, Fritz H 1990 Studies for revealing a possible sensitization to hirudin after 4 intravenous injections on baboon. Submitted for publication.

Blombäck B 1967 Substrate specificity of thrombin on proteins and synthetic substrates. In: Seegers W H (ed) Blood clotting enzymology. Academic Press, New York, pp 143–215

Blombäck J G, Hessel B, Hogg D, Claesen G 1977 Substrate specificity of thrombin on proteins and synthetic substrates. In: Lundblad R L, Fenton J W II, Mann K G (eds) Chemistry and biology of thrombin. Ann Arbor Science, Ann Arbor, pp 275–290

Brace L D, Fareed J 1985 An objective assessment of the interaction of heparin and its fractions with human platelets. Sem Thromb Haemostasis 11: 190–198

Brace L D, Fareed J, Walenga J 1989 Heparin-induced platelet aggregation (H-IPA) is not observed in hirudin antiaggregated platelet-rich plasma. Thromb Haemostasis 61 (suppl 1): 109 (Abstract)

Braun P J, Dennis S, Hofsteenge J, Stone S R 1988 Use of site directed mutagenesis to investigate the basis for the specificity of hirudin. Biochemistry 27: 6517–6522

Braunstein K M, Eurenius K 1976 Minimal heparin cofactor activity in disseminated intravascular coagulation and cirrhosis. Am J Clin Pathol 66: 488–494

Bucha E, Nowak G, Markwardt F 1988 Prevention of experimental coronary thrombosis by hirudin. Folia Haematol, Leipzig 115: 52–58

Buchanan M R, Boneu B, Ofosu F A, Hirsh J 1985 The relative importance of thrombin inhibition and factor Xa inhibition to the antithrombotic effects of heparin. Blood 65: 198–200

Carrell R W, Christey P B, Baswell D R 1987 Serpins: antithrombin and other inhibitors of coagulation and fibrinolysis. Evidence from amino acid sequences. In: Verstraete M, Vermylen J, Lijnen H R, Arnout J (eds) Thrombosis and haemostasis 1987. Leuven University Press, Leuven, pp 1–15

Chang J Y 1983 The functional domains of hirudin, a thrombin specific inhibitor. FEBS Lett 164: 307–313

Chang J Y 1989 The hirudin-binding site of human α-thrombin. Identification of lysyl residues which participate in the combining site of hirudin–thrombin complex. J Biol Chem 264: 7141–7146

Clore G M, Sukumaran D K, Nilges M, Zarbock J, Gronenborn A G 1987 The conformations of hirudin in solution: a study using nuclear magnetic resonance, distance geometry and restrained molecular dynamics. EMBO J 6: 529–537

Colman R W, Robboy S J, Minna J D 1972 Disseminated intravascular coagulation (DIC): an approach. Am J Med 52: 679–689

Courtney M, Loison G, Lemoine Y et al 1987 Production and evaluation of recombinant hirudin. Semin Thromb Haemostasis 15: 288–301

Degryse E, Acher M, Defreyn G et al 1989 Point mutations modifying the thrombin inhibition kinetics and antithrombotic activity in vivo of recombinant hirudin. Protein Eng 2: 459–465

Dejana E, Villa S, de Gaetano G 1982 Bleeding time in rats: a comparison of different experimental conditions. Thromb Haemostasis 48: 108–111

de Prost 1986 Heparin fractions and analogues: a new therapeutic possibility for thrombosis. Trends Pharm Sci 7: 496–500

Dodt J 1984 Hirudine, die Thromboinhibitoren des Blutegels 'Hirudo medicinalis'. Dissertation zur Erlangung der Doktorwürde am Fachbereich Chemie und Pharmazie des Ludwig-Maximilian Universität München, München

Dodt J, Müller H-P, Seemüller U, Chang J-Y 1984 The complete amino acid sequence of hirudin, a thrombin specific inhibitor. FEBS Lett 165: 180–183

Dodt J, Seemüller U, Maschler R, Fritz H 1985 The complete covalent structure of hirudin. Biol Chem Hoppe-Seyler 366: 379–385

Dodt J, Machleidt W, Seemüller U, Maschler R, Fritz H 1986 Isolation and characterization of hirudin isoinhibitors and sequence analysis of hirudin PA. Biol Chem Hoppe-Seyler 367: 803–811

Dodt J, Kohler S, Raici A 1988 Interaction of site specific hirudin variants with alpha-thrombin. FEBS Lett 229: 87–90

Fareed J, Walenga J M, Hoppenstead D A, Pifarre R 1989 Development perspectives for recombinant hirudin as an antithrombotic agent. Biol Clin Hematol 11: 143–152

Fenton J W 1981 Thrombin specificity. Ann NY Acad Sci 370: 468–495

Fenton J W 1989 Thrombin interactions with hirudin. Semin Thromb Haemostasis 15: 265–267

Fink E 1989 Comparison of hirudins. Semin Thromb Haemostasis 15: 283–287

Fortkamp E, Rieger M, Heisterberg-Moutses G, Schwezier S, Sommer R 1986 Cloning and expression in Escherichia coli of a synthetic DNA for hirudin, the blood coagulation inhibitor in the leech. DNA 5: 511–517

Glusa E, Urban U 1988 Studies on platelet functions in hirudin plasma. Folia Haematol, Leipzig 115: 88–93

Glusa E, Wolfram U 1988 The contractile response of vascular smooth muscle to thrombin and its inhibition by thrombin inhibitors. Folia Haematol, Leipzig 115: 94–100

Gray E, Watton J, Barrowcliffe T W, Thomas D P 1989 Anticoagulant and antithrombotic effects of recombinant hirudin. Thromb Haemostasis 62(suppl 1): 187 (Abstract)

Grossenbacher H H, Auden J A L, Bill K, Liersch M, Maerki W, Mäschler R 1987 Isolation and characterization of recombinant desulphato-hirudin from yeast, a highly selective thrombin inhibitor. Thromb Res (suppl 7): 34 (Abstract)

Harvey R P, Degryse E, Stefani L et al 1986 Cloning and expression of a cDNA coding for the anticoagulant hirudin from the bloodsucking leech, Hirudo medicinalis. Proc Natl Acad Sci USA 83: 1084–1088

Haycraft J B 1884 On the action of secretion obtained from the medicinal leech on the coagulation of the blood. Proc R Soc London 36: 478–487

Henschen A, Markwardt F, Walsmann P 1987 Identification by HPLC analysis of the unaltered forms of hirudin and desulated hirudin after kidney passage. Thromb Res (suppl 7): 37 (Abstract)

Henschen A, Markwardt F, Walsmann P 1988 Evidence for the identity of hirudin isolated after kidney passage with the starting material. Folia Haematol, Leipzig 115: 59–63

Heras M, Chesebro J H, Penny W J, Bailey K R, Badimon L, Fuster V 1989 Effects of thrombin inhibition on the development of acute platelet-thrombus deposition during angioplasty in pigs: heparin versus recombinant hirudin, a specific thrombin inhibitor. Circulation 79: 657–665

Hirsh J 1984 Heparin induced bleeding. Nouv Rev Fr Hematol 26: 261–266

Hoffmann A, Markwardt F 1984 Inhibition of the thrombin-platelet reaction by hirudin. Haemostasis 14: 164–169

Hofsteenge J, Taguchi H, Stone S R 1986 Effect of thrombomodulin on the kinetics of the interaction of thrombin with substrates and inhibitors. Biochem J 237: 243–251

Ishikawa A, Hafter R, Graeff H 1979 The effect of heparinized blood exchange transfusion on endotoxin induced disseminated intravascular coagulation (DIC). J Perinat Med 7: 250–256

Ishikawa A, Hafter R, Seemüller U, Gokel J M, Graeff H 1980 The effect of hirudin on endotoxin induced disseminated intravascular coagulation (DIC). Thromb Res 19: 351–358

Jacoby C 1904 Dtsch Med Wochenschr 30: 1786

Jakubowski H V, Kline M D, Owen W G 1986 The effect of bovine thrombomodulin on the specificity of bovine thrombin. J Biol Chem 261: 3876–3882

Johnson P, Sze P, Winant R, Payne P W, Lazar J B 1989 Biochemistry and genetic engineering of hirudin. Semin Thromb Haemostasis 15: 302–315

Kaiser B, Markwardt F 1986 Antithrombotic and haemorrhagic effects of synthetic and naturally occurring thrombin inhibitors. Thromb Res 43: 613–620

Kawabata S-L, Morita T, Miyata T, Kaida S, Igarashi H, Iwanaga S 1986 Difference in enzymatic properties between 'staphylothrombin' and free α-thrombin. Ann NY Acad Sci USA 485: 27–40

Klöcking H-P, Güttner J, Fink E 1988 Toxicological studies with recombinant hirudin. Folia Haematol, Leipzig 115: 75–82

Krstenansky J L, Mao S J T 1987 Antithrombin properties of C-terminus of hirudin using synthetic insulfated N^{α}-acetyl-hirudin 46–65. FEBS Lett 211: 10–16

Krstenansky J L, Owen T J, Yates M T, Mao S J T 1987 Anticoagulant peptides: nature of the interaction of the C-terminal region of hirudin with a non-catalytic binding site on thrombin. J Med Chem 30: 1688–1691

Krstenansky J L, Owen T J, Yates M T, Mao S J T 1988 Comparison of hirudin and hirudin PA C-terminal fragments and related analogs as antithrombin agents. Thromb Res 52: 137–141

Lasch H G, Heene D H 1975 Heparin therapy of diffuse intravascular coagulation (DIC). Thromb Diathes Haemorrh 33: 105–106

Loison G, Findeli A, Bernard S et al 1988 Expression and secretion in S. cerevisiae of biologically active leech hirudin. Biotechnology 6: 72

Maffrand J P, Bernat A, Delebassee D, Courtney M, Roitsch C, Defreyn G 1989 Antithrombotic and haemorrhagic effects of $2HV_2$-Lys^{47} hirudin compared with standard heparin in rabbits. Thromb Haemostasis 62(suppl 1): 1395 (Abstract)

Mann K G, Lundblad R L 1982 Biochemistry of thrombin. In: Colman R W, Hirsh J, Marder V J, Salzman E W (eds) Haemostasis and thrombosis. JB Lippincott, Philadelphia, pp 112–116

Mann K G, Tracy P B, Nesheim M E 1985 Assembly and function of prothrombinase complex on synthetic and natural membranes. In: Oates J A, Hawiger J, Ross R (eds) Interaction of platelets with the vessel wall. Mol Am Physiol Soc, Bethesda, pp 47–57.

Mao S J T, Yates M T, Owen T J, Krstenansky J L 1988 Interaction of hirudin with thrombin: identification of a minimal binding domain that inhibits clotting activity. Biochemistry 27: 8170–8173

Maraganore J M, Chao B, Joseph M L, Jablonski J, Ramachandran K L 1989 Anticoagulant activity of synthetic hirudin peptides. J Biol Chem 265: 8692–8698

Markwardt F 1955 Untersuchungen über Hirudin. Naturwissenschaften 52: 537–538

Markwardt F 1958 Versuche zur pharmakologischen Charakterisierung des Hirudins. Naunyn-Schmiedebergs Arch Pharmacol 234: 516–529

Markwardt F 1970 Hirudin as an inhibitor of thrombin. In: Perlman G E, Lorand L (eds) Methods in enzymology: proteolytic enzymes, vol 19. Academic Press, New York, pp 924–932

Markwardt F 1989 Development of hirudin as an antithrombotic agent. Semin Thromb Haemostasis 15: 269–282

Markwardt F, Walsmann P 1967 Reindardstellung und Analyse des Thrombininhibitors Hirudin. Hoppe Seylers Z Physiol Chem 348: 1381–1386

Markwardt F, Nowak G, Hoffman J 1977 The influence of drugs on disseminated intravascular coagulation (DIC). II. Effects of naturally occurring and synthetic thrombin inhibitors. Thromb Res 11: 275–283

Markwardt F, Hauptmann J, Nowak G, Klessen C, Walsmann P 1982 Pharmacological studies on the antithrombotic action of hirudin in experimental animals. Thromb Haemostasis 47: 226–229

Markwardt F, Hoffmann A, Stürzebecher J 1983 Influence of thrombin inhibitors on the thrombin-induced activation of human blood platelets. Haemostasis 13: 227–233

Markwardt F, Nowak G, Stürzebecher J, Griessbach U, Walsmann P, Vogel G 1984 Pharmacokinetics and anticoagulant effect of hirudin in man. Thromb Haemostasis 52: 160–163

Markwardt F, Nowak G, Stürzebecher U, Walsmann P 1987 Studies on the pharmacokinetics of hirudin. Biomed Biochim Acta 46: 237–244

Markwardt F, Fink G, Kaiser B, Klöcking H-P, Nowak G, Richter M, Stürzebecher J 1988a Pharmacological survey of recombinant hirudin. Pharmazie 43: 202–207

Markwardt F, Nowak G, Stürzebecher J, Vogel G 1988b Clinico-pharmacological studies with recombinant hirudin. Thromb Res 52: 393–400

Markwardt F, Kaiser B, Nowak G 1989 Studies on antithrombotic effects of recombinant hirudin. Thromb Res 54: 377–388

Marsh H C Jr, Meinwald Y C, Lee S, Martinelli R A, Scheraga H A 1985 Mechanism of action of thrombin on fibrinogen, NMR evidence for a β bend at or near fibrinogen Aα Gly (P$_5$)–Gly (P$_4$). Biochemistry 24: 2806–2812

Meinwald Y C, Martinelli R A, van Nispen J W, Sheraga H A 1980 Mechanism of action of thrombin on fibrinogen: size of the Aα fibrinogen like peptide that contacts the active site of thrombin. Biochemistry 19: 3820–3825

Meyhack B, Heim J, Rink H, Zimmermann W, Maerki W 1987 Desulphatohirudin, a specific thrombin inhibitor: expression and secretion in yeast. Thromb Res (suppl 7): 33 (Abstract)

Mirshahi M, Soria J, Soria C et al 1989 Evaluation of the inhibition by heparin and hirudin of coagulation activation during rt-PA-induced thrombolysis. Blood 74: 1025–1030

Noe G, Hofsteenge J, Rovelli G, Stone S R 1988 Use of sequence specific antibodies to identify a secondary binding site in thrombin. J Biol Chem 263: 11729–11735

Nowak G, Markwardt F 1987 Pharmacokinetic studies with hirudin. Thromb Res (suppl 7): 36 (Abstract)

Nowak G, Markwardt F, Fink E 1988 Pharmacokinetic studies with recombinant hirudin in dogs. Folia Haematol, Leipzig 115: 70–74

Perdue J F, Lubensky W, Kivity E, Sonder S A, Fenton II J W 1981 Protease mitogenic response of chick embryo fibroblasts and receptor binding processing of human α-thrombin. J Biol Chem 256: 2767–2776

Petersen E T, Roberts H R, Soltrup-Jensen L, Magnusson S, Bogdy D 1976 Primary structure of hirudin, a thrombin-specific inhibitor. In: Peeters H (ed) Protides of the biological fluids (Proceedings of the 23rd collegium held in Brugge, 1975). Pergamon Press, Oxford, pp 145–149

Pieters J, Lindhout T, Hemker H C 1989 In situ-generated thrombin is the only enzyme that effectively activates factor VIII and factor V in thromboplastin-activated plasma. Blood 74: 1021–1024

Richter M, Walsmann P, Cyranka U, Markwardt F 1986 ^{125}I-Markierung von Hirudin. Pharmazie 41: 510

Richter M, Cyranka U, Nowak G, Walsmann P 1988 Pharmacokinetics of ^{125}I-hirudin in rats and dogs. Folia Haematol 115: 64–69

Riehl-Bellon N, Carvallo D, Acker M et al 1989 Purification and biochemical characterization of recombinant hirudin produced by *Saccharomyces cerevisiae*. Biochemistry 28: 2941–2949

Roitsch C, Riehl-Bellon N, Carvallo D et al 1987 Characterization of hirudin isolated from *Hirudo medicinalis*. Thromb Res (suppl 7): 32 (Abstract)

Saba H I, Saba S R, Morelli G A 1984 Effect of heparin on platelet aggregation. Am J Hematol 17: 295–306

Salzman E W, Rosenberg R D, Smith M H, Lindon J N, Favreau L 1980 Effects of heparin and heparin fractions on platelet aggregation. J Clin Invest 65: 64–73

Scharf M, Engels J, Tripier D 1989 Primary structures of new 'iso-hirudins'. FEBS Lett 225: 105–110

Seemüller U, Dodt J, Fink E, Fritz H 1986 Proteinase inhibitor of the leech *Hirudo medicinalis* (hirudins, bdellins, eglins). In: Barett A J, Salvesen G (eds) Proteinase inhibitors. Elsevier, Amsterdam, pp 337–359

Smith J R, White A M 1982 Fibrin, red cell and platelet interactions in an experimental model of thrombosis. Br J Pharmacol 77: 29–39

Snider R M 1986 Thrombin effects on cultured nerve cells: clinical implications and evidence for novel mechanism of neuronal activation. Ann NY Acad Sci USA 485: 310–313

Spinner S, Stöffler G, Fink E 1986 Quantitative enzyme-linked immunosorbent assay (ELISA) for hirudin. J Immunol Methods 87: 79–83

Spinner S, Scheffauer F, Maschler R, Stöffler G 1988 A hirudin catching ELISA for quantitating the anticoagulant in biological fluids. Thromb Res 51: 617–625

Stone S, Hofsteenge J 1986 The kinetics of the inhibition of thrombin by hirudin. Biochemistry 25: 4622–4628

Stone S, Braun P J, Hofsteenge J 1987 Identification of regions of α thrombin involved in its interaction with hirudin. Biochemistry 26: 4617–4624

Sukumaran D K, Clare G M, Presus A, Zarbock J, Gronenborn A M 1987 Proton nuclear magnetic resonance study of hirudin: resonance assignment and secondary structure. Biochemistry 26: 333–338

Talbot M 1989 Biology of recombinant hirudin (CGP 39393): a new prospect in the treatment of thrombosis. Semin Thromb Haemostasis 15: 293–301

Talbot M, Ambler J, Butler K D et al 1989a Recombinant desulfatohirudin (CGP 39393): anticoagulant and antithrombotic properties in vivo. Thromb Haemostasis 61: 77–80

Talbot M, Ambler J, Butler K D et al 1989b Recombinant desulphatohirudin (CGP 39393): comparative studies with standard and low molecular weight heparin. Thromb Haemostasis 62 (suppl 1): 647 (Abstract)

Tertrin C, de la Llosa P, Jutisz M 1967 Effet des modifications chimiques de l'hirudine sur son action inhibitrice de l'activité enzymatique de la thrombine. Bull Soc Chim Biol Paris 49: 1837–1843

Tripier D 1987 Isolation and sequence analysis of new hirudin. Thromb Res (suppl 7): 31 (Abstract)

Tripier D 1988 Hirudin: a family of iso-proteins isolation and sequence determination of new hirudins. Folia Haematol, Leipzig 115: 30–35

van Obberghen-Schilling E, Perez-Rodriquez R 1982 Hirudin, a probe to analyze the growth-promoting activity of thrombin in fibroblasts: reevaluation of the temporal action of competence factors. Biochem Biophys Res Comm 106: 79–86

Villanueva G B, Konno S, Fenton J 1987 Evidence for multiple binding sites of hirudin in thrombin. Thromb Res (suppl 7): 35 (Abstract)

Vogel G, Markwardt F 1987 Preclinical reports on the antithrombotic action of hirudin. Thromb Res (suppl 7): 42 (Abstract)

Vogel G, Markwardt F 1988 Clinical use of hirudin. Folia Haematol, Leipzig 115: 113–118

Walenga J M, Pifarre R, Hoppensteadt D A, Fareed J 1989 Development of recombinant hirudin as a therapeutic anticoagulant and antithrombotic agent: some objective considerations. Semin Thromb Haemostasis 15: 316–333

Wallace A, Dennis S, Hofsteenge J, Stone S R 1989 Contribution of the N-terminal region of hirudin to its interaction with thrombin. Biochemistry 28: 10079–10084

Walsmann P 1988 Hirudin as a diagnostic agent. Folia Haematol, Leipzig 115: 36–40

Walsmann P, Markwardt F 1981 Biochemische und pharmakologische Aspekte des Thrombininhibitors Hirudin. Pharmazie 26: 653–660

Williams D O, Borer J, Braunwald E et al 1986 Intravenous recombinant tissue type plasminogen activator in patients with acute myocardial infarction: a report from the NHLBI, 1986, thrombolysis in myocardial infarction trial. Circulation 73: 338–346

Yeo K-T, Detwiler T C 1985 Analysis of the fate of platelet-bound thrombin. Arch Biochem Biophys 236: 399–410

12

Optimal therapeutic range for oral anticoagulation

L. Poller

The aim of oral anticoagulant treatment is to prevent the occurrence or the spread of thrombotic disease while preserving adequate haemostasis. The clinical indications for oral anticoagulant treatment and the intensity of anticoagulation required to achieve this aim have been the subject of prolonged controversy.

The debate has arisen from two main causes. First, until recently the various clinical decisions have not been based on scientifically based randomized studies which are essential for valid recommendations. Second, the problems associated with dose adjustment by the prothrombin time (PT) have been considerable. Nearly 50 years after the introduction of oral anticoagulant treatment in routine medical practice many of these matters are still not resolved despite great progress in the last few years. In the present chapter an assessment is attempted of the optimal therapeutic ranges to be used for the various conditions and of the strength of the evidence on which these recommendations have been based.

Advice on the correct therapeutic intervals prompted by the introduction of the international normalized ratio (INR) system of prothrombin standardization has emanated in recent years from three different groups, i.e. the British Society for Haematology (BSH) (1984, 1990), a conference in Leuven (Loeliger et al 1985), and the American College of Chest Physicians/National Heart, Lung and Blood Institute (ACCP/NHLBI) Consensus Meetings (Hirsh et al 1986, 1989). The source material and reliability of these recommendations will be discussed.

Evidence of the difficulties of oral anticoagulant control continuing into the 1980s was provided by an international survey of dosage in different geographical locations (Poller & Taberner 1982). This showed that although one oral anticoagulant drug, warfarin, was almost universally the most popular, being used by most participants in the survey, the mean dosage of warfarin varied considerably between different centres. Extremes were a requirement for less than 2 mg in the Hong Kong Chinese to over 8 mg in some North American hospitals. In the UK and Netherlands the dosage schedules were intermediate between the Hong Kong and North American levels. Returns from North America, parts of Europe and other countries which employed the most widely used commercial thromboplastin reagents tended to employ much larger doses of the warfarin than those whose prothrombin time incorporated hospital-made thromboplastins of human brain origin which were invariably more responsive to the coumarin-induced coagulation defect.

The scale of the differences in resulting intensity of anticoagulation can perhaps be gauged from the respective mean doses. In fact they are even more considerable than is apparent because even a small blood concentration of free warfarin above the threshold of the albumin binding capacity for the drug makes a great difference to the individual patient's PT response. Furthermore it has long been apparent from the medical literature that the incidence of bleeding side-effects encountered in North America and many other parts of the world was higher than experienced in the UK and the Netherlands where dosage was known to be relatively conservative. Hirsh et al (1989) pointed out that there was a change in North America in the 1950s from responsive types of thromboplastin of human origin to less responsive reagents of commercial manufacture without adjustment of the therapeutic range in PT ratios or activities. This led some physicians inadvertently to use more intensive treatment.

Clinicians were often not only largely unaware of the effects of the laboratory differences and the disagreement between measurements of the PT but also confused by the various methods of expressing PT results. The alternatives in common usage included simple PT, percentage activities from various types of dilution curves which as a consequence gave different results, prothrombin ratios, i.e. the relation of the patient's PT to the normal control and indices, the reciprocal of the ratio. These terms were often used incorrectly, with activity in particular often referred to as the prothrombin index and vice versa in routine work and publications.

The first published report of measures to standardize PT control and its method of reporting was by the provision of a standardized thromboplastin, Manchester comparative reagent, for use over a large geographical area (Poller 1964). It was almost 20 years before an acceptable international scheme of PT standardization based on international reference thromboplastin preparations (IRP) and a uniform method of expression of results was introduced. The international normalized ratio (INR) system is based on a quantitative assessment of the responsiveness of a thromboplastin, i.e. the international sensitivity index (ISI). From the ISI the INR is obtained as follows: $INR = prothrombin\ ratio^{ISI}$. This is obtained by testing normal and coumarin-treated patients' plasma samples in parallel with the local reagent and the IRP. The ISI is derived from the slope of the orthogonal regression line of the calibration. The INR system was approved by the World Health Organization and the international scientific committees in 1983. It resulted from the collaborative endeavours from many countries. The list of contributors includes Biggs & Denson (1967), Zucker et al (1970), ICSH/ICTH (1979), Loeliger et al (1979), van den Besselaar et al (1980), Kirkwood (1983) and many others.

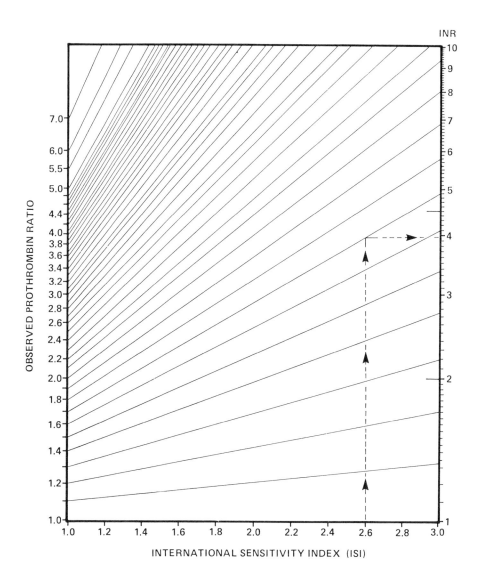

Fig. 12.1   A simple nomogram for the derivation of international normalized ratios for the standardization of prothrombin times.
Example:

Observed ratio 1.7 with thromboplastin ISI 2.6: INR = 4.0.
Reproduced with permission of the Department of Medical Illustration, Withington Hospital, Manchester.

The introduction of INR facilitated application of uniform oral anticoagulant therapy on a world scale. As a result of the greater refinement and definition of therapeutic intervals resulting from INR, it has also permitted the treatment to be tailored to the type of case, by segmentation of the therapeutic range in INR according to the different clinical situations. The three expert groups referred to earlier made recommendations on therapeutic ranges in INR to be used according to the clinical condition (Table 12.1).

The British Society for Haematology (BSH) ranges, originally promulgated in 1984, were slightly revised in 1990. A second set of INR recommendations for the various clinical disorders which took into account the 1984 BSH proposals and the evidence from which they were derived came from a group of European consultants who met later in Leuven in 1984 (Loeliger

Table 12.1   INR recommendations of the three expert groups

	British Society for Haematology (1984, 1990)	Leuven Conference (1985)	ACCP/ NHLBI Consensus (1989)	Recom- mendation grade
Prophylaxis of postoperative DVT (general surgery)	2.0–2.5	1.5–2.5	2.0–3.0	A
Prophylaxis of postoperative DVT in hip surgery and fractures	2.0–3.0	2.0–3.0	2.0–3.0	A
Myocardial infarction prevention of venous thromboembolism	2.0–3.0	2.0–3.0	2.0–3.0	B
Treatment of venous thrombosis	2.0–3.0	2.0–4.0	2.0–3.0	A
Treatment of pulmonary embolism	2.0–3.0	2.0–4.0	2.0–3.0	A
Transient ischaemic attacks	2.0–3.0			C
Tissue heart valves	2.0–3.0	?	2.0–3.0	A
Atrial fibrillation	2.0–3.0	?	2.0–3.0	C
Valvular heart disease	2.0–3.0	?	2.0–3.0	C
Recurrent deep vein thrombosis and pulmonary embolism	3.0–4.5	2.0–4.0	2.0–3.0	C
Arterial disease including myocardial infarction	3.0–4.5	3.0–4.5	2.0–3.0	C
Mechanical prosthetic valves	3.0–4.5	3.0–4.5	3.0–4.5	C
Recurrent systemic embolism	3.0–4.5	3.0–4.0	3.0–4.5	

et al 1985). A third series arose from two consensus meetings of the American College of Chest Physicians/National Heart and Lung Institute (ACCP/NHLBI) in 1986 and 1989. The full reports of the consensus conferences have been published in two special supplements to *Chest* (Hirsh et al 1986, 1989). In these the ACCP/NHLBI group categorized in detail the evidence from published clinical trials according to different levels of confidence graded I to V in decreasing order of dependability (Sackett 1989) as follows:

Confidence level:

Level I	Large randomized trials with clear-cut results
Level II	Small randomized trials with uncertain results
Level III	Non-randomized contemporaneous controls
Level IV	Non-randomized historical controls
Level V	No control, case series only

Recommendations:

Grade A	Supported by at least one level I study
Grade B	Supported by at least one level II study
Grade C	Supported only by level III, IV or V evidence

This useful system of classification has been used in the present review. An assessment of the reliability of the respective decisions has been made and it is indicated where further studies are still required to confirm or define the recommended optimal therapeutic ranges for the different conditions. The overall and continuing trend is to a progressive diminution of the intensity of anticoagulation (lower warfarin dose) in the various conditions with consequent reduction in bleeding complications, i.e. an improved benefit/risk ratio.

PREVENTION OF VENOUS THROMBOSIS IN GENERAL SURGERY

There was great enthusiasm for the use of heparin and oral anticoagulation in prophylaxis of deep venous thrombosis (DVT) during general surgery in the early days of anticoagulation. This was based on enthusiastic claims from uncontrolled trials. Surgeons largely have been unwilling to accept the risk of bleeding from heparin and oral anticoagulation and the inconvenience of the mandatory laboratory testing. In a questionnaire survey Brenkel & Clancy (1990) reported that currently less than one in 12 UK orthopaedic surgeons ever use warfarin prophylaxis.

With oral anticoagulation there is the need for a preparatory induction period of several days prior to surgery to achieve the necessary coagulation defect. The greater effectiveness of oral anticoagulants in DVT prophylaxis when given before operation rather than postoperatively for major gynaecological procedures has been demonstrated (Taberner et al 1978) (Table 12.2). The Vroonhoven study where treatment was induced after operation was considerably less successful than in the group of patients given heparin.

All three groups made recommendations on the INR range required for prophylaxis of DVT in general surgery. The North American 2.0–3.0 range was slightly more intense whereas the recommended Leuven therapeutic interval of 1.5–2.5 was the least, the BSH range of 2.0–2.5 INR being intermediate. The last two levels have the support of the two studies from Manchester (Taberner et al 1978, Poller et al 1987). There is, however, little practical difference between these two treatment levels. The Consensus Group recommended dosage may be more intense particularly in view of the relative unresponsiveness of North American thromboplastins with their tendency to underestimate the INR in the early days of treatment.

Over the years, the surgeon's natural reluctance to employ any prophylactic procedures which may induce bleeding at operation has increasingly militated against the administration of heparin and oral anticoagulant prophylaxis. A new approach which is based on a fixed minidose of warfarin (1 mg a day started preoperatively), may prove acceptable if the first reports (Poller et al 1987, Bern et al 1990) of its effectiveness are confirmed. This produces no evident disturbance of haemostasis at operation, and appears to cause no additional bleeding (Poller et al 1987). The fixed minidose warfarin regime was developed from an observation by Bern et al (1986) that a small fixed dose of warfarin (2 mg daily) prevented thrombosis of indwelling catheters in patients with malignancy. However, this dose proved excessive in some patients and necessitated reversal by vitamin K_1. The smaller fixed dose of

Table 12.2 DVT in major gynaecological surgery

Level I studies	Oral anti-coagulant	INR range	Untreated control group	Low-dose heparin
Taberner et al (1978) (5 days pre-op. induction)		2.0–2.5 preop. 2.0–4.0 postop.		
Total no.	48		48	49
DVT incidence	3		11	3
Vroonhoven et al (1974) (induction postop.)		2.4 postop.		
Total no.	50		–	50
DVT incidence	9		–	1
Poller et al (1987) (inductions 5 days preop.)		1.5–2.5 preop. 2.0–3.0 postop.		
Total no.	35		37	
DVT incidence	1		11	

1 mg daily began before gynaecological surgery had been shown to prevent DVT (Poller et al 1987) (level I). The mechanism of action of minidose warfarin is not clear although the drug exaggerates the normal postoperative depression of the PT. The maximum PT depression with minidose warfarin did not occur, however, until the second day after operation and even then the INR was only 1.2. This is well below the minimum INR of the conventional dose warfarin range for prophylaxis of DVT (i.e. 1.5) set by the three expert groups. A possible explanation for the protective action is enhanced fibrinolysis. Increased fibrinolysis with warfarin may be due to inhibition of the normal postoperative rise of plasminogen activator (PAI), the most important fibrinolytic inhibitory enzyme (MacCallum et al in press). A subsequent report by Bern et al (1990) ((level I) in patients with central vein catheters used a 1-mg daily regime started 3 days before the insertion. There was a significant reduction in the incidence of thrombosis, supporting the value of minidose warfarin.

PROPHYLAXIS IN HIP SURGERY

Elective and emergency hip operations are associated with a high incidence of DVT and pulmonary embolism (40–70% venographically proved DVT in most reports with 20% proximal vein DVT resulting in an incidence of 1–5% pulmonary embolism). Level I studies described by Francis et al (1983) and Powers et al (1989) (see Table 12.3) indicate that this DVT incidence can be more than halved by the administration of warfarin. There is a fundamental agreement between the recommendations from the three groups in INR terms. The need for slightly more intense treatment in hip than in general surgery, i.e. INR 2.0–3.0, was emphasized. The advice is largely dependent on the level I study by Francis et al (1983) in which an observed PT ratio range of 1.3–1.5 was the target.

The study by Powers et al (1989) was published after the ACCP/NHLBI proposals. In this study of hip fractures PT ratios were based on a relatively unresponsive North American type thromboplastin with an ISI of 2.4. It is of interest that despite postoperative induction of warfarin the incidence of DVT was approximately halved and similar to the study by Francis and co-workers when treatment was started before operation.

Effective prophylaxis in hip surgery is necessarily short term, covering the

Table 12.3 Warfarin prophylaxis in hip surgery

	Time of induction	Warfarin no.	PT ratio	INR	DVT/PE	Control no.	DVT
Powers et al (1989)	Postop.	65		2.0–2.7	13 (20%)	63	29 (46%)
Francis et al (1983)	Preop.	53	1.3–1.5	2.0–2.6	11 (21%)	57	30 (53%)

perioperative period and the first few days after operation. The observed PT ratios (hence INR) in the McMaster study (Powers et al) are likely therefore to be somewhat smaller than the PT ratios which would have been obtained with a more responsive type (lower ISI) thromboplastin on the same test plasmas. Therefore the INR values extrapolated from their data may underestimate the intensity of the true coagulation defect. In the early days of anticoagulation high ISI thromboplastin reagents of the type used by Francis and coworkers may not reflect the full coagulation defect as they are relatively unresponsive to depression of coagulation factors VII and X reduced first by warfarin. Continuing reluctance to use warfarin in hip surgery has been emphasized by the recent questionnaire survey described by Brenkel & Clancy (1990). They showed that over half of 690 UK orthopaedic surgeons who completed the questionnaire use no pharmacological prophylaxis in hip surgery and of these only a small proportion (8.1%) give warfarin.

TREATMENT OF ESTABLISHED DVT AND PULMONARY EMBOLISM

For many years oral anticoagulant administration following several days' intravenous heparin has been the conventional approach to treatment for DVT. The acceptance of this regime antedated the statistical requirements of modern clinical trials. Until recently there was in fact little firm statistical data to support this procedure, reliance being on early uncontrolled case report studies, indirect evidence and clinical impressions.

The only well-planned level I trial of heparin and oral anticoagulation for treatment of venous thrombosis and prevention of pulmonary embolism was undertaken in Bristol, UK, in the late 1950s but was abandoned on ethical grounds (Barritt & Jordan 1960). The study is the classical investigation on which the decision to treat with oral anticoagulation has been based. It has, however, been criticized, mainly because of the small numbers, and for an apparently excessive benefit in the anticoagulant-treated group. Since that time the incorporation of an untreated control group with DVT or pulmonary embolism has never been thought to be justified. The closest to the use of a control group has been the indirect evidence from a level I investigation reported by Hull et al (1979) (see Table 12.4). After 14 days intravenous heparin, patients with acute DVT were randomized to receive either low-dose heparin (5000 units twice daily) or warfarin (INR 3.0–4.5). After 12 weeks therapy the 9 of 35 patients receiving subcutaneous heparin had new episodes of objectively documented venous thromboembolism but none of the 33 receiving warfarin ($P = 0.001$). Warfarin was obviously effective at an observed prothrombin ratio range of 1.5–2.0 using a North American type thromboplastin (INR 3.0–4.5) but nevertheless this intensity of anticoagulation resulted in an excess of bleeding complications (21%).

Table 12.4   Treatment of DVT (randomized studies)

Level I	Ratio	INR	Incidence of haemorrhage (%)	Recurrence of venous thrombosis (%)
Hull et al (1979)	1.5–2.0	3.0–4.5	21	0
Warfarin	–	–		25.7
S.c. heparin				
Hull et al (1982)				
Simplastin control	1.5–2.0	3.0–4.5	22.4	2.0
Manchester comparative reagent control	2.0–2.5	2.0–2.5	4.3	2.1

A further (level I) trial was then undertaken to elucidate the optimum therapeutic range for oral anticoagulants in DVT and whether the benefit/ risk ratio could be improved by a so-called 'low-dose' treatment with warfarin, this being the conventional dosage used in the UK and the Netherlands. In the subsequent McMaster University study (Hull et al 1982) two intensities of treatment were undertaken. The INR was based on a therapeutic range of 1.5–2.0 PT ratio (INR 3.0–4.5) using a typical North American thromboplastin, and the other, a less intense treatment with a 2.0–2.5 ratio (INR 2.0–2.5), used the more responsive human brain Manchester comparative reagent (ISI = 1.0). The results indicated that protection from thrombosis was equal in the two groups but the less intensive therapy resulting from control by the Manchester reagent reduced the incidence of bleeding complications to less than a fifth. These two studies therefore have been the basis for the levels of warfarin recommended by all three groups for the management of established venous thrombosis.

MYOCARDIAL INFARCTION (MI)

Whereas the value of oral anticoagulants in the prevention and the treatment of venous thromboembolic disorders is not questionable the situation does not apply to arterial disease, particularly myocardial infarction. Initial claims made in the 1940s and 1950s for the benefit afforded by oral anticoagulant treatment after MI proved to be exaggerated. These studies, like the early venous thrombosis studies, lack scientific control groups and often were simply compared with the norms established in the same institutions before the anticoagulant era (level IV).

By the early 1960s a more critical approach was adopted. New published studies were undertaken but were undermined by problems with regard to laboratory control. Modifications of the PT test had been introduced which caused organizers of these trials unsuspectingly to provide a less intense coagulation defect. The studies all shared a common tendency to undertreatment. The Danish level III cohort study reported by Hilden et al

(1961) employed the dilute prothrombin time 'P and P' test of Owren to control dosage, whereas the level II, British Medical Research Council study (MRC 1969) substituted a less marked coagulation defect with a target value of 15% Thrombotest (1.8 INR approximately) instead of the 2.0–3.0 INR employed in the earlier (level II) Medical Research Council long-term study (1964) in which the Quick test PT had been used to monitor dosage. Confirmation of the reduced anticoagulation comes from the fact that the phenindione dose per patient was significantly less compared with that of the earlier MRC study, although the organizers did not appreciate the reason.

The overall verdict from the main studies in the 1960s was that there was a slight but significant reduction in mortality with short-term anticoagulation (e.g. Hilden et al 1961, MRC 1969). Of over 30 reports listed by Chalmers et al (1977) only three were of sufficient size to have an 80% chance of demonstrating a 50% difference in death or reinfarction. Furthermore in only one study was a statistically significant reduction in mortality reported (Drapkin & Merskey 1972). Two level II studies, the MRC (1964) and the US Veterans Administration Co-operative Study (1973), found a significant reduction in morbidity from strokes and venous thromboembolism.

With the MRC (1964) study there was a non-significant reduction in mortality. A significant reduction in MI recurrence and significantly less thromboembolism was found with anticoagulant treatment. The MRC (1964), the US Veteran's Cooperative Study (1973), the German Austrian study (Breddin et al 1980) and the Danish level III study (Hilden et al 1961) all showed, however, a reduction in the incidence of venous thromboembolism. The present increasing evidence of the effectiveness of less intense anticoagulation for the prophylaxis of venous thromboembolism provides an explanation for the discrepant findings.

For more than 20 years following the results of these trials progressively fewer physicians have advocated a potentially dangerous form of therapy where the benefit was considered doubtful or marginal. Arguments for the importance of prevention of secondary venous thromboembolic complications were still made. The 1970s provided debate but few clinical trials. In 1981 the results of the 'Sixty-Plus' Reinfarction Study of the Netherlands Thrombosis Service were published and provided a challenge to the clinicians who had discarded the routine use of oral anticoagulants. Using an INR range of 2.7–4.5 there was a significant reduction in mortality and of recurrent myocardial infarction in the group continued on long-term oral anticoagulation versus a group discontinued after 6 months' treatment. It could be argued, however, that this study of patients over 60 years might only be demonstrating that long-term anticoagulant treatment, whilst not beneficial, once instituted on a long-term basis in MI was dangerous when stopped. It is of interest, however, that the benefit was demonstrated in an age group which might be expected to be the least promising, i.e. the over-sixties. The 'Sixty-Plus' study was, however, well planned, organized and skilfully managed. It established a need to reassess the value of oral anticoagulation in myocardial infarction. A group of investigators from Norway (Smith et al 1990) in a level I study has recently provided a report on their long-term study which has indicated significant reduction in both mortality and morbidity from oral anticoagulation compared with placebo. The Norwegian MI study (Smith et al 1989, 1990) involved 1214 patients, and showed a reduction in mortality and morbidity with oral anticoagulants using an INR treatment range of 2.0–4.8. There were 94 deaths on warfarin and 123 on placebo on an intention-to-treat basis. Recurrently myocardial infarctions were 70 with warfarin and 122 with placebo. The results of this large, carefully performed and controlled study may lead to a reappraisal of the present almost universal policy not to prescribe warfarin, long term, for patients with acute MI. Another long-term multicentre study is in progress in the Netherlands and the results are awaited with interest.

A summary of the main studies in MI is given in Table 12.5 related to the INR ranges. Table 5 shows that where benefit proved substantial there is a tendency to a more pronounced coagulation defect in INR.

Table 12.5   Myocardial infarction

| | | Level | INR | Mortality | Reduction in | |
					Recurrence	Embolism
Long term						
Medical Research Council	1959	II	2.0–2.5	–	+	+
Medical Research Council	1964					
Sixty Plus Reinfarction	1981	I	2.7–4.5	+	+	+
Norwegian Study (Smith et al)	1990	I	2.8–4.8	+	+	+
US Veterans (Ebert et al)	1965 1969	II II	2.0–2.5	?	–	–
Short term						
Hilden et al	1961	III	1.2–1.5	–	–	+
Medical Research Council	1969	II	1.6–2.0	–	–	+
US Veterans	1973	II	2.0–2.5	–	–	+
Drapkin & Merskey	1972	II	2.0–2.5	+	–	–

Before the availability of the Norwegian results, on the basis of the available evidence, the ACCP/NHLBI consensus conference (Resnekow et al 1989) strongly recommended short-term anticoagulation only for MI in patients with acute myocardial infarction at increased risk of systemic embolism on the findings of the MRC (1969) and US Veterans Administration Study (1973). Patients with anterior transmural myocardial infarction were recommended to receive initial heparin therapy followed by warfarin for three months at INR between 2.0 and 3.0. The Consensus Group also recommended that warfarin should be continued on a long-term basis in the presence of continuation of defined risk factors. This recommendation was based on level V studies. Long-term anticoagulant therapy was in general not recommended by the Consensus Group for survivors of acute myocardial infarction despite favourable reports from notably the US Veterans Administration Study (1965) and the German Austrian Study (1980). The Consensus Group felt that the trends were too small and the risk and inconvenience of long-term anticoagulant therapy were too considerable. Long-term warfarin therapy with an INR between 2.0 and 3.0 was recommended, however, for acute MI with any of the following risk factors: systemic or pulmonary embolism, atrial fibrillation, previous systemic embolism, venous thromboembolism, significant left ventricular dysfunction or severe heart failure; although these policies only had the support of level V studies.

The INR ranges used in the respective MI studies which showed benefit and those where results were not encouraging are given in Table 12.5. It has been possible to derive the INR values retrospectively for the respective studies because the reference reagent British comparative thromboplastin and its routine counterpart Manchester comparative reagent (ISI of 1.0) had been used to characterize the therapeutic intervals of many other thromboplastins used in these studies years before the introduction of the INR system. It will be seen that in general where benefit proved substantial a more pronounced coagulation effect in INR terms had been the target of the study. All three sets of INR recommendations from the three groups agree on the 2.0–3.0 INR range for the prevention of the venous thromboembolic complications of myocardial infarction but the British and Leuven recommendations influenced largely by the Netherlands 'Sixty-Plus' study differ from those of the ACCP/NHLBI in recommending a more intense range for the long-term management of MI. Both the BSH and the Leuven group based their proposals largely on the indirect evidence of the '60 Plus' Netherlands study which employed a similar INR range to that used in the later Norwegian study (Smith et al 1989). This is in agreement with the recommendations of the BSH and the Leuven Group (3.0–4.5 INR) but is more intense than the Consensus Group recommendation of 2.0–3.0 INR which according to BSH advice should be used only for the prevention of secondary venous thromboembolism in MI.

VALVULAR HEART DISEASE

The risk of thromboembolism with rheumatic heart disease is greater than in any other common form of heart disease and increases dramatically with the development of atrial fibrillation. Levine et al (1989) in the report of the Consensus Conference strongly recommended that patients at risk for thromboembolism from rheumatic mitral valve disease be given warfarin at an INR of 3.0–4.5. This should be given for one year, after which time the INR should be reduced to 2.0–3.0. The recommendation is more conservative after 12 months and the same as the range of the other two groups but is based only on level III studies by Fleming & Bailey (1971) and Adams et al (1974).

The Consensus recommendation on aortic valve disease was that this does not merit warfarin treatment because of the low risk of thromboembolism. If recurrent systemic embolism occurred in mitral valve disease despite warfarin, dipyridamole should be considered as an additional treatment but there was no substantive evidence of benefit.

Where rheumatic heart disease is associated with chronic or paroxysmal atrial fibrillation it was strongly recommended that warfarin be prescribed at the INR of 2.0–3.0 on the basis of level IV and V studies.

PROSTHETIC HEART VALVES

Increasing numbers of patients have undergone heart valve replacements. Patients given a mitral mechanical prosthetic valve are generally believed to require life-long anticoagulant therapy to reduce the incidence of thromboembolic complications. The risks of thromboembolism, particularly cerebral embolism, were greater with the older type of mechanical heart valves. Experience with the recent types of prosthesis and particularly tissue valves has shown that the incidence of such complications is considerably reduced. Furthermore the thromboembolic risk associated with replacement aortic valves alone is much less than with mitral valve replacements. Life-long anticoagulation is generally regarded as mandatory in patients with mitral valve mechanical prostheses, but the indications are less strong after tissue valve replacement, and particularly with aortic valves (Oakley & Doherty 1976). In the absence of adequate randomized clinical studies it is unlikely that the precise clinical benefit from coumarin drugs in prevention of embolism from mechanical valves will ever be precisely quantified although from level V reports and from clinical impressions it is regarded as substantial. For review of the relative risks of thromboembolism from the different types of prosthetic valve and the value of combined warfarin and dipyridamole administration see Cheseboro et al (1986). The ACCP/NHLBI Consensus (Stein & Kantrovitz 1989) conclusion was that all patients with mechanical prosthetic heart valves should be treated with long-term warfarin to an INR of 3.0–4.5, on the basis of level III studies. The ACCP/

NHLBI Group also recommended that patients with bioprosthetic valves in a mitral position be treated for the first three months after valve insertion with warfarin, at an INR of 2.0–3.0. This proposal was based on the important level I randomized study by Turpie et al (1988) which showed that a conservative range with Manchester reagent control (INR 2.0–3.0) gave the same protection from thromboembolism as more intense treatment (INR 3.0–4.5) with a North American type thromboplastin (ISI 2.3). Bleeding was significantly higher with the more intense dosage (see Table 12.6). The ACCP/NHLBI Consensus recommended that patients with bioprosthetic valves who had a history of systemic embolism, left atrial thrombus at surgery or atrial fibrillation be treated with long-term warfarin, although these recommendations were based on non-randomized historical control results only (level IV).

All three of the groups making recommendations agreed on the 3.0–4.5 INR range for mechanical heart valves, although this was based on clinical experience and non-randomized studies only (level IV and V). The question of whether the intensity of treatment really needs to be so great has not been established by randomized study. There have only been two recent randomized controlled trials in patients with heart valve prostheses involving different treatment intensities. The Turpie study (1988) was a two-level trial, for the insertion of prosthetic tissue valves. A recent study from Saudi Arabia (Saour et al 1990) gave two levels of treatment based on laboratory control with a poorly responsive North American type thromboplastin reagent (ISI = 2.3) (see Table 12.6). Although from the title it might be presumed that the purpose of this study was to decide whether the relatively intense treatment with 3.0–4.5 range was really necessary, it did not provide the answer. One group received treatment less intense than the 3.0–4.5 INR scale but was compared with a much more intensely treated group with higher INR values (7.4–10.8) which can only be regarded as representing gross overdosage on the basis of the recommendations of the three expert groups (see Table 12.1). An important finding although not appreciated by the authors is that there was no therapeutic gain in protection from embolism in the over-treated group but, as might have been an-

Table 12.6 Prosthetic heart valves: different intensities of anticoagulation

Study	Valve type	INR		Thrombo-embolism (%)		Bleeding (%)	
		Low dose	High dose	Low dose	High dose	Low dose	High dose
Turpie et al (1989)	Tissue	2.0–2.5	3.0–4.5	1.2	1.2	5.7	20.6
Saour et al (1990)	Mechanical	1.9–3.6	7.4–10.8	1.4	1.3	21.3	42.4

ticipated on first principles, there was a gross increase of haemorrhage. It is noteworthy that the incidence of bleeding in the Saour et al study in the less intensely treated group was about identical to that of the intensely dosed patients in the study by Turpie et al. The trial which really is needed in heart valves is to determine whether a more conservative treatment (e.g. 2.5–3.5 INR) would reduce the incidence of bleeding complications but still be effective compared with the more intense present 3.0–4.5 INR range. In other words this would show whether it is possible to achieve a reduced risk of haemorrhagic complications whilst retaining adequate protection from embolism. Perhaps the less thrombogenic types of mechanical valves should be studied first. Patients with mechanical prosthetic valves have been shown in a new important randomized study (Altman et al, in press) to receive equal protection from embolism at 2.0–3.0 INR but suffer less bleeding than patients kept between 3.0 and 4.5 INR. However both groups also received a combination of aspirin and dipyridamole in addition to the oral anticoagulant which undoubtedly influenced the findings.

ATRIAL FIBRILLATION

The ACCP/NHLBI Consensus recommendations (Dunn et al 1989) were that long-term warfarin administration (INR 3.0–4.5) should be given to patients with atrial fibrillation who suffered documented systemic embolism, but after one year the therapeutic range could be reduced to 2.0–3.0 INR if there had been no recurrences. This recommendation was based on case series reports (levels III, IV, V). Since these recommendations were made two scientific randomized studies on the effect of warfarin on atrial fibrillation have been published from Denmark and the United States (Petersen et al 1989 and Stroke Prevention Study 1990) (See Table 12.7).

Table 12.7 Atrial fibrillation

		Warfarin v Aspirin v Placebo			
	Total	Inclusion (%)	INR range	Strokes (n)	
				Treated	Placebo
Petersen et al (1989)	1007	37	2.4–4.2	5	21
Stroke Prevention Study (1990)	1224	47	2.0–3.5*	7	18

	Range
*Claimed INR range	2.0–3.5
Assumed ISI = 2.0	1.7–3.25
2.3	1.8–3.9
2.6	2.0–4.6

A more intense treatment level has the support of the first investigation study (2.4–4.2 INR) (Petersen et al 1989). This was the first level I study performed in this area. In 2546 patients with chronic non-rheumatic atrial fibrillation, with an INR range of 2.4–4.2, the yearly incidence of thromboembolism was 2% on warfarin but 5.5% on aspirin and placebo. A similar incidence of thromboembolism (1.6% per year) was found in the Preliminary Report of the US Stroke Prevention on Atrial Fibrillation Study (1990). In the latter whereas the placebo arm gave an even rate of 8.3% per year in the study of 1244 patients, the second randomized study of this group had to be terminated because of the higher incidence of stroke compared with the antithrombotic treated group. The INR quoted of 2.0–3.5 in the preliminary report of this study unfortunately were misleading as they purported to be the equivalent of 1.3–1.8 ratio with a 'typical North American thromboplastin'. Simple INR calculations or a reference to the INR nomogram on p. 247 will show that these values cannot be correct. It is hoped that this matter will be clarified in the final report. In the interim it must be assumed that both the Peterson and Stroke Prevention studies demonstrate the need for a higher INR than 2.0–3.0 advocated by all three groups for atrial fibrillation. An intensity of anticoagulation (2.0–3.0 INR) was recommended by BSH in this condition, again on the basis of clinical consensus but not randomized study (level III). It would be difficult now to substantiate the need for further randomized studies in this area with a placebo group in view of the strong clinical agreement on the value of warfarin. For patients without embolism in the presence of atrial fibrillation and valvular heart disease the ACCP/NHLBI Consensus recommendation was that long-term warfarin (INR 2.0–3.0) be given to patients with atrial fibrillation associated with mitral valve disease, but this was again only on the basis of historical data and uncontrolled case series (level V). With atrial fibrillation associated with non-valvular heart disease the situation is not clear-cut. In patients with atrial fibrillation and dilated and hypertrophic cardiomyopathy, long-term warfarin with an INR of 2.0–3.0 was recommended by the ACCP/NHLBI Consensus on the basis of uncontrolled clinical data (level V). With other forms of non-valvular disease and atrial fibrillation definite recommendations were not made but young patients who are not at increased risk of haemorrhagic complications could be considered for long-term warfarin. With congestive cardiac failure in patients complicated by atrial fibrillation and non-valvular heart disease warfarin may be preferred because of the risk of pulmonary embolism and left ventricular thrombi, but this decision is based only on level V evidence.

For patients with atrial fibrillation and thyrotoxic heart disease the ACCP/NHLBI group made a strong recommendation for warfarin therapy with an INR 2.0–3.0 being instituted, and continued short term, 2–4 weeks, after conversion to sinus rhythm and the euthyroid state is regained. This was recommended by level V study.

On the basis of a non-randomized controlled study it was recommended that patients with atrial fibrillation and cardioversion should be given warfarin for 3 weeks before elective cardioversion and maintained for 2–4 weeks, at an INR at 2.0–3.0 (level III).

CEREBROVASCULAR DISEASE

Oral anticoagulants might protect patients with an established stroke following cerebral thrombosis or embolism from extension of the thrombus. But it has been shown that anticoagulant treatment is of no value in the established thrombotic cerebral infarction, and in fact that prognosis may be made worse by the increased risk of cerebral haemorrhage.

The value of oral anticoagulation in cerebral embolism and in the prevention of further transient ischaemic attacks (TIAS) was claimed in a level II study by Carter (1961) and in level II and III studies to reduce morbidity and mortality in a slowly progressive stroke. The conclusion from the Consensus Group (Sherman et al 1989) was then that anticoagulants should not be given routinely to patients with TIAS. With regard to progressing thrombotic strokes the Consensus opinion was that the decision to give oral anticoagulant should be based on individual clinical judgement. For cardiogenic brain embolus see the section on heart valves. For recurrent thromboembolism to the brain, heparin followed by warfarin (INR 3.0–4.5) was recommended in non-hypertensive patients where a CT scan showed no haemorrhage transformation (level III, IV and V studies).

PERIPHERAL VASCULAR DISEASE

Peripheral arterial occlusion may be due to embolism or thrombosis of a stenosed artery. In peripheral arterial occlusion the purpose of anticoagulants is to improve the local circulation and to reduce the associated high mortality from cerebral and cardiac disease.

Evidence from retrospective studies (level III) suggest that heparin or oral anticoagulants in patients with embolic occlusion reduce the frequency of systemic embolism (Elliot et al 1980, Holm & Schersten 1972). Whereas other studies have suggested oral anticoagulants are of no value in protecting against thrombosis following arterial reconstruction, one recent level I randomized study of patients with reversed saphenous vein femoro-popliteal bypasses demonstrated significant benefit of warfarin in patency, (18% occlusions were found in treated compared to 37% in controls), and patients survival (Kretschmer et al 1988).

CORONARY BYPASS GRAFTS

Warfarin may be given after coronary bypass operations. Serial angiographic studies have shown that about one-half of the occlusions observed 12 months after operation occur within the first 4 weeks. Most occlusions are due to thrombosis. A level I trial from West Germany reported improved graft patency with phenprocoumon in a study of 89 patients contrasted with 84 controls (Kretschmer et al 1988). All subjects received heparin and dipryridamole for 7 days before randomization into the two groups. Graft patency after 8 weeks was 90.4% in the coumarin-tested group and 83.4% in the control group. The study does not answer the questions of how long anticoagulants need to be administered, as the benefit might extend beyond the period of the study, or indeed whether there is delayed or 'rebound' occlusion when coumarin drugs are discontinued. In contrast, longer studies for six months and two years have indicated no benefit.

SUMMARY – THE MAIN TRENDS OF ORAL ANTICOAGULANT TREATMENT

The trends are currently to wider administration of warfarin in lower doses to improve the benefit/risk ratio by reducing bleeding, to segment the therapeutic range in INR according to clinical state and to improve the safety and effectiveness of laboratory monitoring of drug administration with increasing application of the INR system.

REFERENCES

ACCP/NHLBI 1986 National conference on antithrombotic therapy. Chest 89(suppl): S1–169

Adams C F, Merret J D, Hutchinson W M et al 1974 Cerebral embolism and mitral valve stenosis. J Neural Neurosurg Psychiatry 37: 378–383

Altman R, Rouvier J, Gurfinkel E et al 1990 Comparison of two levels of anticoagulant therapy in patients with substitute heart valves. J Thorac Cardiovasc Surg (in press)

Barritt D W, Jordan S C 1960 Anticoagulant drugs in the treatment of pulmonary embolism. Lancet i: 1309–1312

Bern M M, Bothe A, Bistrian B et al 1986 Prophylaxis against central vein thrombosis with very low dose warfarin. Surgery 99: 216–221

Bern M M, Lokich J L, Wallach S A et al 1990 Very low doses of warfarin can present thrombosis in central venous catheters. Ann Int Med 112: 423–428

Biggs R, Denson K W E 1967 Standardisation of the one-stage prothrombin time for the control of anticoagulant therapy. Br Med J 1: 84–88

Breddin D, Loew D, Lechner K 1980 The German Austrian aspirin trial comparison of acetyl salicylic acid, placebo and phenprocoumon in secondary prevention of myocardial infarction. Circulation 62(suppl): 63

Brenkel I J, Clancy M J 1990 Total hip replacement and antithrombotic prophylaxis. Br J Hosp Med 42: 282–284

British Society for Haematology 1984 Guidelines on oral anticoagulation, quoted by Poller L, Br Med J 1985 290: 1683–1686

British Society for Haematology 1990 Guidelines on oral anticoagulation, 2nd edn. J Clin Pathol 43: 177–183

Carter A B 1961 Anticoagulant treatment in progressing strokes. Br Med J 2: 70–73

Chalmers T C, Martta R, Smith H, Kunzler A M 1977 Use of anticoagulants in acute myocardial infarction. N Engl J Med 297: 1091–1095

Cheseboro J H, Adams P C, Fuster V 1986 Antithrombotic therapy in patients with valvular heart disease and prosthetic valves. J Am Cell 8: 41B–56B

Drapkin A, Merskey C 1972 Anticoagulant therapy after acute myocardial infarction. JAMA 222: 541–543

Dunn M, Alexander J, Silva R de, Hildner F 1989 Antithrombotic therapy in atrial fibrillation. Chest 95: S118–127

Ebert R V, Borden C V, Hipp H R 1969 Long term anticoagulant therapy after myocardial infarction. Final report of Veterans' Administration Cooperative Study. JAMA 207: 2263

Elliot J P, Hageman J H, Szilagyi E et al 1980 Arterial embolisation, problems of source, multiplicity recurrence and delayed treatment. Surgery 88: 883

Fleming H A, Bailey S M 1971 Mitral valve disease. Postgrad Med J 47: 509–604

Francis C W, Marder V J, McCollister C et al 1983 Two step warfarin therapy. JAMA 249: 374–378

Hilden T, Iversen K, Raaschou F 1961 Anticoagulants in myocardial infarction. Lancet 2: 327–331

Hirsh J, Deykin D, Poller L 1986 Therapeutic range for oral anticoagulant therapy. Chest 5: 11–15

Hirsh J, Poller L, Deykin D et al 1989 Optimal therapeutic range for oral anticoagulants. Chest 95: S5–11

Holm J, Schersten J 1972 Anticoagulant treatment during and after embolectomy. Acta Clin Scand 138: 683

Hull R, Delmore T, Carter C et al 1979 Warfarin sodium versus low dose heparin in the long term treatment of venous thrombosis. N Engl J Med 301: 855–858

Hull R, Hirsh J, Carter C et al 1982 Different intensities of oral anticoagulant therapy in the treatment of proximal vein thrombosis. N Engl J Med 307: 1676–1681

ICSH/ICTH 1979 Prothrombin time standardisation. Report of expert panel on oral anticoagulant control. Thromb Haemostasis 42: 1073–1100

Kirkwood T B L 1983 Calibration of reference thromboplastins and standardisation of the prothrombin time ratio. Thromb Haemostasis 49: 238–244

Kretschmer G, Schemper M, Ehringer H et al 1988 Influence of postoperative anticoagulant treatment on patient survival after femoro popliteal by-pass surgery. Lancet 1: 797

Levine H J, Pauker G P, Salzman E W 1989 Antithrombotic therapy in valvular heart disease. Chest 95: 985–1065

Loeliger E A, Halem Visser L P van 1979 Results of calibration by Dutch national reference laboratory of the thromboplastins included in the ICSH/ICTH collaborative study. Thromb Haemostasis 42: 1128–1131

Loeliger E A, Poller L, Samama M et al 1985 Questions and answers on prothrombin time standardisation in oral anticoagulant control. Thromb Haemostasis 54: 515–518

MacCallum P K, Thomson J M, Poller L 1990 Effects of fixed minidose warfarin on coagulation and fibrinolysis following major gynaecological surgery. Thromb Haemostasis (in press)

Medical Research Council 1964 Second report of the working party on anticoagulant therapy after myocardial infarction. Br Med J 2: 837–843

Medical Research Council 1969 Assessment of short term anticoagulant administration after cardiac infarction. Br Med J 1: 335–342

Oakley C, Doherty P 1976 Pregnancy in patients after valve replacement. Br Heart J 38: 1140

Petersen P, Boysen G, Godtfredsen E et al 1989 Placebo controlled randomised trial of warfarin and aspirin for prevention of thromboembolic complications in chronic atrial fibrillation. Lancet 1: 175–178

Poller L 1964 Standardisation of anticoagulant treatment: the Manchester regional thromboplastin scheme. Br Med J 2: 565–566

Poller L, Taberner D A 1982 Dosage and control of oral anticoagulants: an international survey. Br J Haematol 51: 479–485

Poller L, McKernan A, Thomson J M 1987 Fixed minidose warfarin: a new approach to prophylaxis against venous thrombosis after major surgery. Br Med J 295: 1309–1312

Powers P J, Gent M, Jay K M et al 1989 A randomized trial of less intense post operative warfarin or aspirin therapy in the prevention of venous thromboembolism after surgery for fractured hip. Arch Int Med 149: 771–774

Report of the Sixty Plus Reinfarction Study Research Group 1980 A double blind trial to assess long term oral anticoagulant therapy in elderly patients after myocardial infarction. Lancet 2: 989–994

Resnekow L, Chediak J, Hirsh J, Lewis H D 1989 Antithrombotic agents in coronary artery disease. Chest 95: S52–72

Sackett D L 1989 Rules of evidence and clinical recommendations on the use of antithrombotic agents. Chest 95: S2–5

Saour J N, Sieck J O, Maimo A R, Gallus A S 1990 Trial of different intensities of anticoagulation in patients with prosthetic heart valves. N Engl J Med 322: 428–431

Sherman D G, Dyken M L, Fisher M et al 1989 Antithrombotic therapy for cardiovascular disorders. Chest 95: S140–155

Smith P, Arnesen H, Holme I 1989 Effects of oral anticoagulants on mortality, recurrent infarction and cerebrovascular attacks in survivors of acute myocardial infarction. Thromb Haemostasis 62: 327 (Abstract)

Smith P, Arnesen H, Holme I 1990 The effect of warfarin on mortality, and re-infarction after acute myocardial infarction. N Engl J Med 323: 147–152

Stein P D, Kantrovitz A 1989 Antithrombotic therapy in mechanical biological prosthetic heart valves and sapheous by pass grafts. Chest 95: S107–117

Stroke Prevention Study 1990 Preliminary report of the Stroke Prevention in Atrial Fibrillation Study. N Engl J Med 322: 863–868

Taberner D A, Poller L, Burslem R W, Jones J B 1978 Oral anticoagulants controlled by British Comparative Thromboplastin versus low dose heparin in prophylaxis of deep vein thrombosis. Br Med J 1: 272–274

Turpie A G G, Gunstensen J, Hirsh J et al 1988 Randomized comparison of two intensities of oral anticoagulant therapy after tissue heart valve replacement. Lancet 1: 1242–1245

US Veterans Administration 1965 Long term anticoagulant therapy after myocardial infarction. JAMA 193: 157

US Veterans Administration Co-operative Study 1973 Anticoagulants in myocardial infarction. JAMA 225: 724–726

van den Besselaar A M H P, Halem Visser L P van, Hoekstra-Schuman M et al 1980 Simplified thromboplastin calibration. Thromb Haemostasis 43: 53–57

Vroonhoven T J M V, van Ziijl J, Muller H 1974 Low-dose subcutaneous heparin versus oral anticoagulants in the prevention of postoperative deep-venous thrombosis. Lancet 1: 375–377

Zucker S, Brosius E, Cooper G R 1970 One stage prothrombin time survey. Am J Clin Path 53: 340–347

13

Clinical and laboratory aspects of thrombolytic therapy

G.D.O. Lowe

INTRODUCTION

The major advance in thrombolytic therapy in recent years has been a clinical one: the demonstration by large, randomized trials that such treatment reduces mortality in evolving myocardial infarction. The synergistic effect of aspirin and streptokinase on mortality (ISIS-2 Collaborative Group 1988), as well as the persistence of clinical benefit of treatment up to 24 hours from onset of symptoms (ISIS-2 Collaborative Group 1988), have shown the clinical importance of both the platelet and the fibrin components of coronary thrombi, as well as the dynamic, evolving nature of coronary thrombosis and myocardial infarction. Thrombolytic therapy is now routine management in acute myocardial infarction and is now by far its commonest clinical use. While the clinical use of thrombolytic therapy in acute myocardial infarction will therefore form the major part of this update, the other possible indications for thrombolytic therapy will be briefly considered, as will newer thrombolytic agents and some laboratory aspects of their use.

ACUTE MYOCARDIAL INFARCTION

Herrick (1912) gave a clinical description of acute myocardial infarction and suggested that 'hope for the damaged myocardium lies in the direction of securing a supply of blood ... so as to restore as far as possible its functional integrity'. Fletcher and colleagues (1959) performed pilot studies of streptokinase in acute myocardial infarction, and following a number of smaller studies a larger (764 patients), multicentre, randomized controlled trial found a statistically and clinically significant reduction in hospital mortality in patients randomized to streptokinase (18.5%) compared to heparin (26.3%) (European Working Party 1971). However, despite a sound rationale (fibrin-rich coronary artery thrombi precipitate myocardial infarction, and are lysed by streptokinase which may restore arterial patency and limit infarct size, which is a major determinant of mortality) and a good trial by the standards of the day, streptokinase did not become generally accepted treatment in acute myocardial infarction. Thus 'with the benefit of hindsight it is now evident that until very recently patients with acute myocardial infarction have been deprived of the benefits of a treatment that was shown to be effective nearly 20 years ago' (Hampton 1989).

The lack of acceptance probably reflected doubts about the causal connection between coronary thrombosis and infarction; the reporting of 'negative' as well as 'positive' trials; the cost and complications of thrombolytic therapy; and the interest of cardiologists in other aspects of infarction. However, from about 1979 several developments promoted a renaissance of interest in the prime role of coronary thrombosis in myocardial infarction, and in thrombolytic therapy as the prime treatment. Firstly, careful pathological studies (using radiolabelled fibrinogen, serial sections, and post-mortem angiography) strongly supported a causal role for coronary thrombosis not only in myocardial infarction, but also in unstable angina and sudden coronary death (Davies et al 1979, Falk 1983, Davies 1989, De Wood 1989). The current concept is illustrated in Figures 13.1 and 13.2 (Davies 1989). Secondly, these pathological associations were supported

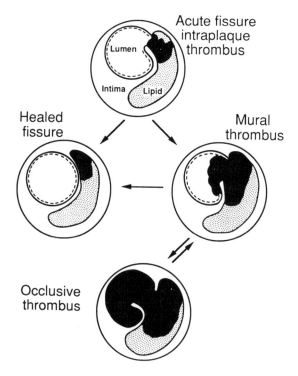

Fig. 13.1 Diagrammatic representation in a coronary artery of the relation between plaque fissuring with intra-plaque thrombosis and subsequent healing, or formation of intraluminal thrombosis (mural or occlusive). Mural thrombi may precipitate unstable angina; occlusive thrombi may precipitate myocardial infarction; and sudden death may follow either large vessel occlusion or microvascular ischaemia from distal microthromboembolism. (Reproduced with permission from Davies 1989.)

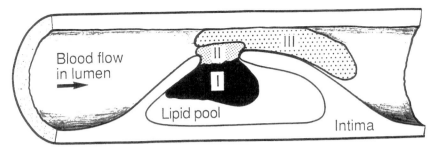

Fig. 13.2   Diagrammatic representation in a coronary artery of a reconstruction in longitudinal section of an occluding thrombus due to plaque fissuring. The thrombus within the plaque labelled I is rich in platelets, stage II contains both platelets and fibrin, while stage III thrombus which has propagated in the lumen is predominantly fibrin and red cells with a minimal platelet component. (Reproduced with permission from Davies 1989.)

by studies of coronary angiography, embolectomy and most recently angioscopy in vivo, which showed high prevalences of occlusive thrombi during the evolution of acute myocardial infarction (especially if transmural) or unstable angina, or following resuscitation from 'sudden coronary death' (De Wood et al 1980, Davies 1989, De Wood 1989).

Thirdly, there developed in the early 1980s a vogue for intracoronary thrombolysis (Rentrop et al 1981) which was readily combined with serial angiography, which showed a high incidence of reperfusion of the infarct-related artery, as well as a reduction in mortality (Simoons et al 1985). The non-availability of acute cardiac catheterization in most hospitals, and its logistic and economic problems, led to re-examination of intravenous thrombolysis, which can be initiated much more rapidly.

Fourthly, as well as investigation of high-dose, short-term intravenous streptokinase (Schroeder et al 1983), there was increasing clinical and commercial interest in newer, potentially 'fibrin-specific' plasminogen activators such as anistreplase, alteplase and saruplase (see below). It was hoped that these agents might be more effective in lysing fibrin thrombi, while at the same time having a lesser risk of bleeding due to a lesser degree of plasminogen activation and fibrinogen digestion in the circulation.

Finally, while all these agents have been shown to be effective in causing coronary reperfusion, and streptokinase and alteplase have been shown to thus reduce infarct size and preserve left ventricular function (Cairns et al 1989, White & Norris 1989), the most important patient-related endpoint is reduction in mortality. A meta-analysis of 24 randomized studies of intravenous streptokinase or urokinase performed between 1959 and 1979 found a pooled odds reduction in mortality of $22 \pm 5\%$ ($P < 0.001$; Yusuf et al 1985a). Subsequently, several larger, randomized, placebo-controlled trials have shown significant reductions in mortality for intravenous streptokinase (GISSI 1986, ISAM Study Group 1986, ISIS-2 Collaborative Group 1988), anistreplase (AIMS Study Group 1990) and alteplase (the

ASSET Study: Wilcox et al 1988). This reduction in mortality is maintained for at least a year after therapy; it outweighs the risks of thrombolytic therapy in patients without significant contraindications; it justifies its cost; and it is now standard recommended therapy in evolving myocardial infarction (British Heart Foundation Working Group 1989, Cairns et al 1989, Petch 1990). Further studies (including the ISIS-3 study which compares streptokinase, anistreplase and alteplase, as well as the addition of early heparin therapy) are awaited to establish the optimal thrombolytic agent and regimen of adjunctive therapy. Meanwhile, aspirin has a synergistic effect with streptokinase (ISIS-2 Collaborative Group 1988), and alteplase appears similar to streptokinase (Table 13.1).

Choice of patient

Because of the evidence now available that early intravenous thrombolytic therapy reduces mortality for up to one year, it is recommended that it be considered in every patient with suspected evolving acute myocardial infarction (Cairns et al 1989). Such a diagnosis is likely in patients with at least 30 minutes of ischaemic cardiac pain, and at least 1 mm of ST segment elevation in at least two adjacent limb leads or precordial leads on the ECG. However, some physicians do not wait for such ECG changes, e.g. in the ISIS-3 study (Petch 1990). The benefits of treatment are greatest when given early (less than 6 hours from onset of symptoms), hence every effort should be made to admit patients as soon as possible to coronary care units, insert an intravenous cannula and commence ECG monitoring, and assess patients for thrombolytic therapy. While relative benefit is less in patients treated 6–24 hours after onset of symptoms, it is still significant and thrombolytic therapy may again be indicated (ISIS-2 Collaborative

Table 13.1   Comparison of in-hospital mortality and clinical events in a randomized trial of alteplase versus streptokinase in 20 891 patients with suspected acute myocardial infarction of less than 6 hours duration. (Data from International Study Group 1990; 12 490 patients were in the GISSI-2 trial 1990). Alteplase therapy was associated with higher incidences of stroke and total bleeding, and with lower incidences of major bleeds (requiring transfusion of 2 or more blood units), allergic reactions and hypotension

	Alteplase	Streptokinase	Relative risk (95% CI)
Number	10 372	10 396	
Death	8.9%	8.5%	1.05 (0.95–1.16)
Ventricular fibrillation	6.8%	6.5%	1.06 (0.95–1.18)
Shock	5.6%	5.9%	0.94 (0.84–1.06)
Reinfarction	2.6%	3.0%	0.87 (0.74–1.03)
Stroke	1.3%	0.9%	1.41 (1.06–1.83)
Major bleeds	0.6%	0.9%	0.67 (0.49–0.91)
All bleeds	4.2%	3.3%	1.26 (1.09–1.45)
Allergic reactions	0.2%	1.7%	0.20 (0.15–0.27)
Hypotension	1.7%	3.8%	0.45 (0.38–0.53)

Group 1988; Cairns et al 1989), for example in patients with ongoing ischaemic pain, or a 'stuttering' course suggesting intermittent coronary occlusion (Fuster et al 1989). The risk of death in acute myocardial infarction is highest in older patients, those with previous myocardial infarctions, and those with anterior infarctions. These factors, as well as the relative risks and contraindications to thrombolytic therapy, should all be weighed by the assessing physician for the individual patient. Particular care should be taken to exclude patients with causes of chest pain which mimic myocardial infarction, but in whom thrombolytic therapy may cause fatal bleeding, i.e. aortic dissection, acute pericarditis and oesophagitis (Petch 1990).

Choice of drug

Streptokinase

Streptokinase is produced by β-haemolytic streptococci. It forms a 1 : 1 stoichiometric complex with plasminogen, in which it exposes an active site conferring plasminogen activator activity upon the complex. It is currently the 'gold standard' drug for thrombolytic therapy in acute myocardial infarction for three reasons: there is more experience than with newer agents; it is clinically as effective (GISSI-2 1990, International Study Group 1990); and it is the cheapest. (The cost of the standard dose of 1.5 million units in the UK in 1990 was about £80, and the cost per life 'saved' was about £3000). Its disadvantages are a higher risk of hypotension and allergic reactions (Table 13.1), as well as antibody formation which may complicate further thrombolytic therapy in the subsequent year (see below). Streptokinase should be given in a dose of 1.5 million units, diluted in 50–200 ml isotonic saline or 5% glucose, over 1 hour. Aspirin (150–300 mg/day) should be given concurrently because of its synergistic effects on mortality (ISIS-2 Collaborative Group 1988) and continued long term unless contraindicated. Streptokinase has a half-life of about 25 minutes. Infusion produces rapid falls in plasma levels of plasminogen, α_2-antiplasmin, fibrinogen (and hence plasma and whole-blood viscosity) and factors V and VIII; and rapid increases in free plasmin and plasmin-derived degradation products of fibrinogen ($B\beta_{1-42}$ fragment and low-molecular-weight products) and of cross-linked fibrin ($B\beta_{15-42}$ fragment and low-molecular-weight products including cross-linked degradation products) (Fig. 13.3).

Anistreplase

Anistreplase (anisoylated streptokinase–plasminogen activator complex, APSAC) is a pro-enzyme, whose catalytic serine active site is temporarily masked by an anisoyl group. Following intravenous infusion it is slowly activated by sustained deacylation and release of the anisoyl group, and has

Fig. 13.3   Systemic effects of thrombolytic therapy. (Modified from Lowe & Douglas in press.)

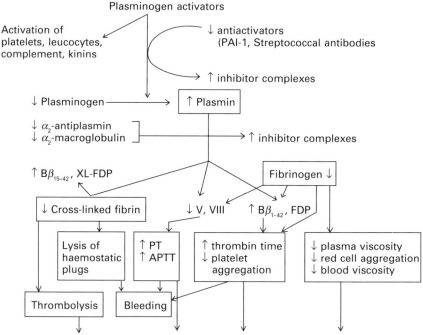

Restoration of blood flow, tissue salvage, clinical benefit

a half-life of about 90 minutes. Unlike streptokinase, it can be given as a bolus infusion over 5 minutes (the dose is 30 units). This is not an advantage in hospitalized patients, but offers the potential for earlier administration prior to hospital admission (e.g. by trained general practitioners or ambulancemen). The benefits and risks of such outpatient administration are currently under evaluation (British Heart Foundation Working Group 1989). The systemic effects, adverse effects, and coronary reperfusion rates in acute myocardial infarction appear comparable for anistreplase and streptokinase, as do the effects on the blood (Fig. 13.3). Its current cost in the UK in 1990 was about five times higher than streptokinase. Anistreplase significantly reduces mortality in acute myocardial infarction compared to placebo (AIMS Study Group 1990). Its risks and benefits relative to streptokinase and alteplase are currently being assessed in the ISIS-3 study.

Alteplase

Alteplase (recombinant tissue-type plasminogen activator, rt-PA) is an endogenous serine protease plasminogen activator of physiological importance (see Ch. 2) which is now produced by recombinant biotechnology for pharmaceutical use. The dose of single-chain alteplase is 100 mg (or 1.5 mg/kg for patients weighing under 67 kg), diluted in isotonic saline and given by intravenous infusion over 3 hours. The first 10% of the drug is given over 2 minutes; a further 50% over 1 hour; and the final 40% over the next 2 hours. The half-life in the circulation is about 5 minutes, but as it binds specifically to fibrin and activates plasminogen at the fibrin surface several hundred times more efficiently than in the circulation, its effects on fibrin thrombi (or on fibrin haemostatic plugs) may be prolonged for several hours. It has fewer systemic effects on blood coagulation and viscosity than streptokinase, although such effects are still substantial (Marder & Sherry 1988) (Fig. 13.3). Possibly because of its relative 'fibrin specificity' compared to streptokinase, it produces higher early coronary patency rates (Verstraete et al 1985, Chesebro et al 1987). On the other hand, comparable early patency rates were achieved by higher doses of streptokinase (3 million units; Six et al 1988); 24 hour patency rates are similar for the two drugs (Chesebro et al 1987); and differences in 90-minute patency rates were less striking in patients treated early (Rapaport 1989). In two large randomized trials, anistreplase and streptokinase had similar effects on death plus severe left ventricular damage (23.1% and 22.5%; relative risk 1.04, 95% CI 0.95–1.13; GISSI-2 1990) and on hospital mortality (8.9% and 8.5%; relative risk 1.05, 95% CI 0.96–1.16; International Study Group 1990). In the latter study, the alteplase group had fewer allergic reactions, hypotensive episodes and major bleeds than the streptokinase group, but more total bleeds (major plus minor) and strokes (but not confirmed haemorrhagic strokes) (Table 13.1). Hence these two agents appear comparable in terms of clinical benefits and overall complications. However, the GISSI-2 study (1990) and International Study Group (1990) used alteplase with or without subcutaneous heparin, and there is some evidence that early intravenous heparin may improve coronary patency rates after alteplase therapy (International Study Group 1990). Hence the results of the ISIS-3 study in which heparin is started earlier will be of interest. In 1990 in the UK, the cost of alteplase was about ten times higher than streptokinase.

Urokinase

Urokinase has been produced commercially from human urine and latterly from tissue culture of kidney cells: both forms have similar activities and are less antigenic than streptokinase in man. Its systemic effects are similar to those of streptokinase, but slower in onset. It is not currently licensed for use in acute myocardial infarction in the UK, but studies are in progress.

Saruplase

Saruplase (recombinant urinary-type plasminogen activator, rscu-PA) is another endogenous plasminogen activator (see Ch. 2) which has recently been produced by recombinant biotechnology for pharmaceutical use. Like alteplase, it shows enhanced plasminogen activation in the presence of fibrin, although the mechanisms are different. It is currently under evaluation in treatment of acute myocardial infarction (PRIMI Trial Study Group 1989).

How does thrombolytic therapy reduce mortality in acute myocardial infarction?

There are two common causes of death in acute myocardial infarction: dysrhythmias (especially ventricular fibrillation) and deaths from heart failure which are related to infarct size. Reduction in mortality by thrombolytic therapy appears due largely to reduction in deaths from heart failure. This follows restoration of myocardial blood flow, reduction in infarct size and improvement in left ventricular function (White & Norris 1989). In contrast, there may be an early *increase* in dysrhythmic deaths. In the GISSI–1 study, a little-known finding was the *increased* fatality rate on the first day in the streptokinase group compared to the placebo group (Mauri et al 1987). This may reflect ventricular fibrillation due to reperfusion injury (see below) or to platelet–fibrin microaggregates, released from lysed coronary thrombi, impacting in the myocardial microcirculation. The latter mechanism may be analogous to that of sudden coronary death. It is interesting that aspirin has a synergistic effect with streptokinase in reducing mortality after acute myocardial infarction (ISIS-2 Collaborative Group 1988): this may partly reflect a protective effect of aspirin against such streptokinase-induced microemboli.

While lysis of coronary artery thrombi is probably the major mechanism by which thrombolytic therapy reduces infarct size and mortality, other mechanisms also merit consideration. With the standard dose of streptokinase, plasma fibrinogen falls by about 80% on average: this produces a rapid fall in plasma and whole-blood viscosity (Theiss et al 1980, personal unpublished observations; Fig. 13.3). The viscosity reduction may increase myocardial blood flow in ischaemic areas and thus also reduce infarct size. Because of the low blood flow rates in ischaemic areas, local shear rates may fall, causing red cell aggregation by fibrinogen and hence local increases in whole blood viscosity. Fibrinogen depletion by thrombolytic therapy may therefore cause a greater reduction in blood viscosity, and increase in flow, in the ischaemic microcirculation. The fall in viscosity may also maintain blood flow in the recanalized coronary artery (reducing the risk of rethrombosis) and also may reduce cardiac workload: this latter effect may also decrease infarct size. Blood viscosity is a determinant of peripheral resistance, and reduction in blood pressure after streptokinase (European Collaborative Study 1979) or anistreplase (AIMS Trial Study Group 1990) may reflect fall in viscosity, or alternatively vasodilatation due to activation of the complement or kallikrein–kinin systems by free plasmin (AIMS Trial Study Group 1990).

Thrombolytic therapy also produces systemic anticoagulation by digesting fibrinogen, factor V and factor VIII, and by producing high plasma levels of low-molecular-weight fibrin(ogen) degradation products (Fig. 13.3). The decrease in fibrinogen and increase in degradation products also inhibit platelet aggregation (Coller 1990). These antiplatelet and anticoagulant effects may be additive to viscosity reduction and vasodilatation in reducing the risk of rethrombosis. Alteplase, which causes less systemic effects, may carry a higher risk of rethrombosis, hence early intravenous heparin has been suggested after therapy (Ross et al 1990). It may be that the greater systemic effects of streptokinase (vasodilatation, viscosity reduction, anticoagulant and antiplatelet effects) counteract the higher initial coronary patency rates of alteplase, resulting in similar clinical benefit (GISSI-2 1990, International Study Group 1990).

Adverse effects

These include hypotension, allergic reactions and antibody formation (all of which are commoner with streptokinase or anistreplase than with urokinase or alteplase), reperfusion dysrhythmias, rethrombosis and bleeding (Table 13.2).

Hypotension

This occurs in about 4% of patients receiving streptokinase, and is more likely the more rapidly it is infused (Table 13.1). In patients who are already hypotensive (e.g. systolic blood pressure under 90 mmHg) alteplase might therefore be preferred (Verstraete et al 1985). Severe hypotension is managed by interrupting the infusion, tilting the patient, and infusion of fluid or atropine (Cairns et al 1989).

Allergic reactions

These are most commonly immediate anaphylactic (Coombs type I) reactions

Table 13.2   Some adverse effects of thrombolytic therapy

Hypotension[a]
Allergic reactions (types I and III)[a]
Antibody formation[a]
Reperfusion injury (heart, brain)
Rethrombosis
Thromboembolism ('trash foot', Stafford et al 1989)
Bleeding

[a] Commoner with streptokinase or antistreplase than with urokinase or alteplase.

to foreign proteins by pre-existing antibodies to streptococci in patients treated with streptokinase or anistreplase. Possible allergic reactions (fever, rash, rigor, bronchospasm, hypotension) occur in about 2% of patients receiving streptokinase, and are about five times more common than in patients receiving alteplase or placebo (Table 13.1). Severe anaphylactic reactions to streptokinase were reported in 0.1% of patients in the GISSI-1 study (GISSI 1986) and in 0.2% of patients in the ISIS-2 study (ISIS-2 Collaborative Group 1988). Less common are delayed (6–21 days) immune complex-mediated vasculitic (Coombs type III) reactions. These may resemble Henoch-Schönlein purpura, with vasculitic purpura, arthralgia, abdominal pain and microscopic haematuria. Glomerulonephritis rarely occurs, and may indicate treatment with steroids or plasmapheresis (Payne et al 1989). To avoid allergic reactions, it may be wise to use alteplase rather than streptokinase or anistreplase in patients with documented allergy to streptokinase or anistreplase, or who have been treated with these drugs in the previous year. Prophylactic steroids did not reduce the risk of allergic reactions in the ISIS-2 study (ISIS-2 Collaborative Group 1988). However, steroids may be used in treatment of severe reactions.

Antibody formation

Surprisingly little information is available on the natural history of anti-streptococcal antibody titres after streptokinase treatment. However, in view of its routine use in acute myocardial infarction and the increasingly common problem of reinfarction in the several months after hospital discharge following streptokinase therapy, it is important to study this. According to the recent study of Jalihal & Morris (1990), reviewed in chapter 14, there is a high risk that the standard dose of streptokinase (1.5 million units) will be ineffective in patients treated within the previous year; hence alteplase may be preferred in such patients.

Reperfusion dysrhythmias

As already noted, streptokinase increased early hospital mortality in the GISSI-1 study (Mauri et al 1987), possibly due to reperfusion injury and dysrhythmias. The incidence of reperfusion dysrhythmias is probably impossible to determine, because it would require both continuous ECG monitoring and repeated angiography in both control and active treatment groups (Goldberg et al 1983). The 'disadvantage' of reperfusion dysrhythmias is transient, and is more than compensated by the later benefit of reduced infarct size and decreased risk of later dysrhythmias which complicate large infarcts (de Bono 1989). The possibility of reperfusion dysrhythmias is therefore not a contraindication to thrombolysis in myocardial infarction, but patients should have ECG monitoring as well as facilities and skilled personnel readily available for defibrillation and other management of dysrhythmias (Anonymous 1989, British Heart Foundation Working Group 1989).

Other aspects of reperfusion injury include mechanical 'stunning' (contractility impairment) of myocardial cells, microvascular damage resulting in the 'no-reflow' phenomenon, and myocardial necrosis or haemorrhage. The 'no-reflow' phenomenon may result from interactions between neutrophil leucocytes and vascular endothelium, with ischaemia–reperfusion changes in intracellular calcium ions and formation of toxic oxygen free radicals (Lucchesi 1989). Changes in intracellular calcium and free radical formation may also play causal roles in myocardial damage, hence there is a rationale for the addition of calcium antagonists, free radical scavengers, or β-adrenergic blockers to thrombolytic therapy of acute myocardial infarction (Anonymous 1989). The TIMI-II study has suggested that concomitant β-blockade improves the results of thrombolysis with alteplase (TIMI Study Group 1989). In view of the evidence that β-blockers reduce mortality after myocardial infarction (Yusuf et al 1985b) they should be considered in all patients after thrombolytic therapy (Cairns et al 1989), as indeed they were in the GISSI-2 Study (1990) and International Study Group Trial (1990).

Rethrombosis and reinfarction

Removal of the acute fibrin-rich occlusive thrombus which is precipitating acute myocardial infarction usually leaves a stenotic, deeply fissured plaque with both intra-plaque and mural platelet-rich thrombus (Figs 13.1 and 13.2). Rethrombosis is therefore favoured chemically by continued exposure of flowing blood to plaque lipid, collagen, von Willebrand factor and tissue factor; as well as to high local concentrations of adenosine diphosphate (ADP) released from red cells and tissue cells; and also to high local concentrations of thromboxane A_2 and serotonin from activated platelets. The latter two compounds (and possibly endothelial-derived constricting factor and endothelin) may cause local arterial vasospasm, which combines with the residual arterial stenosis to cause high local shear forces, which may also mechanically activate platelets (O'Brien 1990). Local platelet aggregation and generation of thrombin may then promote rethrombosis (Heras et al 1989).

Coronary angiographic studies over the past ten years have shown the presence of an occlusive thrombus in 85% of cases of acute transmural infarction during the first 6 hours of evolution; spontaneous reperfusion in about 10% of cases during acute angiographic observation; spontaneous patency rates of about 35% by 24 hours and up to 67% by 2 weeks; and reocclusion in about 20% of vessels which initially reperfuse, mostly by 24 hours but with further reocclusions over subsequent days (Cairns et al 1989). The reinfarction rate is doubled after intravenous streptokinase therapy (Cairns et al 1989).

Approaches to prevention of rethrombosis and reinfarction include choice of thrombolytic drug; adjunctive drug therapy with antiplatelet agents, anticoagulants, vasodilators or rheological agents; and angioplasty. To date, only the addition of aspirin to streptokinase therapy has been proven to be clinically useful in further reducing mortality (ISIS-2 Collaborative Group 1988). This combined effect may reflect suppression of the platelet component of coronary artery rethrombosis (Fig. 13.2); effects on platelet microemboli (as discussed above); or possibly stimulation of endogenous fibrinolysis in whole blood (Moroz 1977). In respect of the latter possibility, it is worth noting that activated platelets release plasminogen activator inhibitor type 1 (PAI-1; see Ch. 2), high local concentrations of which may promote rethrombosis. The possible roles of platelets in limiting thrombolysis, promoting rethrombosis, and promoting haemorrhage after thrombolytic therapy are reviewed by Coller (1990) (see Ch. 14), who also reviews other antiplatelet drugs.

In contrast to the proven role of aspirin as adjunctive therapy, there is as yet little evidence that reinfarction or hospital mortality is any different with streptokinase or alteplase (Table 13.1), or reduced by adjunctive heparin (GISSI-2 1990, International Study Group 1990). However, as previously noted, the results of the ISIS-3 study, which includes randomization to early heparin therapy, may clarify the role of early anticoagulation. Meanwhile it should be remembered that full-dose heparin may be indicated in patients with large (especially anterior) infarcts as prophylaxis of mural thromboembolism; while low-dose subcutaneous heparin may be indicated as prophylaxis of venous thromboembolism in at-risk patients (e.g. large infarcts, previous myocardial infarction or venous thromboembolism, heart failure, shock, immobility, obesity) (Cairns et al 1989, Fuster et al 1989).

Studies are in progress to study the possible benefits of other adjunctive therapies, including vasodilators (Hackett et al 1987), rheological therapies such as haemodilution (Merzx et al 1981) or defibrinogenation with ancrod (Hossmann et al 1990), and low-molecular-weight heparins. It should be noted that intravenous nitroglycerine antagonizes the anticoagulant effect of intravenous heparin (Habbab & Haft 1986).

Three randomized studies have all suggested that immediate percutaneous transluminal coronary angioplasty (PTCA) is not advantageous after thrombolytic therapy, and may be associated with increased risks of reinfarction and mortality (Passamani et al 1987, Topol et al 1987, Simoons et al 1988). Hence, despite the importance of residual arterial stenosis in rethrombosis (Harrison et al 1984), this may be outweighed by the vascular trauma of PTCA as a stimulus to rethrombosis.

Bleeding

Haemorrhage is an inevitable side effect of thrombolytic therapy in any series of patients, because invariably a percentage of patients have recently formed platelet–fibrin haemostatic plugs, which (despite the hopes of many ingenious biochemists and molecular biologists) I doubt that any plasminogen activator can distinguish from platelet–fibrin thrombi. While bleeding may also be promoted by systemic effects of hyperplasminaemia (Fig. 13.3), several lines of evidence suggest that dissolution of fibrin plugs is the most important mechanism of bleeding (Marder & Sherry 1988, Lowe & Douglas in press):

1. Streptokinase (marked systemic effects) and alteplase (less systemic effects) have similar risks of bleeding (Table 13.1).

2. Anticoagulant or defibrinogenating drugs, which do not digest haemostatic plugs, have lower risks of bleeding than thrombolytic therapy.

3. The relationship of anticoagulant effects (e.g. clotting times, fibrinogen level, levels of fibrin(ogen) degradation products) to bleeding is very poor.

4. In contrast, the effects of thrombolytic therapy on haemostatic plugs may be more important as a determinant of bleeding (Marder & Sherry 1988), and recently Gimple et al (1989) correlated prolongation of the skin bleeding time with clinical bleeding during alteplase therapy. The role of platelets in bleeding during and after thrombolytic therapy is further considered by Coller (1990) – see postscript to this chapter.

5. Bleeding after thrombolytic therapy is commonly due to vascular trauma, which is largely iatrogenic and must be minimized (Tables 13.3 and 13.4; Fig. 13.4). Useful guidelines for minimizing puncture site bleeding during and after thrombolytic therapy of acute myocardial infarction are given by de Bono (1989) and are summarized in Table 13.4.

In studies of myocardial infarction involving early angiography to determine coronary artery patency, bleeding occurred in 20-70% of patients following treatment with streptokinase or alteplase. In contrast, recent, larger studies not involving early angiography (GISSI 1986, ISIS-2 Collaborative Group 1988, Wilcox et al 1988, AIMS Study Group 1990, GISSI 1990, International Study Group 1990) had much lower incidences of bleeding (3–8%) following treatment with streptokinase, anistreplase or alteplase (de Bono 1989). This compares favourably with the incidence of bleeding of 1–3% in patients in the placebo groups of these studies (de Bono 1989), especially as in many patients in these studies thrombolytic therapy was given with aspirin and/or anticoagulant therapy, which increase the risk of post-thrombolytic bleeding. Major bleeds (e.g. intracranial haemorrhage or bleeds requiring transfusion) occur in less than 1% of patients receiving thrombolytic therapy for acute myocardial infarction (Cairns et al 1989, de Bono 1989, International Study Group 1990; Table 13.1). They are, however, outweighed by the beneficial effects of thrombolytic therapy on mortality: for every patient with a major bleed, between two and five patients will have their lives saved by thrombolytic therapy. Nevertheless, to optimize the ratio of benefit to risk, it is important to consider contraindications to thrombolytic therapy (Table 13.3) in all patients, and to weigh these against the anticipated benefit.

Bleeding may occur during thrombolytic therapy, but more commonly occurs in the succeeding hours, days or even weeks (Fig. 13.5). The addition of aspirin has little effect on bleeding risk (ISIS-2 Collaborative Group 1988), whereas the addition of heparin significantly increases the risk (Cairns et al 1989, GISSI-2 1990, International Study Group 1990). In the latter study, subcutaneous heparin increased the risk of major bleeds

Table 13.3   Some contraindications to thrombolytic therapy (see also National Institutes of Health Consensus Development Conference 1980, Cairns et al 1989, and manufacturer's data sheets). NB: many contraindications are relative rather than absolute; e.g. life-threatening PTE in a pregnant (or elderly) patient may well justify thrombolytic therapy despite the increased risk of placental (or intracranial) bleeds

---

Current or recent (6 months) internal bleeding or stroke

Known bleeding disorder	(e.g. thrombocytopenia, haemophilias, severe liver or kidney disease)
Possible aortic dissection } Acute pericarditis, oesophagitis }	NB: may mimic acute myocardial infarction or pulmonary embolism

Oesophageal varices

Active peptic ulcer, ulcerative colitis or gastrointestinal neoplasm; acute pancreatitis

Previous intracranial haemorrhage (at any time)

Severe arterial hypertension (risk of intracranial haemorrhage): systolic > 200 mmHg or diastolic > 120 mmHg

Haemorrhagic retinopathy (e.g. diabetic)

Bacterial endocarditis

Left heart thrombus (e.g. in mitral valve disease, atrial fibrillation: risk of thromboembolism)

Active genitourinary lesion

Active lung cavitation (e.g. tuberculous)

Active intracranial disease (e.g. neoplasm)

Recent (2–4 weeks):
 surgery or trauma (especially cranial or ocular)
 organ biopsy
 puncture of non-compressible vessels (e.g. subclavian)
 prolonged cardiopulmonary resuscitation
 abortion or obstetric delivery

Pregnancy (risk of retroplacental haemorrhage)

Age over 75 years

Contraindications to streptokinase or anistreplase
(consider alteplase or urokinase)

Known hypersensitivity

Recent streptococcal infection

Recent (6–12 months) treatment with either drug (unless clinical situation can await measurement of streptokinase resistance)

Table 13.4 Minimizing iatrogenic bleeding complications in thrombolytic therapy (with acknowledgements to de Bono 1989)

1   *Intramuscular injection sites*
    Avoid intramuscular injections: use intravenous or subcutaneous routes

2. *Peripheral venepuncture sites*
    Avoid multiple venepunctures. Use a large cannula in each arm, flushed with heparin–saline (one for blood sampling, and one for intravenous medication including thrombolytic drug, heparin etc.)

3   *Central venous access sites* (e.g. for central venous pressure measurements or temporary electrical pacing)
    Avoid subclavian vein (Fig. 13.4) if possible, which cannot be compressed. Use basilic vein in antecubital fossa; or jugular or femoral vein (if expert)

4. *Arterial puncture sites*
    Avoid if possible. If essential, seal during thrombolytic therapy by indwelling cannula, sheath or suture

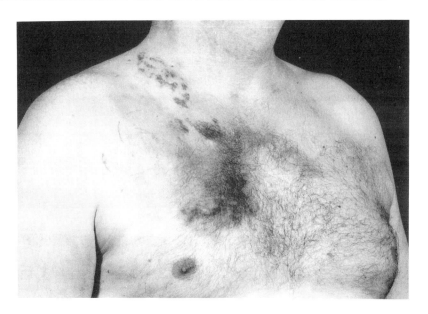

Fig. 13.4 Bruising following subclavian venous puncture for central venous access in a patient who had received thrombolytic therapy for acute myocardial infarction.

from 0.5% to 1% (relative risk 1.79; 95% CI 1.31–2.45), but did not affect the incidence of stroke or hospital mortality. As noted above, there are several subgroups of patients with acute myocardial infarction in whom heparin may be positively indicated as prophylaxis of mural or venous thromboembolism.

Bleeding may be iatrogenic (Table 13.4) or spontaneous. Spontaneous bleeding may be intracranial (Fig. 13.5), aortic or pericardial, retroperitoneal,

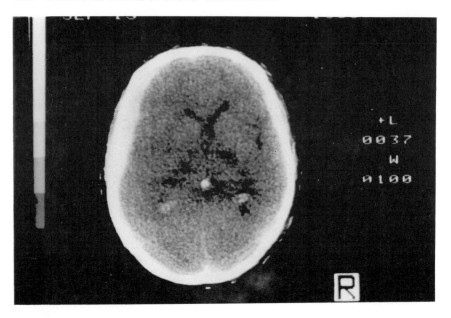

Fig. 13.5 CT brain scan showing subdural haematoma in a patient who received thrombolytic therapy for acute myocardial infarction, followed by anticoagulants and aspirin. Symptoms started more than a week after thrombolytic therapy.

or occur from the mouth, stomach, bowel, kidney or bladder or into the muscles or skin.

Intracranial bleeding. This is the most feared complication, and must be suspected in all patients with headache, vomiting, drowsiness or focal signs. Lumbar puncture should be avoided as it wastes time and carries a bleeding risk. Urgent management involves reversal of thrombolytic therapy, and neurosurgical consultation regarding CT brain scanning and evacuation of intracranial haematomas (Fig. 13.5). There is a dose–response relationship for alteplase and risk of intracranial bleeding, which is unacceptably high above a dose of 100 mg (or 1.5 mg/kg body weight) (Braunwald et al 1987). Furthermore, alteplase carries a higher risk of stroke than streptokinase (Table 13.1): this may reflect either its efficacy in digesting intracranial haemostatic plugs, or else its lesser effect in reducing the risk of thromboembolic stroke through systemic effects (Fig. 13.3). The importance of the latter effect is suggested by the findings of the ISIS-2 Collaborative Group (1988) that, compared to placebo, streptokinase reduced the incidence of non-haemorrhagic stroke, which outweighed the increased risk of haemorrhagic stroke, resulting in an overall decrease in total stroke incidence.

Aortic or pericardial bleeding. This can be lethal in patients whose chest pain is misdiagnosed as acute myocardial infarction, when it is in fact due to aortic dissection or pericarditis, which are contraindications to thrombolysis (Petch 1990). Diagnosis is by ultrasound.

Retroperitoneal bleeding. This may follow cardiac resuscitation or twisting movements of the trunk, and should be suspected in patients with pain in the abdomen, loin or shoulder tip, or unexplained hypotension or anaemia. Abdominal ultrasound, laparoscopy or paracentesis may reveal the bleeding and urgent surgical consultation is required.

Gastrointestinal bleeding. This may reflect previous peptic ulcer or acute stress ulceration. Active peptic ulcer or gastrointestinal bleeding in the past 6 months contraindicate thrombolysis; past history of ulcer or dyspepsia need not contraindicate therapy, but prophylactic H_2-antagonist drugs may be wise (de Bono 1989).

Haematuria. This is common, and if heavy or persistent merits intravenous urography and cystoscopy to exclude an underlying lesion.

Reversal of thrombolytic therapy. This may be indicated, either for serious bleeding or for urgent surgery. The infusion should be stopped: however, plasminogen activators which are highly fibrin-bound (e.g. alteplase) may continue to exert local lytic effects on fibrin haemostatic plugs for some hours. Circulating plasmin can be inhibited by infusions of the protease inhibitor aprotinin (500 000 units over 10 minutes, then 200 000 units over 4 hours) or by tranexamic acid (10 mg/kg, repeated if necessary after 6–8 hours), which blocks the binding of plasminogen to fibrin via its lysine binding sites. Administration of the latter drug carries an increased risk of arterial thrombosis (Lowe & Small 1988). If clotting times or fibrinogen concentration suggest substantial depletion of fibrinogen, administration of fresh frozen plasma may be indicated. Because this also replenishes plasma plasminogen, concurrent administration of tranexamic acid or aprotinin has been suggested (de Bono 1989).

Delivery of thrombolysis to patients with evolving myocardial infarction

Speedy thrombolysis is now the treatment of choice in suspected myocardial infarction (British Heart Foundation Working Group 1989): however, many patients do not receive it (Burrell et al 1990). To ensure optimal delivery of effective treatment will require improvements in public education about symptoms of evolving myocardial infarction; improvements in acute medical services in the population including education and training of general practitioners; evaluation in controlled studies of pre-hospital thrombolysis; and reorganization of coronary care units to maximize immediate assessment of potentially benefitting patients on hospital admission.

OTHER POSSIBLE INDICATIONS FOR THROMBOLYTIC TREATMENT

Clinicians prescribing thrombolytic therapy for evolving myocardial infarction do so in the knowledge that this treatment significantly reduces morbidity and mortality. Provided that they have weighed indications and contraindications (Table 13.3) appropriately, they may confidently defend their therapeutic decision either in court (should they face litigation as a result of a major complication such as a fatal bleed), or to a hospital manager (should they face challenge on use of expensive therapies). In contrast, clinicians are on softer ground in prescribing thrombolytic therapy in other clinical situations, because they cannot at present justify routine thrombolytic treatment by randomized controlled trials of adequate size which show clinical benefit (morbidity or mortality). They must ask themselves: do the unproven benefits justify the proven risks, as well as the cost? (I do not mean to sound pejorative against either physicians or thrombolytic therapy: after all, surgeons can perform an operation without the constraints of regulatory authorities or controlled trials.) The recently reported studies in acute myocardial infarction should perhaps inspire clinicians to enrol patients into similarly large, multicentre randomized controlled trials of acute management of other thrombotic diseases. Future reviewers may then be able to offer more confident guidance than the present author!

Unstable angina pectoris

Patients with unstable angina frequently have non-occlusive mural coronary thrombi overlying a fissured atheromatous plaque, and are at risk of complete thrombotic occlusion, myocardial infarction and sudden death. It is therefore logical to treat such patients with antithrombotic therapy (Gold 1989). Antiplatelet therapy with aspirin has a proven place in management, reducing the risks of myocardial infarction and death (Hennekens et al 1989). Heparin infusions also appear clinically effective (Theroux et al 1988, Neri Serneri et al 1990). While several studies of thrombolytic therapy in unstable angina have been performed, there is as yet no evidence that they are more effective than antiplatelet and/or anticoagulant therapy, which may be sufficient to inhibit further platelet–fibrin thrombosis in the coronary artery (Gold 1989, Neri Serneri et al 1990).

Peripheral arterial occlusion

Intravenous infusion of streptokinase in patients with peripheral arterial occlusion was initially reported by Fletcher et al (1959), and several series reported during the 1960s and 1970s reported reperfusion rates of about 50%. However, there was a high incidence of bleeding and mortality, especially from intracranial bleeding, hence systemic thrombolysis is now seldom used (Graor & Olin 1989, Martin 1989). Martin (1989) has advocated a high-dose, short-duration regimen (9 million units of streptokinase over 6 hours) which requires further study.

Local infusion of streptokinase into a thrombosed peripheral artery was initially reported from Glasgow Royal Infirmary (McNicol et al 1963) and later developed and popularized by Dotter et al (1974). The potential advantage of local infusion is that lower doses can be used, thus minimizing the risk of general bleeding: however, systemic effects are often observed in practice (Fig. 13.3), especially after reperfusion. While catheter-related bleeding is common, it can usually be controlled, and arteriography is usually indicated anyway to determine management of peripheral arterial thromboembolism. The recent success of thrombolysis in acute myocardial infarction, as well as the availability of newer thrombolytic agents, has stimulated renewed interest (Anonymous 1990), not only in acute thromboembolism of limb arteries (or thrombosed grafts) but also in subacute or chronic critical limb ischaemia, i.e. rest pain and/or skin necrosis of the foot. It is widely believed that lysable thrombus may be present for up to 12 months in the iliac arteries, up to 6 months in the superficial femoral artery, and up to 1 month in the crural arteries (Dormandy & Stock 1990, Krings & Peters 1990).

The selection of patients for local thrombolysis, as well as the practical aspects of treatment, have been reviewed recently (Graor & Olin 1989, Krings & Peters 1990, Martin 1989, Anonymous 1990). The usual contraindications to systemic thrombolysis should be considered (Table 13.3). In addition, thrombosed peripheral aneurysms and thrombosis of bypass grafts within 48 hours of surgery carry increased risks of bleeding, and surgical management may be preferred. Patients presenting with acute ischaemia which threatens limb viability within a few hours should be considered for whichever reopening procedure is most expeditious: this is again often surgery rather than thrombolytic therapy (Graor & Olin 1989).

There is no doubt that local thrombolytic therapy can restore limb arterial patency (Fig. 13.6). In a recent review of reported series, Graor & Olin (1989) found in pooled data 67% success in 474 infusions of streptokinase, 81% in 162 infusions of urokinase, and 90% in 105 infusions of alteplase. Major complications were reported in 19%, 12% and 9% of patients respectively in these treatment groups. This trend for benefit-to-risk ratios to increase with the newer thrombolytic drugs should, however, be interpreted cautiously, because there is a lack of randomized controlled trials (Graor & Olin 1989). Further studies are required to establish the clinical benefits and risks of thrombolytic drugs compared to other treatments of peripheral arterial thrombosis, but in the meantime the results are promising, and thrombolysis has a role in treatment of selected patients, with close cooperation between surgeons, radiologists and angiologists (Anonymous 1990).

Stroke

The success story of thrombolysis in myocardial infarction and the development of new plasminogen activators has also renewed interest in thrombolytic treatment of acute thromboembolic stroke. Thromboembolism

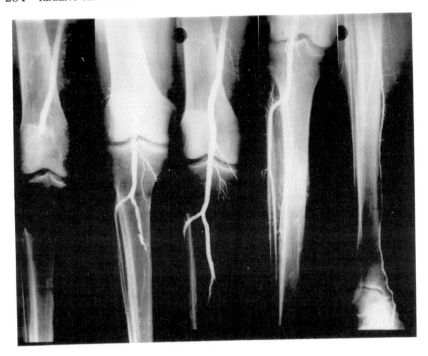

Fig. 13.6 Serial angiograms showing progressive reperfusion following local infusion of streptokinase in a patient with recent peripheral arterial thromboembolism. (Reproduced with kind permission of Drs A Reid, D Reid and J G Pollock.)

accounts for 80–85% of acute strokes, for which there is no proven specific treatment. Several studies of streptokinase, urokinase or alteplase are currently in progress (Sloan et al 1989, Anonymous 1990). While promising results have been shown in some studies (especially for patients with several vertebrobasilar occlusion, who have a poor prognosis), there remain many problems. These include the need for rapid hospital admission of patients with evolving thrombotic stroke and diagnosis by CT brain scanning; the risk of intracranial bleeding; and the development in some patients of fatal cerebral oedema, possibly due to reperfusion injury (Koudstaal et al 1988). At present, therefore, the use of thrombolytic therapy in stroke remains experimental.

Venous thromboembolism

A National Institutes of Health Consensus Development Conference (1980) recommended that thrombolytic therapy be considered more frequently by clinicians treating patients with venous thromboembolism. However, in a recent report from the Second American College of Chest Physicians Conference on Antithrombotic Therapy, Hyers et al (1989) concluded: 'The use of thrombolytic agents in the treatment of venous thromboembolism continues to be highly individualized. Further clinical investigation is needed before more definite recommendations can be made.'

There is no doubt that thrombolytic therapy increases the occurrence and extent of lysis of both deep vein thrombosis and pulmonary embolism, compared to conventional anticoagulant therapy (heparin and oral anticoagulants). In a pooled analysis of the six properly randomized trials of streptokinase versus heparin for initial treatment of deep vein thrombosis, Goldhaber et al (1984) found that patients receiving streptokinase achieved significant angiographic lysis 3.7 times more often than patients receiving heparin (95% CI 2.5–5.7; $p<0.0001$). Similar rates of angiographic lysis in deep vein thrombosis to streptokinase have also been reported for urokinase (National Institutes of Health Consensus Development Conference 1980) and for alteplase (Turpie 1989). In the Urokinase Pulmonary Embolism Trial (1973), patients randomized to urokinase showed significantly greater angiographic and haemodynamic improvement than patients randomized to heparin, after 24 hours of treatment. Similar rates of angiographic and haemodynamic improvement in pulmonary embolism to urokinase have also been reported for streptokinase, anistreplase and alteplase (Meyer et al 1989).

Why then is the use of thrombolytic therapy controversial? Firstly, the increased rates of *angiographic* lysis have not been shown in large controlled trials to result in significant *clinical* benefit (morbidity or mortality). Whether or not thrombolytic therapy of deep vein thrombosis prevents the chronic post-thrombotic syndrome of leg pains, swelling and ulceration is unclear (Browse et al 1988, Hyers et al 1989, Turpie 1989). In the Urokinase Pulmonary Embolism Trial (1973), the difference in haemodynamic improvement between urokinase and heparin at 24 hours was not sustained after a few days; and in general, trials of thrombolytic therapy in acute pulmonary embolism have been of insufficient size to establish whether or not it reduces mortality (Hyers et al 1989, Meyer et al 1989). Furthermore there is little evidence that the initial treatment of pulmonary embolism has any influence on long-term prognosis (Meyer et al 1989).

Secondly, thrombolytic therapy carries a higher risk of bleeding than conventional treatment of venous thromboembolism with heparin and oral anticoagulants (Goldhaber et al 1984, Fennerty et al 1989, Meyer et al 1989, Turpie 1989). In deep vein thrombosis, the incidence of major bleeding is about threefold higher with thrombolytic therapy compared to heparin therapy (Goldhaber et al 1984, Fennerty et al 1989). The incidence of major bleeds in patients with pulmonary embolism treated with thrombolytic therapy following diagnostic pulmonary angiography is even higher (over 20%) and is related to invasive procedures (angiography, arterial punctures for blood gas estimations), which should therefore be minimized (Fennerty et al 1989; Table 13.4). At present, there is little evidence that bleeding complications are less with newer agents (anistreplase, alteplase) than with older drugs (streptokinase, urokinase).

Many clinicians therefore feel that in most cases of deep vein thrombosis or pulmonary embolism anticoagulant therapy is adequate, and that the additional bleeding risks of thrombolytic therapy, as well as the other complications (Table 13.2) and the cost, are not justified in the absence of demonstrable clinical benefit in randomized controlled trials. However, thrombolytic therapy is more often used in the minority of patients with severe clinical symptoms due to massive thromboembolism which threatens life or limb, e.g. impending venous gangrene (phlegmasia dolens) or massive pulmonary embolism with haemodynamic instability. The case for consideration of thrombolytic therapy in such patients, provided that they have little or no contraindications (Table 13.4) is logical and reasonable, and many clinicians have been impressed by the clinical response to thrombolysis in individual patients. Because of the rarity of such patients, as well as the differences in diagnostic and therapeutic facilities and management policies between hospitals, the performance of large randomized controlled trials of thrombolysis appears difficult (but perhaps not impossible in view of the enthusiastic recruitment of patients in recent large, multicentre studies of thrombolysis in acute myocardial infarction). Furthermore, in such patients thrombolytic therapy has to compete not only with conventional anticoagulant therapy, but also with surgery (venous thrombectomy for impending venous gangrene, and pulmonary embolectomy for unstable, massive pulmonary embolism), which is also controversial (Browse et al 1988, Kwaan & Samama 1989, Meyer et al 1989). The final choice of treatment may well depend therefore on local expertise and facilities (e.g. availability of venography, lung scanning, pulmonary arteriography, intensive care, vascular surgeons, cardiothoracic surgeons, and distance from referral centres). For fuller discussions of the place of thrombolytic therapy in management of venous thromboembolism, the reader is referred to recent reviews (Browse et al 1988, Marder & Sherry 1988, Hyers et al 1989, Kwaan & Samama 1989, Meyer et al 1989, Turpie 1989). Its place in the treatment of rarer forms of venous thrombosis (retinal, visceral, superior vena caval) has been reviewed recently in Kwaan & Samama (1989).

Laboratory monitoring of thrombolytic therapy in venous thromboembolism is summarized in Table 13.5. While it is important to exclude baseline haemostatic defects, and to determine whether or not a systemic thrombolytic effect is occurring early in treatment (particularly with streptokinase and anistreplase, because of the wide variation in levels of anti-streptococcal antibodies), there is little evidence that either efficacy of thrombolysis, or risk of bleeding, is associated with laboratory test results (Marder & Sherry 1988, Lowe & Douglas in press). Frequent monitoring of the systemic anticoagulant effects after cessation of thrombolytic therapy is required (e.g. with the APTT and/or thrombin time), to determine the time of initiation of maintenance heparin therapy. This is important following thrombolytic therapy to prevent rethrombosis by fibrin, which may be poorly lysable because of its low plasminogen content.

Table 13.5 Guidelines for monitoring of sustained thrombolytic therapy with streptokinase or urokinase (e.g. for peripheral arterial occlusion, deep vein thrombosis, pulmonary embolism) (see also National Institutes of Health Consensus Development Conference 1980, Marder & Sherry 1988, Lowe & Douglas in press)

---

1 *Patent selection*
Confirm recent, potentially lysable thrombus by objective test

Carefully evaluate potential benefit of thrombolysis against contraindications (Table 13.3)

Minimize iatrogenic bleeding (Table 13.4)

2. *Baseline haemostatic screen*
Haematocrit or haemoglobin, platelet count

APTT, prothrombin time, thrombin time

Save plasma for fibrinogen, fibrin degradation products, euglobulin clot lysis time and streptokinase resistance test if required

Save serum for blood group and cross-match

3. *Initiate thrombolytic treatment with standard dose*

4. *Establish systemic fibrinolytic state (2–4 hours)* Repeat thrombin time (most sensitive) and/or APTT

If no lytic state (less than 1.5 times baseline):
measure fibrinogen, FDP, ECLT (pre- and post-treatment) ± streptokinase resistance test
consider $\left\{\begin{array}{l}\text{(repetition of tests after short interval}\\ \text{(increasing dose}\\ \text{(changing thrombolytic agent}\\ \text{(stopping thrombolytic therapy}\end{array}\right.$

5. *After cessation of thrombolytic therapy*
Monitor thrombin time and/or APTT

Do not start heparin until less than twice control value

REFERENCES

AIMS Trial Study Group 1990 Long-term effects of intravenous anistreplase in acute myocardial infarction: final report of the AIMS study. Lancet 335: 427–431
Anonymous 1989 Reperfusion injury after thrombolytic therapy for acute myocardial infarction. Lancet 2: 655–657
Anonymous 1990 Non-coronary thrombolysis. Lancet 335: 691–693
Braunwald E, Knatterud G L, Passamani E et al 1987 Update from the Thrombolysis in Myocardial Infarction Trial (Letter). J Am Coll Cardiol 10: 970
British Heart Foundation Working Group 1989 Role of the general practitioner in managing patients with myocardial infarction: impact of thrombolytic treatment. Br Med J 299: 555–557
Browse N L, Burnand K G, Lea Thomas M L 1988 Diseases of the veins: pathology, diagnosis and treatment. Edward Arnold, London
Burrell C J, Skehan V D, Cowley M L et al 1990 Districts' use of thrombolytic agents. Br Med J 300: 237–238
Cairns J A, Collins R, Fuster V et al 1989 Coronary thrombolysis. Chest 95(suppl): 73S–87S
Chesebro J H, Knatterud G, Roberts R et al 1987 Thrombolysis in myocardial infarction (TIMI) trial, phase I: a comparison between intravenous tissue plasminogen activator and intravenous streptokinase. Circulation 76: 142–154

Coller B S 1990 Platelets and thrombolytic therapy. N Engl J Med 322: 33–42

Davies M J 1989 Thrombosis and coronary atherosclerosis. In: Julian D, Kübler W, Norris R M, Swan H J C, Collen D, Verstraete M (eds) Thrombolysis in cardiovascular disease. Marcel Dekker, Basel, pp 25–43

Davies M J, Fulton W F M, Robertson W B 1979 The relation of coronary thrombus to ischaemic myocardial necrosis. J Pathol 127: 99–110

de Bono D 1989 Problems in thrombolysis. In: Julian D, Kübler W, Norris R M, Swan H J C, Collen D, Verstraete M (eds) Thrombolysis in cardiovascular disease. Marcel Dekker, Basel, pp 279–292

De Wood M A 1989 Coronary thrombosis and myocardial necrosis. In: Julian D, Kübler W, Norris R M, Swan H J C, Collen D, Verstraete M (eds) Thrombolysis in cardiovascular disease. Marcel Dekker, Basel, pp 1–24

De Wood M A, Spores J, Notske R et al 1980 Prevalence of total coronary occlusion during the early hours of transmural myocardial infarction. N Engl J Med 303: 897–902

Dormandy J A, Stock G (eds) 1990 Critical limb ischaemia: its pathophysiology and management. Springer-Verlag, Berlin

Dotter C T, Rosch J, Seamen A J 1974 Selective clot lysis with low dose streptokinase. Radiology 111: 31–37

European Collaborative Study Group 1979 Streptokinase in acute myocardial infarction. N Engl J Med 301: 797–802

European Working Party 1971 Streptokinase in recent myocardial infarction: a controlled multicentre trial. Br Med J 3: 325–331

Falk E 1983 Plaque rupture with severe pre-existing stenosis precipitating coronary thrombosis: characteristics of coronary atherosclerotic plaques underlying fatal occlusive thrombi. Br Heart J 50: 127–134

Fennerty A G, Levine M N, Hirsh K 1989 Haemorrhagic complications of thrombolytic therapy in the treatment of myocardial infarction and venous thromboembolism. Chest 95(suppl): 88S–97S

Fletcher A P, Sherry S, Alkjaersig N et al 1959 Maintenance of a sustained thrombolytic state in man. II. Clinical observations on patients with myocardial infarction and other thromboembolic disorders. J Clin Invest 38: 1111–1119

Fuster V, Israel D, Badimon L et al 1989 Coronary artery disease: role of antithrombotic therapy. In: Kwaan H C, Samama M M (eds) Clinical thrombosis. CRC Press, Boca Raton, FL, pp 151–179

Gimple L W, Gold H K, Leinbach R C et al 1989 Correlation between template bleeding times and spontaneous bleeding during treatment of acute myocardial infarction with recombinant tissue-type plasminogen activator. Circulation 80: 581–588

GISSI (Gruppo Italiano per Lo Studio della Streptochinasi nell' Infarto Miocardio) 1986 Effectiveness of intravenous thrombolytic treatment in acute myocardial infarction. Lancet 1: 397–402

GISSI (Gruppo Italiano per Lo Studio della Sopravvivenza nell' Infarto Miocardio) 1990 GISSI-2: a factorial randomised trial of alteplase versus streptokinase and heparin versus no heparin among 12,490 patients with acute myocardial infarction. Lancet 336: 65–71

Gold H K 1989 Thrombolysis in patients with unstable angina pectoris. In: Julian D, Kübler W, Norris R M, Swan H J C, Collen D, Verstraete M (eds) Thrombolysis in cardiovascular disease. Marcel Dekker, Basel, pp 325–335

Goldberg S, Greenspoon A J, Urban P L et al 1983 Reperfusion arrhythmia: a marker for restoration of antegrade flow during intracoronary thrombolysis for acute myocardial infarction. Am Heart J: 105–132

Goldhaber S Z, Buring J E, Lipnick R J et al 1984 Pooled analyses of randomized trials of streptokinase and heparin in phlebographically documented acute deep venous thrombosis. Am J Med 76: 393–397

Graor R A, Olin J W 1989 Regional thrombolysis in peripheral arterial occlusions. In: Julian D, Kübler W, Norris R M, Swan H J C, Collen D, Verstraete M (eds) Thrombolysis in cardiovascular disease. Marcel Dekker, Basel, pp 381–395

Habbab M A, Haft J I 1986 Heparin resistance induced by intravenous nitroglycerin. Circulation 74(suppl II): II-321 (Abstract)

Hackett D, Davies G, Chierchia S, Maseri A 1987 Intermittent coronary occlusion in acute myocardial infarction. N Engl J Med 317: 1055–1059

Hampton J R 1989 Thrombolytic treatment and survival rates of patients with acute myocardial infarction. In: Julian D, Kübler W, Norris R M, Swan H J C, Collen D, Verstraete M (eds) Thrombolysis in cardiovascular disease. Marcel Dekker, Basel, pp 163–177

Harrison D G, Ferguson D W, Collins S M et al 1984 Rethrombosis after reperfusion with streptokinase: importance of geometry of residual lesions. Circulation 69: 991–999

Hennekens C H, Buring J E, Sandercock P, Collins R, Peto R 1989 Aspirin and other antiplatelet agents in the secondary and primary prevention of cardiovascular disease. Circulation 80: 749–756

Heras M, Chesebro J H, Thompson P L et al 1989 Prevention of early and late rethrombosis and further strategies after coronary reperfusion. In: Julian D, Kübler W, Norris R M, Swan H J C, Collen D, Verstraete M (eds) Thrombolysis in cardiovascular disease. Marcel Dekker, Basel pp 203–229

Herrick J B 1912 Clinical features of sudden obstruction of the coronary arteries. JAMA 59: 2015–2020

Hossmann V, Mertens E, Auel H, Valdivieso E, Burkhardt W 1990 Haemostasiology and haemorrheology in acute myocardial infarction treated by heparin, streptokinase and ancrod. Blut 60: 130

Hyers T M, Hull R D, Weg J G 1989 Antithrombotic therapy for venous thromboembolic disease. Chest 95(suppl): 37S–51S

International Study Group 1990 In-hospital mortality and clinical course of 20,891 patients with suspected acute myocardial infarction randomised between alteplase and streptokinase with or without heparin. Lancet 336: 71–75

ISAM Study Group 1986 A prospective trial of intravenous streptokinase in acute myocardial infarction (ISAM). N Engl J Med 314: 1465–1471

ISIS-2 (Second International Study of Infarct Survival) Collaborative Group 1988 Randomised trial of intravenous streptokinase, oral aspirin, both, or neither among 17, 187 cases of suspected acute myocardial infarction: ISIS-2. Lancet 2: 349–360

Jalihal S, Morris G K 1990 Antistreptokinase titres after intravenous streptokinase. Lancet 335: 184–185

Koudstaal P J, Stibbe J, Vermeulen M 1988 Fatal ischaemic brain oedema after early thrombolysis with tissue plasminogen activator in acute stroke. Br Med J 297: 1571–1574

Krings W, Peters P 1990 Percutaneous opening procedures. In: Dormandy J, Stock G (eds) Critical leg ischaemia: its pathophysiology and management. Springer-Verlag, Berlin, pp 53–68

Kwaan H C, Samama M M (eds) 1989 Clinical thrombosis. CRC Press, Boca Raton, FL

Lowe G D O, Douglas J T (in press) Haematological aspects of thrombosis and thrombolysis. In: Hillis W S, Dunn F (eds) Thrombolytic therapy in acute myocardial infarction. MTM Press, Lancaster

Lowe, G D O, Small M 1988 Stimulation of endogenous fibrinolysis. In: Kluft C (ed) Tissue-type plasminogen activator (t-PA): physiology and clinical importance, vol II. CRC Press, Boca Raton, FL, pp 129–169

Lucchesi B 1989 Synergistic mechanisms for limitation of infarct size during thrombolysis: reduction of myocardial demand, metabolic support, and prevention of reperfusion injury. In: Julian D, Kübler W, Norris R M, Swan H J C, Collen D, Verstraete M (eds) Thrombolysis in cardiovascular disease. Marcel Dekker, Basel, pp 203–229

Marder V J, Sherry S 1988 Thrombolytic therapy: current status. N Engl J Med 318: 1512–1520, 1585–1595

Martin M M 1989 Peripheral arterial thromboembolic disorders. In: Kwaan H C, Samama M M (eds) Clinical thrombosis. CRC Press, Boca Raton, FL, pp 181–205

Mauri F, De Biase A M, Franzosi M G et al 1987 In-hospital causes of death in the patients admitted to the GISSI study. G Ital Cardiol 17: 37–44

McNicol G P, Reid W, Bain W H et al 1963 Treatment of peripheral arterial occlusion by streptokinase perfusion. Br Med J 1: 1508–1509

Merz W, Betge C, Effert S, von Essen R, Dörr R, Schmid-Schönbein H 1981 Supraselective fibrinolysis in acute myocardial infarction. Bibl Haematol 47: 205–212

Meyer G, Charbonnier B, Stern M et al 1989 Thrombolysis in acute pulmonary embolism. In: Julian D, Kübler W, Norris R M, Swan H J C, Collen D, Verstraete M (eds) Thrombolysis in cardiovascular disease. Marcel Dekker, Basel, pp 337–360

Moroz L A 1977 Increased blood fibrinolytic activity after aspirin ingestion. N Engl J Med 296: 525–529

National Institutes of Health Consensus Development Conference 1980 Thrombolytic therapy in thrombosis. Ann Intern Med 93: 141–144

Neri Serneri G G, Gensini G F, Poggesi L et al 1990 Effect of heparin, aspirin, or alteplase in reduction of myocardial ischaemia in refractory unstable angina. Lancet 335: 615–618

O'Brien J R 1990 Shear-induced platelet aggregation. Lancet 335: 711–713

Passamani E, Hodges M, Herman M et al 1987 The thrombolysis in myocardial infarction (TIMI) phase II pilot study: tissue plasminogen activator followed by percutaneous transluminal coronary angioplasty. J Am Coll Cardiol 10: 51B–64B

Payne S T, Hosker H S R, Allen M B et al 1989 Transient impairment of renal function after streptokinase therapy. Lancet 2: 1398

Petch M C 1990 Dangers of thrombolysis. Br Med J 300: 483–484

PRIMI Trial Study Group 1989 Randomised double-blind trial of recombinant pro-urokinase against streptokinase in acute myocardial infarction. Lancet 1: 863–868

Rapaport E 1989 Thrombolytic agents in acute myocardial infarction. N Engl J Med 320: 861–864

Rentrop P, Blanke H, Karsch K R et al 1981 Selective intracoronary thrombolysis in acute myocardial infarction and unstable angina. Circulation 63: 307–317

Ross A M, Hoia J, Hamilton W et al 1990 Heparin versus aspirin after recombinant tissue plasminogen activator and early intravenous heparin in acute myocardial infarction: a randomised trial. J Am Coll Cardiol 15(suppl A): 64A (Abstract)

Schroeder R, Biamino G, Leitner E R et al 1983 Intravenous short-term infusion of streptokinase in acute myocardial infarction. Circulation 67: 536–548

Simoons M L, Serruys P W, Brand M et al 1985 Improved survival after early thrombolysis in acute myocardial infarction. Lancet 2: 578–581

Simoons M L, Arnold A E R, Betrui A et al 1988 Thrombolysis with tissue plasminogen activator in acute myocardial infarction: no additional benefit from immediate percutaneous coronary angioplasty. Lancet 1: 197–203

Six A J, Louwerenburg J W, Braams R et al 1988 Early results of a randomized, double-blind, dose-ranging study of intravenous streptokinase for acute myocardial infarction. In: Kakkar V V, Kennedy J W, Mettinger K L (eds) Coronary thrombolysis. Current Medical Literature, London, pp 18–23

Sloan M A, del Zoppo G J, Brott T G 1989 Thrombolysis and stroke. In: Julian D, Kübler W, Norris R M, Swan H J C, Collen D, Verstraete M (eds) Thrombolysis in cardiovascular disease. Marcel Dekker, Basel, pp 361–380

Stafford P J, Strachan C J L, Vincent R et al 1989 Multiple microemboli after disintegration of clot during thrombolysis for acute myocardial infarction. Br Med J 299: 1310–1312

Theiss W, Volger E, Wirtzfeld A et al 1980 Coagulation studies and rheological measurements during streptokinase treatment of myocardial infarction. Klin Wochenschr 58: 607–615

Theroux P, Ouimet H, McCans J et al 1988 Aspirin, heparin or both to treat acute unstable angina? N Engl J Med 319: 1105–1111

TIMI Study Group 1989 Comparison of invasive and conservative strategies after treatment with intravenous plasminogen activator in acute myocardial infarction: results of the thrombolysis in myocardial infarction (TIMI) phase II trial. N Engl J Med 320: 618–627

Topol E J, Califf R M, George B S et al 1987 A randomised trial of immediate versus delayed elective angioplasty after intravenous tissue plasminogen activator in acute myocardial infarction. N Engl J Med 317: 581–588

Turpie A G G 1989 Thrombolysis in deep vein thrombosis. In: Julian D, Kübler W, Norris R M, Swan H J C, Collen D, Verstraete M (eds) Thrombolysis in cardiovascular disease. Marcel Dekker, Basel, pp 397–408

Urokinase Pulmonary Embolism Trial 1973 A national cooperative study. Circulation 47(suppl 2): 1–108

Verstraete M, Bernard R, Bory M et al 1985 Randomised trial of intravenous recombinant tissue-type plasminogen activator versus intravenous streptokinase in acute myocardial infarction. Lancet 1: 842–847

White H D, Norris R M 1989 Left ventricular function in patients with myocardial infarction treated with intracoronary or systemic thrombolysis. In: Julian D, Kübler W, Norris R M, Swan H J C, Collen D, Verstraete M (eds) Thrombolysis in cardiovascular disease. Marcel Dekker, Basel, pp 129–139

Wilcox R G, Olsson C G, Skene A M et al 1988 Trial of tissue plasminogen activator for mortality reduction in acute myocardial infarction (ASSET). Lancet 2: 525–530

Yusuf S, Collins R, Peto R et al 1985a Intravenous and intracoronary fibrinolytic therapy in acute myocardial infarction: overview of results on mortality, reinfarction and side effects from 33 randomised controlled trials. Eur Heart J 6: 556–585

Yusuf S, Peto R, Lewis J et al 1985b Beta blockade during and after myocardial infarction: an overview of the randomized trials. Prog Cardiovasc Dis 27: 335–371

14

Reviews of some key papers published in 1989/1990

1. Characterization of a thrombin clearance site mutation in the factor VIII gene

Arai M, Higuchi M, Antonarakis S E, Kazazian H H Jr, Philips J A III, Janco R L, Hoyer L W 1990 Characterization of a thrombin cleavage site mutation (Arg$_{1689}$ to Cys) in the factor VIII gene of two unrelated patients with cross-reacting material-positive haemophilia A. Blood 75: 384–389

The identification of the molecular defect responsible for haemophilia A was reported for two unrelated patients with the cross-reacting material (CRM)-positive form of the disorder. It was found that the immunopurified dysfunctional factor VIII was resistant to cleavage by thrombin at Arg$_{1689}$ in the 80-kDa light chain, and a single base substitution (arginine to cysteine) was found at amino acid residue 1689. The dysfunctional factor VIII was designated 'factor VIII–East Hartford'.

Comment
The cofactor function of factor VIII in the activation of factor X by factor IXa requires proteolytic modification of the factor VIII molecule. Cleavage of both the heavy chain (at Arg$_{372}$) and the light chain (at Arg$_{1689}$) are critical for the activation of factor VIII (p. 3).

Non-functional, immunoreactive factor VIII-like protein at levels comparable to those in normal plasma is seen in around 10% of plasmas from patients with haemophilia A, termed CRM-positive. The molecular abnormality of the non-functional factor VIII protein has been addressed in this and a previous study from the same group (Arai et al 1989) which described a haemophilic patient with CRM-positive plasma whose molecular defect was identified as residing at Arg$_{372}$ in the heavy chain region of factor VIII. Between these two studies three of the 12 CRM-positive plasmas tested have had a mutation, either at Arg$_{372}$ or Arg$_{1689}$, resulting in impaired cleavage and activation by thrombin.

REFERENCE

Arai M, Inaba H, Higuchi M et al 1989 Direct characterization of factor VIII in plasma:

detection of a mutation altering a thrombin cleavage site (arginine-372 to histidine). Proc Natl Acad Sci USA 86: 4277–4281

D.O., B.B.

2. Congenital antithrombin III deficiency

Bauer K A, Rosenberg R D 1989 Congenital antithrombin III deficiency: insights into the pathogenesis of the hypercoaguable state and its management using markers of haemostatic system activation. Am J Med 87(suppl 3b): 39S–43S

The authors hypothesize that small amounts of factor Xa as well as factor Va are continuously formed within the vascular system. These activated clotting factors are components of the prothrombinase complex at the platelet membrane surface. The formation of the prothrombinase complex and also the action of thrombin is opposed by two regulatory systems. These are the endogenous heparan sulphate–antithrombin III and protein C–thrombomodulin mechanisms. Although the enzymes generated by the coagulation cascade cannot be quantified directly, Rosenberg and his colleagues developed a sensitive and specific radioimmunoassay for F_{1+2} that measures the in vivo cleavage of prothrombin by activated factor X.

In this report the investigators have studied the biochemical alterations in the haemostatic mechanism that occur in individuals with familial antithrombin III deficiency. Radioimmunoassays for the prothrombin activation fragment F_{1+2} and fibrinopeptide A were determined in blood samples of 22 asymptomatic individuals from eight separate kindreds with familial antithrombin III deficiency. None of these were receiving oral anticoagulants. Plasma F_{1+2} was significantly elevated in almost all patients with the disorder whereas the concentration of fibrinopeptide A was normal. They also showed that following an infusion of purified antithrombin III concentrate into several affected individuals there was a decrease in the abnormally high concentration of F_{1+2}. The data obtained from this study allowed the investigators to design programmes of daily and weekly antithrombin III infusions to maintain plasma F_{1+2} levels in the normal range.

Rosenberg also evaluated the effects of warfarin on plasma F_{1+2} levels in patients with familial antithrombin deficiency who were receiving long-term oral anticoagulant therapy. At equivalent levels of intensity of oral anticoagulation the mean plasma F_{1+2} levels in patients with antithrombin III deficiency were significantly greater than those of a group of anticoagulated individuals without an inherited thrombotic disorder. The authors speculate that the apparent resistance to warfarin is a consequence of an augmented effect of the drug on the protein C anticoagulant mechanism.

REFERENCES

Bauer K A, Goodman T L, Kass B L, Rosenberg R D 1985 Elevated factor Xa activity in the blood of asymptomatic patients with congenital antithrombin deficiency. J Clin Invest 76: 826–836

Conway E M, Bauer K A, Barzegar S, Rosenberg R D 1987 Suppression of hemostatic system activation by oral anticoagulants in the blood of patients with thrombotic diathyses. J Clin Invest 80: 1535–1544

M.G., F.E.P.

3. Very low doses of warfarin can prevent thrombosis in central venous catheters

Bern M, Lokich J, Wallach S, Bothe A, Benotti P, Arkin C, Greco F, Huberman M, Moore C 1990 Very low doses of warfarin can prevent thrombosis in central venous catheters. Ann Intern Med 112: 423–428

The goal of this study was to determine if very low doses of warfarin might be useful prophylaxis for thrombosis in patients with long-duration central venous catheters. Patients at risk for thrombosis associated with long-term indwelling central venous catheters were assigned in a prospective, random fashion to either 1 mg of warfarin or no warfarin beginning 3 days before catheter insertion and continuing for 90 days. Placebo was not used in the untreated group. Venograms were performed for symptoms or at the end of the study. Eighty-two of the 121 patients who entered the study, finished the study. Four of the 42 patients in the warfarin-treated group had venogram-proven thrombosis compared with 15 of 40 patients in the control group ($p<0.001$). The authors report there were no measurable changes in a variety of coagulation assays.

This study demonstrates an objectively documented improvement in the occurrence of catheter thrombosis. This effect was highly significant and suggests that very low dose warfarin exerts a protective effect even in the absence of changes in the traditional coagulation assays. However, the study would have been strengthened by the use of a placebo in the untreated group since the trigger for early venograms was subjective (e.g. symptoms).

The lack of a measurable effect on the haemostatic system is intriguing and leads to speculation about the utility of monitoring assays and the mechanism of the antithrombotic effect. The traditional view of oral anti-coagulant therapy has been that the levels of vitamin K-dependent proteins must be sufficiently depressed to prolong the prothrombin time to varying degrees. The implication of this view is that the anticoagulant effect requires a lowering of the levels of the procoagulant proteins. Such a lowering effect was not observed and leads one to conjecture whether the combined effect of low levels of abnormal des-carboxy vitamin K-dependent coagulation proteins at multiple levels in the haemostatic mechanism might not inhibit clot formation. The mechanism remains unclear but alternative monitoring strategies can be considered. Three promising monitoring strategies are: (1) the immunochemical assays of normal and functionally distinct des-carboxy isomers of vitamin K-dependent zymogens; (2) immunochemical assays of inhibition of the ongoing level of activation of the haemostatic system (e.g. prothrombin fragment 1.2 and thrombin–antithrombin complex levels); and (3) the measurement of vitamin K metabolites. All of these approaches are presently under investigation.

J.A.S., E.G.B., K.G.M.

4. The role of platelets in thrombolytic therapy

Coller B S 1990 Platelets and thrombolytic therapy. N Engl J Med 322: 33–42

This article reviews the increasing evidence that platelets play an important role in both delaying reperfusion and promoting reocclusion after thrombolytic therapy; and in contributing to the bleeding complications. A review of platelet physiology and pathology is followed by a summary of the complex reciprocal relationships between platelets and fibrinolysis. Animal studies are then reviewed, which in general support the hypotheses that the platelet component of coronary thrombi is resistant to fibrinolysis, and that platelets are important mediators of reocclusion. The clinical benefit of aspirin in the ISIS-2 study is noted, and animal studies of thromboxane synthase inhibitors, thromboxane receptor antagonists, cyclic AMP stimulators, and GPIIb/IIIa receptor blockers are reviewed. Clinical studies of such compounds are now in progress: however, they should be cautious because evidence that platelet dysfunction contributes to bleeding after thrombolytic therapy is also noted.

G.D.O.L.

5. Plasma cofactor necessary for the binding of 'antiphospholipid' antibodies to negatively-charged phospholipid

Galli M, Comfurius P, Maassen C, Hemker H C, de Baets M H, van Breda-Vriesman P J C, Barbui T, Zwaal R F A, Bevers E M 1990 Anticardiolipin antibodies are directed not to cardiolipin but to a plasma protein cofactor. Lancet 335: 1544–1547

In this important paper the authors describe a plasma cofactor necessary for the binding of apparent 'antiphospholipid' antibodies (APA) to negatively charged phospholipid. This provides a possible link between the presence of 'APA' and thrombotic events as well as an explanation for earlier observations that LA activity may occasionally be enhanced when normal plasma is added.

Anticardiolipin antibodies (ACA) were purified from two subjects with a history of thrombosis, using liposomes composed of cardiolipin, phosphatidyl choline and cholesterol. After organic solvent treatment to dissolve the lipids, IgG ACA was separated on a protein A-sepharose column.

These IgG ACA bound strongly to cardiolipin in an ELISA but only in the presence of plasma or serum. Binding to cardiolipin-containing liposomes was also dependent on the presence of a plasma component.

Using these observations a modified ELISA was developed where dilutions of pooled plasma were substituted for bovine serum. In this way the ACA-cofactor could be quantified.

The cofactor was found to be resistant to heat (10 minutes at 90°C) but sensitive to tryptic digestion. It appears to consist of 50-kD polypeptide which increased to 70-kD on reduction. It exhibits calcium-independent binding to negatively charged phospholipids and preliminary work suggests that it interferes with the binding of factor Xa/Va leading to a diminished rate of thrombin formation. It could, then, be a natural anticoagulant and the authors speculate that it may in fact be B_2-glycoprotein I, also known as apolipoprotein H, which is also thought to have anticoagulant properties.

This work is strengthened by that of McNeil et al (1990), who have come to similar conclusions on the presence of a plasma cofactor based on different experimental techniques. The exact nature of the cofactor remains controversial, however.

These discoveries may well alter the approach for screening for so-called antiphospholipid antibodies. The development of specific assays for the polypeptide cofactor can now be developed and the application of these may well result in an increase in our understanding of immune mechanisms in thrombosis.

REFERENCE

McNeil H P, Chesterman C N, Krilis S A 1990 Antiphospholipid antibodies are directed against a complex antigen which includes a lipid-binding plasma glycoprotein. Clin Exp Rheumatol 8: 209

M.G., F.E.P.

6. CpG mutational hotspots

Green P M, Montandon A J, Bentley D R, Ljung R, Nilsson I M, Giannelli F 1990 The incidence and distribution of CpG→TpG transitions in the coagulation factor IX gene: a fresh look at CpG mutational hotspots. Nucl Acids Res 18: 3227–3231

A large part of human genetic disease apparently arises from the deamination of cytosine residues in methylated CpG dinucleotides. The CpG dinucleotide is the preferred site for cytosine methylation in higher eukaryotes and 5-methylcytosine (MeC) is prone to mutate to thymidine by deamination. C→T and G→A (resulting from deamination on the antisense strand) transitions are thus predicted to occur frequently in the heavily methylated human genome. The development of a rapid procedure for the identification of all sequence variations in DNA, namely amplification mismatch detection, has enabled Green et al to undertake the characterization of haemophilia B mutations at a population level and therefore assess the contribution of CpG transitions to haemophilia B mutations. They find that 27 of 51 single-base changes giving rise to haemophilia B were CpG→TpG or CpA transitions. This represents a 38-fold excess over other single-base changes. They hypothesize that this is in part due to the high proportion of CpG dinucleotides at critical positions for the function of the factor IX molecule. The instability of MeC implies that during evolution the position of CpG sites may be prone to change as some are lost and others gained by any given stretch of DNA. Green et al argue that once a CpG dinucleotide occupies a critical site in the factor IX gene it will become fixed, since any detrimental mutation will be subject to strong negative selection through the hemizygosity of the gene in the male. Therefore the marked excess of CpG transitions they find in haemophilia B is in part due to the hypermutability of MeC but is also due to the high proportion of CpG dinucleotides that now occupy critical sites in the factor IX gene.

In support of this interesting evolutionary argument is the fact that the highly homologous but autosomally located genes for factors VII, X and protein C have lower proportions of CpG in their corresponding critical sites. Presumably a similar process accounts for the fact that all three critical arginine residues in factor VIII are encoded by CG containing codons but only one of three homologous arginines in factor V.

J.H.McV., J.K.P., E.G.D.T.

7. Purification of vitamin K-dependent carboxylase from bovine liver

Hubbard B R, Ulrich M M W, Jacobs M, Vermeer C, Walsh C, Furie B, Furie B C 1989 Vitamin K-dependent carboxylase: affinity purification from bovine liver by using a synthetic propeptide containing the γ-carboxylation recognition site. Proc Natl Acad Sci USA 86: 6893–6897

The vitamin K-dependent blood coagulation proteins, prothrombin, factor IX, factor X, factor VII, protein C, and protein S are synthesized in liver as a precursor form. The specific glutamic acid residues in these proteins are converted into γ-carboxyglutamic acid residues (calcium binding residues) by a vitamin K-dependent carboxylase located in rough endoplasmic reticulum. This reaction requires reduced vitamin K, molecular oxygen, and carbon oxide. These precursor proteins contain a propeptide sequence between the signal peptide and the mature protein. The propeptide, which contains the γ-carboxylation recognition site, is required for carboxylation. Synthetic peptides homologous to the propeptide and the NH_2-terminal residues of the mature zymogen or a small peptide such as Phe-Leu-Glu-Glu-Leu (FLEEL) undergo efficient vitamin K-dependent carboxylation in vitro, when a partially purified carboxylase was used. These studies suggested that the γ-carboxylation recognition site in the propeptide binds directly to the carboxylase.

In this study, the vitamin K-dependent carboxylase was purified from bovine liver microsomes after being solubilized with 3-[(3-cholamidopropyl) dimethylammonio]-1-propanesulphonate (CHAPS), followed by ammonium sulphate fractionation and affinity chromatography using a synthetic peptide, HVFLAPQQARSLLQRVRR, of which sequence was based on the structure of the prothrombin propeptide. Elution with 10 mM propeptide yielded a single major band on SDS gel electrophoresis with an M_r of 77 000. Antibodies to the protein inhibited the carboxylase activity in crude preparations. In an alternative affinity purification, the propeptide was coupled through an NH_2-terminal cysteine to an activated thiol-Sepharose column. The carboxylase–propeptide complex was eluted by reductive cleavage of the enzyme–propeptide complex in the presence of detergent and phospholipids. The eluted protein (M_r 77 000) contained both stable vitamin K-dependent carboxylase and vitamin K epoxidase activities. The protein, purified by either method, was detected as a single band (M_r 77 000) in a Western blot using anticarboxylase antibodies. A 10 000-fold purification of carboxylase activity was achieved. Purified vitamin K-dependent carboxylase should facilitate the further studies of its structure and of the mechanism of action of vitamin K as a cofactor in the reaction catalysed by this enzyme.

K.S.

8. Prevention of deep vein thrombosis after total hip replacement – effectiveness of intermittent pneumatic leg compression

Hull R D, Raskob G E, Gent M, McLoughlin D, Julian D, Smith F C, Dale N I, Reed-Davis R, Lofthouse R N, Anderson C 1990 Effectiveness of intermittent pneumatic leg compression for preventing deep vein thrombosis after total hip replacement. JAMA 263: 2313-2317

The objective of this study was to to evaluate the effectiveness of sequential intermittent calf and thigh compression for the prevention of deep vein thrombosis in patients undergoing elective total hip replacement compared with a control given no prophylaxis.

This was a randomized prospective trial using a combination of fibrinogen leg scanning, impedance plethysmography and routine bilateral ascending venography. Deep vein thrombosis was detected in 77 (49%) of 158 control patients compared with 36 (24%) of 152 patients given intermittent pneumatic compression ($P = 0.00001$). Proximal vein thrombosis was present in 42 (27%) of control patients compared with 22 (14%) in patients given intermittent pneumatic compression ($P = 0.008$). Thus, intermittent pneumatic compression gave a clinically and statistically significant reduction in the frequency of both proximal and calf vein thrombosis.

Although this study was not blind, the assessment by ascending venography was highly objective and thus there is unlikely to be any bias in the outcome of the trial. The results are important indicating that pneumatic compression produces a significant reduction in the frequency of deep vein thrombosis in high-risk orthopaedic patients. It is, however, unlikely that pneumatic compression will be the sole method of prophylaxis and will probably complement other forms of prophylaxis such as low-molecular-weight heparin. Intermittent pneumatic compression will, however, have a special role in patients in whom drugs that impair haemostasis are contraindicated.

A.G.G.T.

9. Five- or 10-day course of heparin in the initial treatment of proximal venous thrombosis?

Hull R D, Raskob G E, Rosenbloom D, Panju A A, Brill-Edwards P, Ginsberg J S, Hirsh J, Martin G J, Green D 1990 Heparin for 5 days as compared with 10 days in the initial treatment of proximal venous thrombosis. N Engl J Med 322: 1260–1264

The objective of this study was to compare a five-day course of continuous intravenous heparin with warfarin beginning on the first day with the conventional 10-day course of heparin with warfarin beginning on the fifth day in the initial treatment in patients with acute proximal deep vein thrombosis. The study was randomized double-blind with objectively documented recurrent venous thromboembolism as the outcome assessment. One hundred and ninety-nine patients were randomized in the trial: 100 to the long course and 99 to the short course. There was no difference in the clinical characteristics of the patients in the two groups.

The incidence of recurrent venous thromboembolism was low and virtually identical in the two groups. Seven of the 100 patients who received the long course of heparin (7.0%; 95% confidence interval, 2.9–13.9) and seven of the 99 patients who received the short course (7.1%; 95% confidence interval, 2.9–15.0) had new episodes of symptomatic venous thromboembolism confirmed by objective testing. Major bleeding was infrequent and the rate similar in both groups. Haemorrhagic complications occurred during the initial heparin therapy in 12 of the 100 patients treated with the long course of heparin (12.0%; 95% confidence interval, 6.4–20.0) and in 9 of the 99 patients given the short course (9.1%; 95% confidence interval, 4.2–16.6). Major bleeding occurred in 6 of the 100 patients who received the long course (6%; 95% confidence interval, 2.2–12.6) and 7 of the 99 patients who received the short course (7.1%; 95% confidence interval, 2.9–14.0). The authors concluded that the five-day course of treatment is as effective as the 10-day course in treating acute proximal deep vein thrombosis. This approach to the management of patients with acute deep vein thrombosis will result in a reduced length of stay in hospital and offer substantial cost savings.

A.G.G.T.

The methodology of the study was sound with careful attention paid to eliminate any bias. The trial was well conducted and the method of analysis thoroughly described. The results of the study are consistent with those reported by Gallus et al (1986). This is an important contribution and the results of this study will have a major impact on clinical practice.

REFERENCE

Gallus A, Jackaman J, Tillett J, Mills W, Wycherley W 1986 Safety and efficacy of Warfarin started early after submissive venous thrombosis or pulmonary embolism. Lancet ii: 1293–1296

10. Myocardial infarction and treatment with alteplase and streptokinase with or without heparin

International Study Group 1990 In-hospital mortality and clinical course of 20, 891 patients with suspected acute myocardial infarction randomised between alteplase and streptokinase with or without heparin. Lancet 336: 71–75

With the use of 2×2 factorial design, 12 490 Italian (GISSI-2) and 8401 patients outside Italy were randomly allocated within 6 hours of symptoms to streptokinase (1–5 mU over 30–60 minutes) or alteplase (t-PA 100 mg over 3 hours), and to subcutaneous heparin (12 500 IU administered subcutaneously twice daily) started 12 hours after thrombolytic therapy, or no heparin. All patients were on aspirin and a beta-blocker, unless contraindicated.

The clinically relevant baseline characteristics were similar in each treatment group and the infusion of the thrombolytic drugs was completed in 94.9% of the patients. In 525 of the 4186 patients allocated to subcutaneous heparin, this anticoagulation was not started or had to be reduced or interrupted. Aspirin (325 mg) was given to 96% and intravenous atenol (5–10 mg with oral follow-up) to 23% of the patients. At hospital discharge, the diagnosis of acute myocardial infarction was confirmed in 94.9% of the patients. Coronary angioplasty or coronary bypass surgery was performed in only 2.1% and 1.2% of the patients, respectively. The overall mortality during hospital stay was 8.6%, this figure being high as there was no age limit in the recruitment of patients; about one-quarter of all patients recruited were above 70 years of age. No differences in mortality were found in the comparisons between alteplase versus streptokinase and heparin versus no heparin. The number of deaths in the respective arms of this study with a factorial design were 929/10 372 (8.9%) patients allocated to alteplase, 887/10 396 (8.5%) patients allocated to streptokinase, 884/10 361 (8.5%) patient allocated to heparin and 932/10 407 (8.9%) patients allocated to no heparin.

The in-hospital mortality was 9.2% in 5170 patients treated with alteplase plus SC heparin and 8.7% in 5202 patients treated with alteplase without heparin; the corresponding figures are 7.9% in 5191 patients receiving streptokinase plus SC heparin and 9.2% in 5205 patients treated with streptokinase without heparin. A lower fatality rate is thus observed when heparin was added to streptokinase while the opposite was found for alteplase.

The overall in-hospital stroke rate was 1.3% in the alteplase group and 1.0% in the streptokinase group ($P = 0.007$). The rate of haemorrhagic stroke, which is generally considered to be more closely related to the use of lytic agents, was not significantly different for streptokinase (0.3%) and alteplase (0.4%). There was no difference in overall stroke rate in patients receiving heparin (1.1%) or not (1.2%). There were, however, more major subcutaneous and also significantly more allergic reactions and hypertension with the latter thrombolytic agent.

This well conducted and reported trial is a landmark as it confirms the life-saving influence of thrombolytic treatment in myocardial infarction patients. Furthermore, this study shows that thrombolytic treatment also reduces the mortality in patients above 70 years of age but increases the risk of strokes in this older age group. Analysis of the mortality rates by age, sex, time of treatment, previous infarction or Killip scale did not reveal any significant difference between heparin and no heparin. The bulk of clinical experience with alteplase is a regimen whereby intravenous heparin (1000 IU/h) is given simultaneously with alteplase. The present trial deviates from this regimen by starting heparin late (after 12 hours), by the subcutaneous route or not at all in half of the patients. The importance of concomitant intravenous heparin during alteplase treatment has recently been demonstrated, but at that time this international study was already well under way. Whether immediate intravenous heparin would have modified the results of the present trial can only be tested in a new large-scale trial testing this hypothesis.

M.V.

11. Persistence of streptokinase neutralising antibody titres after streptokinase therapy

Jalihal S, Morris G K 1990 Antistreptokinase titres after intravenous streptokinase. Lancet 335: 184–185

The increasing use of a standard dose of intravenous streptokinase (1.5 million units) as routine treatment of myocardial infarction demands guidelines as to the likely efficacy of streptokinase when readministered in succeeding months (e.g. for reinfarction). The authors developed a method for measurement of streptokinase neutralization titres, and performed serial studies for up to 34 weeks in 25 patients receiving intravenous streptokinase for acute myocardial infarction.

After 12 weeks, 96% of patients would have been able to completely neutralize the standard dose (1.5 million units). Between 17 and 34 weeks, 90% of patients would have been able to neutralize at least 50% of the standard dose. These findings cast doubt on the value of readministration of the standard dose for 8–12 months after streptokinase. The authors recommend measurement of neutralization titres in patients requiring readministration within a year: however, using alteplase would be simpler and quicker.

G.D.O.L.

12. Pitfalls in the interpretation of fibrinolytic parameters

Kooistra T, Bosma P J, Jespersen J, Kluft C 1990 Studies on the mechanism of action of oral contraceptives with regard to fibrinolytic variables. J Obstet Gynaecol (in press)

The introduction of reliable assays of the concentration and activity of t-PA (and u-PA) and their inhibitor (PAI-1) in the blood, after discarding more laborious methods, leads to a false interpretation of the fibrinolytic activity of the blood. Apart from the extremes, changes in the values of t-PA and PAI-1 cannot be translated directly into the capacity to lyse fibrin. In the blood they are sufficiently diluted, and the clearance is fast enough, to prevent the rapid interaction, which has been observed in vitro. Kooistra et al provide evidence that the physiological fibrinolytic capacity in plasma depends on the concentration of circulating t-PA rather than PAI-1. A parallel decrease in t-PA and PAI-1, induced for instance by oral contraceptive drugs, may result in a net decrease in the capacity to lyse a plasma clot.

In the second part of the same article, the authors report on the lack of response of cultured human liver cells, HepG2, and endothelial cells, to oestrogen stimulation with synthesis of t-PA or PAI-1, despite the potential oestrogen response elements in the genes of t-PA and PAI-1, found in a computer search. The changes in circulating levels of t-PA and PAI-1 may be due to indirect effects, or to alterations in the clearance: oestrogens induce several cell surface receptors in hepatocytes.

E. J. P. B., P. B.

13. Purification and characterization of the lipoprotein-associated coagulation inhibitor from human plasma

Novotny W F, Girard T J, Miletich J P, Broze G J Jr 1989 Purification and characterization of the lipoprotein-associated coagulation inhibitor from human plasma. J Biol Chem 264: 18832–18837

The lipoprotein-associated coagulation inhibitor (LACI) was purified from human plasma by successive column chromatographies of hydrophobic, ion-exchange and affinity media. The yield was less than 0.4 mg from 13 litres of plasma with a 13% recovery. The final preparation gave two major bands, 40 and 46 kDa, and four minor, 55, 65, 75, 90 and ~130 kDa on SDS–PAGE gel before reduction, while it migrated as a single band (doublet) of 42 kDa after reduction.

The lowest molecular weight species (42 kDa on reduction) is a free form of LACI corresponding to the 47 kDa species that was previously isolated from the culture of a human hepatoma cell line (HepG2); they have a similar specific activity and a common amino-terminal sequence. The difference in molecular weight is probably due to less glycosylation in the plasma protein. The higher molecular species are complexed with lipoprotein A-II by disulphide bond(s). The 40 kDa is contained primarily in low-density lipoprotein and the 46 kDa in the high-density lipoprotein.

LACI was originally found in human plasma as a potent inhibitor of the intrinsic pathway of blood coagulation. The inhibitory activity requires the presence of factor Xa. It was purified from the culture of HepG2 cells. The purified LACI binds factor Xa and the complex of LACI and factor Xa, in turn, inhibits the catalytic activity of the complex tissue factor and factor VIIa, which converts factor X and IX to their active forms. The primary structure of LACI deduced from the cDNA sequence showed that LACI has a sequence homology with Kunitz-type trypsin inhibitors.

In spite of the excellent progress on the molecular structure, the physiological significance of LACI is not known. It is interesting and important to know if the plasma level of LACI is regulated in regard with certain hyper- or hypothrombotic states.

K.F.

14. Gene transfer as a potential therapy for haemophilia B

Palmer T D, Thompson A R, Miller A D 1989 Production of human factor IX in animals by genetically modified skin fibroblasts: potential therapy for haemophilia B. Blood 73: 438–445

Gene transfer therapy is of two broad types: (a) correction of the genetic defect in the fertilized developing ovum at an early stage of blastogenesis for permanent genetic cure of the individual and his/her descendants; (b) introduction of normal genes or DNA sequences into the patient's somatic tissues to correct the phenotypic defect in that individual. The first, more radical approach will pose many ethical problems even if it becomes a practical proposition. The second approach, in principle, involves no more fundamental ethical dilemmas than organ transplant or even blood transfusion provided that all the usual considerations of possible side effects and informed consent are observed. In this paper the authors describe the insertion of the gene for factor IX into retroviral vectors and hence into normal skin fibroblasts. The infected cells secreted factor IX that was structurally and functionally indistinguishable from normal plasma-derived factor IX as determined by reaction with an antibody which recognized calcium-dependent conformational antigen and by a suitably controlled activity assay. When these cells were transplanted intraperitoneally into rats and intraperitoneally or subcutaneously into mice, human factor IX was produced and could readily be detected in the blood. The authors discuss the possibility that fibroblastic tumours could result from the use of immortalized cell lines but suggest that infected autologous fibroblasts might provide therapeutic levels of factor IX if transplanted into patients suffering from haemophilia B.

Comment
This work points the way to further developments in gene transfer therapy for haemophilia A and B. However, autologous fibroblasts tend to enter a resting phase once their function in healing is complete, whereas a possible alternative, keratinocytes, may require too great a surface area in the recipient. Suitable lymphoid or macrophage progenetors could represent alternative possibilities for future studies.

A.L.B., I.R.P.

15. Atrial fibrillation and stroke prevention

Preliminary report of the stroke prevention in atrial fibrillation study N Engl J Med 322: 863–868

Patients with atrial fibrillation unrelated to rheumatic or prosthetic valvular heart disease have a risk of ischaemic stroke about five times higher than those in normal rhythm. The recommendation for oral anticoagulant therapy in this condition put forward in 1989 by the American College of Chest Physicians Consensus Group had to be based on clinical impressions and the level III evidence of the small cohort study dating from over 20 years ago. The situation has now been changed and clarified by two randomized studies within the last 12 months. The preliminary report of the US Stroke Prevention Study follows the publication of a level I report from Copenhagen in the previous year by Petersen and colleagues. The present US study was a 15-centre randomized trial. In the first phase described in this report a placebo arm is incorporated. Eligible patients had ECG documentation of constant or intermittent atrial fibrillation in the preceding 12 months but no prosthetic heart valves or echocardiograph evidence of rheumatic mitral stenosis. Patients had an equal chance of receiving warfarin, aspirin (325 mg enteric coated daily), or matched placebo in a double-blind fashion. All patients were followed every three months. The diagnosis of ischaemic stroke required the persistence for more than 24 hours of a focal neurological defect of sudden onset confirmed by computerized tomography. Systemic embolism demanded documentation of vascular insufficiency related to acute arterial occlusion.

The report relates to the first 1244 recruited patients, 47% of whom were judged candidates for warfarin. Most exclusions, 335 out of 656, were due to patient or physician refusal or to old age (more than 75 years). After a mean 1.13 patient years of study the incidence of ischaemic stroke, or systemic embolism was 6.3 per 100 patient years in all, in the placebo group. Active treatment with either aspirin or warfarin was significantly superior to placebo ($P < 0.00005$). The rates were 1.6% per year with active treatment contrasted with 8.3% with placebo. Assignment of patients to placebo was then terminated and the trial is continuing to study the relative benefits of warfarin and aspirin. No benefit was apparent from aspirin versus placebo in the group of over 75 years, which was excluded from the warfarin study. Bleeding was 1.7% per year with warfarin, 0.9% with aspirin and 1.2% on placebo.

A minor but important criticism must relate to the interpretation of the prothrombin time results as international normalized ratios (INRs). The authors gave the equivalent of 1.3–1.8 times the control time with a typical North American thromboplastin as 2.0–3.5 INR. This is an obviously incorrect interpretation of the observed prothrombin time range (see p. 247).

L.P.

16. Surprising new function of fibrinolytic inhibitor

Prendergast G C, Diamond L E, Dahl D, Cole M D 1990 The c-*myc*-regulated gene *mrl* encodes plasminogen activator inhibitor 1. Mol Cell Biol 10: 1265–1269

The function of the fast-acting plasminogen activator inhibitor, PAI-1, in the circulation, either free or hidden in platelets, seems obvious. By neutralizing the plasminogen activators t-PA and u-PA, it prevents unrestricted and untimely removal of fibrin, as for instance in the case of haemostatic plugs. However, the involvement of PAI-1 in protecting the cell matrix against breakdown indicates a different function. Some even view the free PAI-1 in the blood simply as a spill-over from the tissue.

Another possible role for PAI-1 is suggested by Prendergast et al. PAI appears to be a target of a cellular oncogene, c-*myc*, that is implicated in the development of many different cancers. C-*myc* can modulate the cellular gene expression of murine PAI-1 at a post-transcriptional level: mRNA export, splicing or mRNA turnover. Since oncogenes often have a function in cell growth and maturation, PAI-1 is possibly also involved in cell growth. Several growth factors turn out to be protease inhibitors. In the case of PAI-1, there may be speculation that it plays a role in the attachment of growing cells to the matrix. The level of PAI-1, and hence of fibrinolysis, in the circulation and in extravascular sites could be regulated by local processes of tissue repair or tumour growth.

E.J.P.B., P.B.

17. A familial factor XIII subunit B deficiency

Saito M, Asakura H, Yoshida T, Ito K, Okafuji K, Yoshida T, Matsuda T 1990 A familial factor XIII subunit B deficiency. Br J Haemat 74: 290–294

Studies on a 32-year-old woman with a bleeding tendency revealed a factor XIII subunit B deficiency. Levels of subunit B were undetectable in the proband and her brother and were reduced in their parents and in her children. The level of subunit A was markedly reduced in the proband and her brother whereas the level in the platelets of the proband was normal. From the shortened half-life of infused factor XIII subunit A it was inferred that this subunit is unstable in plasma deficient in subunit B and that subunit B functions to stabilize the A subunit. The proband was born of a consanguineous marriage and, from the family pedigree, it was concluded that the disorder was inherited as an autosomal recessive trait.

Comment
Congenital deficiency of factor XIII is rare; the homozygous deficiency state presents clinically with a moderate to severe haemorrhagic tendency and an impairment of wound healing.

Factor XIII is found in plasma as a tetramer composed of two A and two B subunits. In the complex the b protein, a long, thin, flexible strand, is wound around the globular a protein. It has been shown that only half of the plasma b protein is complexed with the a protein. Factor XIII is also found in platelets, where it exists solely as the A subunit. It is the subunit A which contains both the thrombin cleavage site and the Ca^{2+} binding site, and which possesses the catalytic activity. The precise function of subunit B has not been clearly defined, but a role in the carriage and stabilization of the subunit A has been postulated.

In cases of factor XIII deficiency reported previously there has been absence of plasma subunit A and diminished levels of subunit B. This family represents the first report of congenital deficiency of factor XIII subunit B, and the findings provide clinical evidence for the essential role of this subunit.

D.O., B.B.

18. Oral anticoagulants and the management of myocardial infarction

Smith P, Arnesen H, Holm I 1990 Effects of oral anticoagulants on mortality, recurrent infarction and cerebral vascular attacks in survivors of acute myocardial infarction. N Engl J Med (in press)

This study represents an important landmark in the evaluation of the role of oral anticoagulation in the management of myocardial infarction. Early reports in the 1950s had been over-enthusiastic and were followed by the reports in the 1960s where the benefit was found to be only marginal, limited to the prevention of thromboembolic sequelae with a small or negligible effect on mortality. The latter studies were criticized as having employed an inadequate intensity of anticoagulation owing to modifications in laboratory control of dosage which led clinicians unsuspectingly to give smaller amounts of the drugs. Nevertheless physicians were discouraged subsequently from using a treatment where the benefit was slight and the efforts in organization, etc., particularly for long-term treatment were so demanding. The publication in 1981 of the Netherlands '60 plus' study re-opened the question by showing that those patients who had continued on oral long-term anticoagulation lived longer and had less recurrences of myocardial infarction than those whose anticoagulant treatment was discontinued. The '60 plus' study was the impetus for the present new study which was reported by the Norwegian team. The WARIS study as it is designated describes the fate of 1214 survivors of acute myocardial infarction who are randomized to receive warfarin or placebo for an average of 37 months. Results were analysed on an intention-to-treat basis. The patients were to be maintained at an international normalized ratio between 2.8 and 4.8 and this was achieved in 64% of the results.

Mortality in the placebo group was 123, but with warfarin was 94, i.e. a 24% reduction ($P = 0.026$). To control the possible adverse effects of rebound thrombosis after oral anticoagulants were stopped, a further analysis was formed for those on treatment and within 28 days of stopping. Ninety-two died on placebo and 60 on warfarin, a risk reduction of 35% ($P = 0.005$). The reinfarction rate was 122 on placebo, but 70 on warfarin, a reduction of 43% ($P = 0.0001$). Surprisingly a significant reduction in cerebrovascular events was observed also with warfarin. There were 16 as opposed to 41 with placebo ($P = 0.001$). Haemorrhagic events occurred in 11 warfarin patients (0.6% per year at risk). This study is probably the most scientific and important one performed in this area for more than two decades. It may result in a reappraisal of the value of routine oral anticoagulation in acute myocardial infarction. When aligned to the benefits of thrombolytic treatment in the acute phase, combination of long-term anticoagulation may further considerably reduce the mortality and morbidity of myocardial infarction.

L.P.

The results of this trial emphasize the importance of thrombin generation in the initiation of thrombus formation in acute myocardial infarction. Dampening the haemostatic response with respect to thrombin generation likely affects platelet activation, as well as fibrin formation. If the propensity to thrombin generation is the important factor mediating the benefits observed in this study, it may prove useful to evaluate alternative laboratory monitoring strategies. The dose chosen by the authors is a based on meta analysis of multiple previous studies. The literature would suggest that long-term warfarin therapy at an INR of 2.8–4.8 may be associated with considerably more haemorrhagic complications than observed by the authors in the environment of a carefully controlled trial at an expert clinical centre. An attractive extension of the present study would be a prospective controlled randomized trial of varied warfarin doses using measures of in vivo thrombin generation to adjust dosage. Such a study would allow optimization of warfarin dose with respect to antithrombotic effect and avoidance of haemorrhagic complications.

J.A.S., E.G.B., K.G.M.

19. Interactions between tissue-type plasminogen activator and platelets

Torr S R, Winters K J, Santoro S A, Sobel B E 1990 The nature of interactions between tissue-type plasminogen activator and platelets. Thromb Res 59: 279–293

Bleeding complications, particularly in the brain, are feared side effects with all thrombolytic agents. Against expectation there is a poor correlation between the fibrinogen levels and bleeding in patients with acute myocardial infarction treated with alteplase.

This in vitro study demonstrates that alteplase does not impair platelet activation induced by ADP or collagen or alter platelet binding of fibrinogen. Furthermore, it shows that the antiaggregatory effects of plasminogen activation by alteplase in whole blood are attributable to plasmin-induced fibrinogen degradation products rather than to intrinsic changes in platelets such as disruption of the glycoproteins IIb/IIIa fibrinogen receptors. If indeed the antiaggregatory effects of alteplase observed in vivo are not a direct effect of alteplase or of plasmin on platelets as the result of fibrinogen degradation products one could imply that these effects and bleeding could be deviated by the use of plasminogen activation with maximal thrombus (fibrin) specificity or with dose regimens of alteplase that do not elicit high circulating plasmin levels and thus avoid the generation of fibrinogen degradation products.

M.V.

20. The detection of point mutations in the factor VIII gene

Traystman M D, Higuchi M, Kasper C K, Antonarakis S E, Kazazian H H 1990 Use of denaturing gradient gel electrophoresis to detect point mutations in the factor VIII gene. Genomics 6: 293–301

Although a large number of molecular defects producing haemophilia A have been characterized, it is unusual to be able to detect the mutation in a particular individual affected by the disease. It has become clear that most unrelated patients have different molecular defects. Large rearrangements and deletions within the gene can easily be identified by classical Southern blot analysis, but account for less than 5% of cases. A further 5% of cases have mutations in Taq I sites and can therefore be detected by Southern blot analysis using that restriction enzyme. Directed-search strategies have also been used to screen for mutations at specific functionally important sites in the factor VIII gene; however, such strategies have only identified the mutation in a further 2% of cases. The mutations in the factor VIII gene responsible for the majority of cases of haemophilia A are single nucleotide substitutions in exons. There is therefore a need for a more generalized, rapid screening method for the identification of the causative mutation in haemophilia A cases. Traystman et al demonstrate the use of the polymerase chain reaction and denaturing gradient gel electrophoresis to characterize single nucleotide substitutions in the factor VIII gene. They analysed five regions of the gene, including 16% of exon and splice junction sequences of the factor VIII gene, and were able to identify ten of 11 previously characterized mutations. They were unable to identify a mutation of the G→C transversion type. Analysis of 52 patients with unknown mutations identified three putative disease-producing mutations. This technique is therefore applicable to mutation screening in the factor VIII gene. However, it will not identify all mutations and must be used in combination with other rapid screening methods such as amplification mismatch cleavage.

J.H.McV., J.K.P., E.G.D.T.

Index